U0276335

本书为国家社科基金项目"中医名词术语英译国际标准化研究"（No.08BYY009）、国家社科基金项目"中医英语翻译理论与方法研究"（No.12BYY024）、国家中医药管理局项目"中国参与世界卫生组织ICTM方案研究"(No.YYS20090010-2)、上海市教委科研创新重点项目"中医英语翻译原则、标准与方法研究"（B-7037-12-000001）、国家外文局重点项目"中医典籍翻译的历史、现状与国际传播调研报告"、上海市教委重点课程建设项目"国学典籍英译"、上海师范大学重点科研项目"国学典籍多译本平行语料库建设"（A-7031-12-002001）的阶段性成果。

汉英对照
Classical Chinese-Modern Chinese-English

Shén Nóng Běn Cǎo Jīng

神农本草经

Agriculture God's Canon of Materia Medica

孙星衍◎考据 Textually Researched by Sun Xingyan

刘希茹◎今译 Translated in Modern Chinese by Liu Xiru

李照国◎英译 Translated in English by Li Zhaoguo

I

上海三联书店

译者例言

神农者,炎帝是也。炎帝者,华夏之始祖,农耕之神灵,本草之厘定者也。《神农本草经》虽成书于秦汉,然其表里本末,皆源自神农。远古之神农,一如五帝之轩辕,志在治国,意在救民。故理政之余,常俯察山谷池泽,以明辨草木、金石、鱼虫之性味,为民生而探路径,为民健而寻良方。

鄙人初入杏林,即闻黄帝之理法、神农之方药。其理法,高不可际;其方药,深不可测。上下求索数载,方知何谓"约而能张,幽而能明,弱而能强,柔而能刚"。学而时习之余,即探索西译岐黄之术,外传国医之法。学古文,读诸子,习国学,研岐黄,译国医,此即鄙人译岐黄之历程也。

历经廿载,《黄帝内经》之译毕矣。其译之难,无以言表。一字一词,即难辨难达,况乎一句一段,一篇一卷?阴者,阳者,气者,精者,神者,即难辨难达之常例也。春夏秋冬,常译常惑。进而退之,退而求之,求而惑之,惑而困之,此即鄙人译《黄帝内经》之体验也。虽困惑如此,然心志却从未移也。所谓"损之而不寡,斫之而不薄,杀之而不残",即鄙人之感验也。

《黄帝内经》者,国医之理法也。虽理奥法博,然方药则鲜矣。《神农本草经》,方药则众,治法则明,故而救民有道,健民有肇。译毕岐黄,即译神农,此乃其缘由是也。历经三载,《神农本草经》之译毕矣,盖因其字简文洁,方药为先,无奥博之理法困之,无奥奇之字词惑之。

西人译《神农本草经》,皆视"神农"之"农"为农人也,故以 Divine Husbandman 译"神农"。以华夏文明观之,"神农"者,实"农神"也,非神圣之农人也。故鄙人所译之"神农",皆 Agriculture God,而非 Divine Husbandman。如此之译,唯求信也,非求雅也。

《神农本草经》者，国医之经典也。何为国医之经典？三代至秦汉所问世之典籍，即国医之经典者也，《黄帝内经》《神农本草经》《难经》《伤寒论》《金匮要略》，即其是也。嗣后历朝历代之国医典籍，皆系国医经典之释难释意者也，抑或补益补充者也。

尘世风雨霜雪，人生寒热温凉，皆为译国医之楼台，译国学之闲阁。此生所欣然者，皆禀于此矣。

李照国
丙申年十月三十于北京永安宾馆

目　录

Content

Volume1　The First Grade

6

9

下卷　下品

Volume 3　The Third Grade

序录

上药一百二十种为君，主养命以应天，无毒，多服久服不伤人。欲轻身，益气，不老，延年者，本上经。

中药一百二十种为臣，主养性以应人，无毒、有毒，斟酌其宜。欲遏病补虚羸者，本中经。

下药一百二十五种为佐使，主治病以应地，多毒，不可久服。欲除寒热邪气，破积聚、愈疾者，本下经。

三品合三百六十五种，法三百六十五度。一度应一日，以成一岁。倍其数合七百三十名也。

药有君臣佐使，以相宣摄合和，宜一君、二臣、三佐、五使，又可一君、三臣、九佐使也。

药有阴阳配合，子母兄弟，根叶华实，草石骨肉。

有单行者，有相须者，有相使者，有相畏者，有相恶者，有相反者，有相杀者。凡此七情，合和视之。当用相须相使者良，勿用相恶相反者。若有毒宜制，可用相畏相杀者；不尔，勿合用也。

药有酸、咸、甘、苦、辛五味，又有寒、热、温、凉四气，及有毒无毒。阴干暴干，采造时月、生熟、土地所出，真伪陈新，并各有法。

药性有宜丸者，宜散者，宜水煮者，宜酒渍者，宜膏煎者，亦有一物兼宜者，亦有不可入汤酒者，并随药性，不得违越。

欲疗病，先察其源，先候病机。五脏未虚，六腑未竭，血脉未乱，精神未散，食药必活。若病已成，可得半愈。病势已过，命将难全。

若用毒药治病，先起如黍粟，病去即止；不去倍之；不去十之，取去为度。

治寒以热药；治热以寒药；饮食不消以吐下药；鬼疰蛊毒以毒药；痈肿疮瘤以疮药；风湿以风湿药，各随其所宜。

病在胸膈以上者，先食后服药；病在心腹以下者，先服药而后食。病在四肢血脉者，宜空腹而在旦；病在骨髓者，宜饱满而在夜。

夫大病之主有中风，伤寒，寒热，温疟，中恶，霍乱，大腹水肿，肠澼，下痢，大小便不通，贲豚上气，咳逆，呕吐，黄胆，消渴，留饮，癖食，坚积，症瘕，惊邪，癫痫、鬼疰，喉痹，齿痛，耳聋，目盲，金疮，踒折，痈肿，恶疮，痔，瘘，瘿，瘤；男子五痨七伤，虚乏羸瘦；女子带下，崩中，血闭，阴蚀；虫蛇蛊毒所伤。此大略宗兆，其间变动枝叶，各依端绪以取之。

Preface

There are one hundred and twenty medicinals in the first grade, [known as] monarch [medicinals in formulae], [which can] cultivate life, corresponding to the sky and [bearing] no toxin. Long-term taking of large dose will not damage the body. [If one] wants to relax the body, replenish Qi, prevent aging and prolong life, [he must] follow [the instructions mentioned in] the first volume.

There are one hundred and twenty medicinals [in the second grade], [known as] minister [medicinals in formulae], [which can effectively] cultivate health, [naturally] corresponding to man and [usually bearing] toxin or no toxin. [To use such medicinals, one must] consider [what is] appropriate [and what is inappropriate]. [If one] wants to prevent disease and improve emaciation, [he must] follow [the instructions mentioned in] the second volume.

There are one hundred and twenty medicinals [in the third grade], [known as] the envoy [medicinals in formulae], [which can effectively] treat diseases, [naturally] corresponding to the earth and [usually bearing] more toxin. [Thus these medicinals] cannot be taken for a long time. To eliminate cold-heat [disease caused by] evil-Qi, to break accumulation [of pathogenic factors] and cure disease, [the instructions mentioned about medicinals in] the third grade [in this] Canon must be followed.

Altogether there are 365 kinds [of medicinals], [which represent] 365 degrees, one corresponding to one day and all to one year. When doubled, the number increases to 730.

[These 365 kinds of] medicinals are [classified into four categories, i. e.] monarch, minister, assistant and envoy, functioning as guidance, assistance, cooperation and companion. [In the formulae, some] contain 1 monarch [medicinal], 2 minister [medicinals], 3 assistant [medicinals] and 5 envoy [medicinals]; [some] contain 1 monarch [medicinal], 3 minister [medicinals], 9 assistant [medicinals] and envoy [medicinals].

[In these] medicinals, [there exists] cooperation between Yin and Yang, and [relationship between] child and mother [as well as] elder brother and younger brother, [such as] root and stalk, flower and fruit, herb and stone, bone and meat.

[Among these medicinals] there are [some that can be] used independently, there are [some that are] used together, there are [some that] support each other, there are [some that] fear each other [and cannot be used together], there are [some that] detest [each other and reduce the effect of each other], there are [some that] function differently, and there are [some that can] remove [toxin from each other]. These seven conditions [should be] noticed [when used together]. [It is] better to use [those that can be] used together and can support each other, [and it is] forbidden to use [those that] detest each other and differ from each other [in function]. [In some cases, those that] fear each other and remove [toxin] from each other can be used [together to formulate certain formulae]. [If it is] not for such a purpose, [these kinds of] medicinals cannot be used together.

[These kinds of] medicinals bear five tastes, i.e. sour, salty, sweet, bitter and pungent; four properties, i.e. cold, heat, warm and cool; and [four differences], i.e. toxic, non-toxic, dried in the shade and dried in the sun. [These medicinals should be] collected in certain seasons and months [and kept] raw [or] processed. [The medicinals] growing [in different] places [are different in action and effect]. [It is also necessary to differentiate whether medicinals are] true or false [according to certain standards and] methods.

[According to] the properties of medicinals, some [can be] made into pills, some [can be] made into powder, some [can be] decocted in water, some [can be] soaked in wine, some [can be] boiled into paste, some [can be] processed in different ways, and some cannot [be boiled] in water [or soaked] in wine. [Hence it is important to process] the medicinals according to the properties, avoiding any violation.

To treat a disease [with certain medicinals], [one must] first be clear about where [these medicinals are collected] and the pathogenesis of the disease. [If] the five Zang-organs are not in deficiency, the six Fu-organs are not exhausted, the blood vessels are not in disorder, the essence and spirit are not dispersed, the disease certainly can be cured [after] taking these medicinals. If the disease is serious, there is half possibility to cure it. [If] the disease is very serious, it is difficult to be cured.

If [one] uses medicinals with toxin to treat disease, [the amount should be] like millet. [When] the disease is eliminated, [use of the medicinals should be] stopped. If [the disease is] not eliminated, [the amount of medicinals can be] doubled. [If the disease is still] not eliminated, [the amount of medicinals can be] increased ten times. The degree [in increasing the amount of medicinals should be adjusted for the purpose of] eliminating [the disease].

To treat cold [disease], medicinals heat [in property can be] used; to treat heat [disease], medicinals cold [in property can be] used; [to resolve] indigestion, medicinals [that can induce] vomiting and diarrhea [can be] used; [to eliminate vicious pathogenic factors like] ghost and worm toxin, medicinals toxic [in property can be] used; [to treat] abscess, sore and tumor, medicinals [for treating] sore [can be] used; [to treat] wind-dampness [disease], medicinals wind-dampness [in property can be] used. [These medicinals should be used] according to the condition [of diseases].

[If] the disease is located in the chest and diaphragm, [the patient should] eat food first and then take the medicinals; [if] the disease is located below the heart and abdomen, [the patient should] take the medicinals first and then eat food; [if] the disease is located in the four limbs and vessels, [the patient should take the medicinals] in the morning with an empty stomach; [if] the disease is located in the bone marrow, [the patient] should eat enough food and take the medicinals at night.

Serious diseases include wind stroke, cold damage, cold-heat [disease], warm malaria, sudden turmoil, severe abdominal edema, diarrhea, dysentery, dysuria, constipation, running piglet, upward counterflow of Qi, cough with dyspnea, vomiting, jaundice, wasting-thirst, fluid retention, retention of cold water [in the bladder], hard accumulation, abdominal lump, infantile convulsion, epilepsy, vicious wandering [disease], throat impediment, toothache, deafness, blurred vision, injury [caused by] metal, fracture, abscess, severe sore, hemorrhoids, cervical ulcer, goiter, tumor, five [kinds of] overstrain and five [kinds of] damages in men, [the disease characterized by] deficiency, fatigue and emaciation, leucorrhea, severe vaginal bleeding, amenorrhea, vulva ulcer and injury [caused by] insect, snake and worm toxin. These are the basic pathological conditions [analyzed in this book] and [there are some] changes about the diseases [mentioned] in this [book]. [The medicinals should be] used according to the conditions [of the diseases].

凡 例

1. 本次所译的《神农本草经》，以清代孙星衍等所考据和编辑的版本为主。该版本是历朝历代对《神农本草经》的研究和考据比较完善的一部，故以此为本进行翻译。在研究和考据的过程中，孙氏将《神农本草经》中一些中药合并在了一起，所以只有 357 种，但内容方面依然是 365 种。

2. 在研究中，孙氏采用了《吴晋本草》《名医别录》《说文》《方言》《证类本草》等文献资料对每个中药从内容到文字进行了较为细致的考据。这些文献资料对于今人学习和了解《神农本草经》的基本精神，颇有启发和指导意义。故此考据部分也纳入到译文之中。其中"葱实"的考据，为译者所补充。

3. 考虑到《神农本草经》基本精神的传播，译文只对考据部分中有关中药的来源、名谓和作用进行了翻译。对于文字考据部分，翻译成英文则缺乏实际的传播意义，故没有纳入译文之中。

4. 为了更明确地传递《神农本草经》的基本信息，孙氏考据和编辑版本中的每一个中药，均按【原文】、【考据】和【今译】予以编排。译文则采用 [Original Text]，[Textual Research] 和 [Notes] 予以编排。

5. 为了避免中药名称的译名出现偏颇，译文采取了"四保险"的翻译方法，即每个中药名称均按拼音、汉字、英语和拉丁语的方式进行翻译。每个中药名称主体上采用音译，音译之后以括号形式附录汉字、英语和拉丁语。如"丹砂"译为 Dansha（丹砂，cinnabar，Cinnabaris），"甘草"译为 Gancao（甘草，licorice，Radix Glycyrrhea Praeparata）。

6. 中药名称如果是一个字（如"术"）、两个字（如"丹砂"）或三个字（如"石钟乳"），其音译则合并在一起，如果是四个字（如"太一余粮"）则前两个字的音译和后两个字的音译分开，以便于阅读。

7.《神农本草经》中,个别中药名称如今已经无法确定究竟指的是什么中药。故在译文中,英语翻译采取音译加 medicinal 的方式进行翻译,拉丁语翻译则采取 materia medica 加音译的方式予以翻译。如"别羁"译作 Bieji（别羁,Bieji medicinal, Materia Medica Bieji）,"屈草"译作 Qucao（屈草,Qucao medicinal, Materia Medica Qucao）,"淮木"译作 Huaimu（淮木,Huaimu medicinal, Materia Medica Huaimu）。

8. 考据部分中的古籍名称,采用音译的形式翻译,括号中附以中文和英语的意译。音译中的每个字独立音译,以区别于中药名称和人名的翻译。如《名医别录》译作 *Ming Yi Bie Lu*（《名医别录》,*Special Record of Great Doctors*）,《列仙传》译作 *Lie Xian Zhuan*（《列仙传》,*Story About Immortals*）。

9. 英译中每个中药的注解,主要包括性味、归经、功效和主治等四个部分,以便西方读者能更好地了解和掌握每个中药的性能和作用。

10. "今译"部分只包括《神农本草经》的原文,不包括孙氏考据的文献资料。

11. 根据中医基本名词术语国际标准化的发展趋势,本书中所涉及到的一些剂量单位均采用音译,基本形式和释义如下:

传统剂量单位	公制剂量单位	音译形式
斤	500 克	*Jin*
丈	3.3333333 米	*Zhang*
尺	0.3333333 米	*Chi*
寸	0.03333333 米	*Cun*

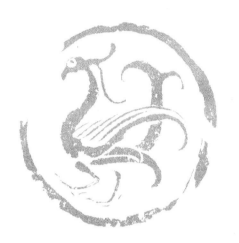

上卷 上品

1. 丹砂

【原文】

味甘,微寒。

主身体五藏百病,养精神,安魂魄,益气,明目,杀精魅邪恶鬼。久服,通神明不老。能化为汞,生山谷。

【考据】

1.《太平御览》引,多有生山谷三字,《大观本》,作生符陵山谷,俱作黑字,考生山谷是经文,后人加郡县耳,宜改为白字,而以郡县为黑字,下皆仿此。

2.《吴普》本草曰:丹沙,神农甘、黄帝苦,有毒。扁鹊苦,李氏大寒,或生武陵,采无时,能化未成水银,畏磁石,恶咸水(《太平御览》)。

3.《名医》曰:作末,名真朱,光色如云母,可折者良,生符陵山谷,采无时。

4. 案《说文》云:丹,巴越之赤石也,象采丹井、象丹形,古文作日,亦作彤、沙、水散石也。澒,丹沙所化为水银也。

5.《管子·地数篇》云:山上有丹沙者,其下有金,《淮南子·地形训》云:赤天七百岁生赤丹,赤丹七百岁生赤澒。高诱云:赤丹,丹沙也。

Volume 1   *The First Grade*

1. Dansha（丹砂，cinnabar，Cinnabaris）[1]

[Original Text]

[Dansha（丹砂，cinnabar，Cinnabaris），] sweet in taste and slightly cold [in property], [is mainly used] to treat all diseases in the five Zang-organs, to cultivate essence and spirit[2], to pacify the ethereal soul and corporeal soul, to replenish Qi, to improve vision, [to eliminate] strange phenomena and to kill ghosts[3]. Long-term taking [of it will enable one] to well improve the mind and live a long life. [It] can transform into mercury and grow in mountains and valleys.

[Textual Research]

[In talking about] medicinal herbs [in the book entitled] *Wu Pu Ben Cao*（《吴普本草》，*Wu Pu's Studies of Materia Medica*），[it] says [that according to] Agriculture God（神农），Dansha（丹砂，cinnabar，Cinnabaris）is] sweet [in taste]；[according to] Yellow Emperor（黄帝），[it is] bitter [in taste] and toxic [in property]；[according to] Bianque（扁鹊），[it is] bitter [in taste]；[according to] Li's（李氏），[it is] very cold [in property]. [It may] grow in Wuling（武陵）[and can be] collected at any time and transformed into Shuiyin（水银，mercury，Hydrargyrum）. [According to the book entitled] *Tai Ping Yu Lan*（《太平御览》，*Imperial Studies in Taiping Times*）[published in the time named] Taiping, [it] fears

6.《山海经》云：丹粟，粟、沙，音之缓急也，沙，旧作砂非，汞，即澒省文。

7.《列仙传》云：赤斧能作水澒，炼丹，与消石服之，按金石之药。古人云久服轻身延年者谓当避谷，绝人道，或服数十年乃效耳。今人和肉食服之，遂多相反，转以成疾，不可疑古书之虚证。

【今译】

味甘、微寒。

主治五脏中的各种疾病，能滋养精神，能安静魂魄，能补益精气，能使眼睛明亮，能杀除妖魔鬼怪。长期服用，能使神志清晰，精神旺盛，能使人长寿不老。能转化为汞，生长在山谷之中。

Cishi (磁石, magnetite ore, Magnetitum) and detests salty water.

Notes

1. Dansha (丹砂, cinnabar, Cinnabaris) refers to Zhusha (朱砂, cinnabar, Cinnabaris) which, also called Chensha (辰砂), is a sort of mineral medicinal, sweet in taste and slightly cold in property with toxin, entering the heart meridian, effective in calming spirit, relieving fright and removing toxin. Clinically it is used to treat convulsive epilepsy, mania, palpitation and insomnia. External application can treat ulcer, swelling, scabies, swelling and pain of the throat.

2. Essence and spirit here actually refer to heart spirit (心神).

3. Ghost here refers to vicious pathogenic factors.

2. 云母

【原文】

味甘,平。

主身皮死肌,中风寒热,如在车船上,除邪气,安五脏,益子精,明目,久服轻身延年。一名云珠,一名云华,一名云英,一名云液,一名云沙,一名磷石,生山谷。

【考据】

1.《名医》曰:生太山,齐卢山,及琅邪,北定山石间,二月采(此录《名医》说者,即是仲景元化,及普所说,但后人合之,无从别耳,亦以补普书不备也)。

2. 案《列仙传》云:方回,炼食云母。

3.《抱朴子·仙药》云:云母有五种,五色并具,而多青者,名云英,宜以春服之。五色并具,而多赤者,名云珠。宜以夏服之。五色并具,而多白者,名云液,宜以秋服之。五色并具,而多黑者,名云母,宜以冬服之。但有青黄二色者,名云沙,宜以季夏服之。晶晶纯白名磷石,可以四时长服之也。李善文选注:引异物志,云母一名云精,人地万岁不

2. Yunmu（云母，muscovite，Muscovitum）[1]

[Original Text]

[Yunmu （云母，muscovite，Muscovitum）] sweet [in] taste [and] mild [in property], [is mainly used] to treat [numbness of] the body and skin, injured muscles, wind stroke, cold [damage] and heat [attack] like staying in a cart or a ship[2], [quite effective in] eliminating evil-Qi, calming the five Zang-organs, replenishing fetal essence[3] and improving vision. Long-term taking [of it will] relax the body and prolong life. [It is also] called Yunzhu （云珠, cloud jade）, Yunhua （云华, cloud flower）, Yunying （云英, cloud blossom）, Yunye （云液, cloud liquid）, Yunshua （云沙, cloud sand） and Linshi （磷石, phosphorus）. [It] grows in mountains and valleys.

[Textual Research]

[In the book entitled] *Lie Xian Zhuan* （《列仙传》, *Story About Immortals* ）, [it] says [that] Yunmu （云母，muscovite，Muscovitum） can be refined for taking.

[In the book entitled] *Bao Pu Zi* （《抱朴子》, *Primitive and Natural View* ） about magic medicinals （仙药）, [it] says [that] Yunmu （云母，muscovite，Muscovitum） includes five categories with five colors, [in which the one that is mainly] blue is called Yunying （云英） [which is] appropriate to be taken in spring, [the one that is

朽,《说文》无磷字。

4. 玉篇云：磷薄也，云母之别名。

【今译】

　　主治身体和皮肤中因失去知觉而类似死亡的肌肉，因感受风邪而导致的疾病，寒热性疾病，如在车上和船上一样眩晕，能清除邪气，能静安五脏，能补益生殖之精，能使眼睛明亮。长期服用能使身体轻盈，能延年益寿。又称为云珠，又称为云华，又称为云英，又称为云液，又称为云沙，又称为磷石，生长在山谷之中。

mainly] red is called Yunzhu（云珠）[which is] appropriate to be taken in summer，[the one that is mainly] white is called Yunye（云液）[which is] appropriate to be taken in autumn，[the one that is mainly] black is called Yunmu（云母）[which is] appropriate to be taken in winter，[and the one that is mainly] blue and yellow is called Yunsha（云沙）[which is] appropriate to be taken in late summer. [If it is] completely white，[it is] called Linshi（磷石）[which] can be taken in the four seasons.

Notes：

1. Yunmu （云母，muscovite，Muscovitum）, also called Yunmushi（云母石），is a mineral medicinal，sweet in taste and mild in property，entering the lung meridian，effective in replenishing the lung，calming panting，relieving fright，ceasing bleeding and resolving sores. Clinically it is used to treat panting，severe palpitation，vertigo，cold malaria，chronic dysentery and morbid leucorrhea. External application can treat bleeding due to traumatic injury.

2. The expression "like staying in a cart or a ship"is a way to describe vertigo.

3. Fetal essence actually refers to the essence responsible for conceiving a baby.

3. 玉泉

【原文】

味甘,平。

主五藏百病,柔筋强骨,安魂魄,长肌肉,益气,久服耐寒暑(《御览》引耐字多作能,古通),不饥渴,不老神仙。人临死服五斤,死三年色不变。一名玉札,生山谷。

【考据】

1.《御览》引作玉浓,初学记引云,玉桃,服之长生不死,《御览》又引云,玉桃,服之长生不死,若不得早服之,临死日服之,其尸毕天地不朽,则杚疑当作桃。

2.《吴普》曰:玉泉,一名玉屑,神农岐伯雷公,甘;李氏,平。畏冬华,恶青竹(《御览》),白玉杚如白头公(同上,事类赋引云,白玉体如白首翁)。

3. 案《周礼》玉府:王斋,则供食玉。郑云:玉是阳精之纯者,食之以御水气。

4. 郑司农云:王斋,当食玉屑。《抱朴子・仙药》云:玉可以乌米

3. Yuquan（玉泉，jade spring，Aqua Giada）[1]

[Original Text]

[Yuquan（玉泉，jade spring，Aqua Giada），] sweet [in] taste [and] mild [in property], [is mainly used] to treat all diseases in the five Zang-organs, to soften sinews, to strengthen bones, to tranquilize the ethereal soul and corporeal soul, to promote muscles and replenish Qi. Long-term taking [of it will enable people] to tolerate cold, summer-heat, hunger and thirst, and to live a long life like a god. [If] a person has taken 5 Jin（斤）[of Yuquan（玉泉，jade spring，Aqua Giada)] before dying, the color [of his body will remain] unchanged in three years [after his] death. [It is also] called Yuzha（玉札，jade letter), existing in mountains and valleys.

[Textual Research]

[In the book entitled] *Wu Pu Ben Cao* (《吴普本草》，*Wu Pu's Studies of Materia Medica*), [it says that] Yuquan（玉泉，jade spring，Aqua Giada) [is also] called Yuxiao（玉屑). [According to] Agriculture God（神农), Qibo（岐伯) and Leigong（雷公), [it is] sweet [in taste]; [according to] Li's（李氏), [it is] mild [in property] [2].

[In the book entitled] *Bao Pu Zi* (《抱朴子》，*Primitive and Natural View*) about Xianyao（仙药，magic medicinals), [it] says [that]) jade can be transformed into water in wine made of Wumi

酒,及地榆酒,化之为水,亦可以葱浆,消之为粙,亦可饵以为丸,亦可烧以为粉,服之,一年以上,入水不沾,入火不灼,刃之不伤,百毒不犯也。不可用已成之器,伤人无益,当得璞玉,乃可用也,得于阗国白玉尤善,其次有南阳徐善亭部界界中玉,及日南,卢容水中玉,亦佳。

【今译】

味甘,性平。

主治五脏中的各种疾病,能柔韧筋,能强健骨,能安静魂魄,能增长肌肉,能补益精气。长期服用能使人耐受寒冷和暑热之气,没有饥渴感,长寿不老,像神仙一样。人临死时服用五斤,死后三年面色不变。又称为玉札,生长在山谷之中。

(乌米, black millet) and Diyu (地榆, root of garden burnet, Radix Sanguisorbae). [It] also can be made into thick liquid with scallion, burnt into soot, produced into pills or burnt into powder. [If one has] taken it for one year, [he will] not be wetted [when] jumping into water, not be burnt [when] touching fire, not be injured [when] attacked by a knife and not be invaded by any toxin. [If it is already] curved into a utensil, [it] cannot be used [as a medicinal otherwise it will] damage the patient. Only natural jade can be used [as medicinal] [3].

Notes

1. Yuquan (玉泉, jade spring, Aqua Giada) was explained quite differently in ancient times. In some books, it was said to be a sort of jade. In some other books, it was said to be spring water in mountains that contain jade. According to traditional medical practice, the second explanation is more natural.

2. This analysis indicates that Yuquan (玉泉, jade spring, Aqua Giada) refers to spring water in mountains that contain jade.

3. This analysis indicates that Yuquan (玉泉, jade spring, Aqua Giada) refers to jade.

4. 石钟乳

【原文】

味甘,温。

主咳逆上气,明目益精,安五藏,通百节,利九窍,下乳汁(《御览》引云,一名留公乳,《大观本》,作一名公乳,黑字)。生山谷。

【考据】

1.《吴普》曰:钟乳,一名虚中,神农辛,桐君黄帝医和甘,扁鹊甘无毒(《御览》引云李氏,大寒)。生山谷(《御览》引云,太山山谷)。阴处岸下,溜汁成(《御览》引作溜汁所成聚),如乳汁,黄白色,空中相通。二月三月采,阴干(凡《吴普》本草,掌禹锡所引者不复注,惟注其出《御览》诸书者)。

2.《名医》曰:一名公乳,一名芦石,一名夏石,生少室及太山,采无时。

3. 案《范子计然》云:石钟乳出武都,黄白者善(凡引计然,多出事文类聚,文选注,《御览》,及《大观本草》)。

4.《列仙传》云:卭疏,煮石髓而服之,谓之石钟乳,钟当为潼,《说

4. Shizhongru（石钟乳，stalactite，Stalactitum）[1]

[Original Text]

[Shizhongru（石钟乳，stalactite，Stalactitum），] sweet [in] taste [and] warm [in property], [is mainly used] to treat paroxysmal cough and difficulty in breath, to improve vision, to replenish essence[2], to calm the five Zang-organs, to unobstruct all joints, to smooth the nine orifices and to promote lactation. [It] grows in mountains and valleys.

[Textual Research]

[In the book entitled] *Wu Pu Ben Cao* (《吴普本草》, *Wu Pu's Studies of Materia Medica*), [it says that] Shizhongru（石钟乳，stalactite，Stalactitum）is also called Xuzhong（虚中）. [According to] Agriculture God（神农），[it is] pungent [in taste]；[according to] Tongjun（桐君），a doctor for Yellow Emperor（黄帝），[it is] gentle [in property and] sweet [in taste]；[according to] Bianque（扁鹊）[3]，[it is] non-toxic, yellow and white in color, appearing like milk. [It could be] collected in February and March and dried in the shade.

[In the book entitled] *Ming Yi Bie Lu* (《名医别录》, *Special Record of Great Doctors*), [it] says [that Shizhongru（石钟乳，stalactite，Stalactitum），also] named Gongru（公乳，public milk），Lushi（芦石，reed stone）and Xiashi（夏石，summer stone），[can be]

文》云乳汁也,钟假音字。

【今译】

味甘,性温。

主治咳嗽并伴有气逆上行,能使眼睛明亮,能补益精气,能安静五脏,能使百节通利,能使九窍通畅,能使乳汁自然通畅。生长在山谷之中。

collected at any time.

［In the book entitled］ *Fan Zi Ji Ran* （《范子计然》，*Studies About Fan Li's Teacher*），［it］ says ［that］ Shizhongru （石钟乳，stalactite，Stalactitum） is produced in Wudu （武都）. ［It is more］ effective ［if it appears］ yellow and white.

Notes：

1. Shizhongru （石钟乳） is another name of Zhongrushi （钟乳石，stalactite，Stalactitum），which is also called Dirushi （滴乳石），Eguanshi （鹅管石） and Rushi （乳石），sweet in taste and warm in property，entering the lung meridian and the kidney meridian，effective in warming the kidney，strengthening Yang and promoting lactation. Clinically it can be used to treat cough and panting due to overstrain，cough due to cold，impotence，pain of the waist and spine and difficulty in lactation.

2. Essence here refers to kidney essence.

3. Bianque （扁鹊，407 BC－310 BC） was a great doctor in the Spring and Autumn Period.

5. 矾石

【原文】

味酸,寒。

主寒热泄利,白沃阴蚀,恶创,目痛,坚筋骨齿。炼饵服之,轻身不老,增年。一名羽涅,生山谷。

【考据】

1.《吴普》曰:矾石一名羽涅,一名羽泽,神农岐伯酸,扁鹊咸,雷公酸,无毒,生河西,或陇西,或武都,石门。采无时,岐伯,久服伤人骨(《御览》)。

2.《名医》曰:一名羽泽,生河西,及陇西,武都,石门,采无时。

3. 案《说文》无矾字,玉篇云:矾石也,涅,矾石也、《西山经》云:女床之山,其阴多涅石。郭璞云即矾石也,楚人名为涅石,秦名为羽涅也,《本草经》,亦名曰涅石也,《范子计然》云:矾石出武都。《淮南子》俶真训云:以涅染缁。高诱云:涅,矾石也,旧,涅石作矾石,羽涅作羽涅非。

5. Fanshi（矾石，alum，Alumen）[1]

[Original Text]

［Fanshi（矾石，alum，Alumen），］sour in taste and cold ［in property］，［is mainly used］to treat cold ［damage］，heat ［attack］，diarrhea，morbid leucorrhea，ulceration of genitals，sore，ulcer，and pain of the eyes. ［It can］strengthen the sinews，bones and teeth. To take refined ［Fanshi（矾石，alum，Alumen）will］relax the body，prevent aging and prolong life. ［It is］also called Yunie（羽涅），growing in mountains and valleys.

[Textual Research]

［In the book entitled］*Wu Pu Ben Cao*（《吴普本草》，*Wu Pu's Studies of Materia Medica*），［it says that］Fanshi（矾石，alum，Alumen) is also called Yunie（羽涅）and Yuze（羽泽）. ［According to］Agriculture God（神农）and Qibo（岐伯），［it is］sour ［in taste］；［according to］Bianque（扁鹊），［it is］salty ［in taste］；［according to］Leigong（雷公），［it is］sour ［in taste］and non-toxic. ［It is］produced either in Hexi（河西）or Longxi（陇西）or Wudu（武都）. ［It can be］collected at any time.

［In the book entitled］*Shan Hai Jing*（《山海经》，*Canon of Mountains and Seas*），it calls Fanshi（矾石，alum，Alumen）Nieshi（涅石）. In the Qing Dynasty，the books about Agriculture God's （神农）Materia Medica all changed Fanshi（矾石，alum，Alumen）

【今译】

味酸,性寒。

主治寒热性疾病,泄泻和痢疾,带下阴部溃疡,恶性痈疮,眼睛肿痛,能使筋骨牙齿坚强。服用烧炼后的涅石,能使身体轻盈,能使人长寿不老,延长寿命。又称为羽涅,生长在山谷之中。

into Nieshi（涅石）.

Notes

1. Fanshi（矾石, alum, Alumen）, also known as Baifan（白矾）
and Mingfan（明矾）, is a mineral medicinal, sour in taste,
astringent and cold in property with slight toxin, entering the
meridians of the lung, stomach and spleen, effective in drying
dampness, dispelling phlegm, ceasing bleeding, stemming prolapse,
killing worms and resolving itching. Clinically it is used to treat
epilepsy, accumulation of phlegm and retained fluid, sore-throat,
stool with blood, vaginal flooding and spotting（metrostaxis and
metrorrhagia）, chronic dysentery, chronic diarrhea and
leukorrhea.

6. 消石

【原文】

味苦,寒。

主五藏积热,胃张闭,涤去蓄结饮食,推陈致新,除邪气。炼之如膏,久服轻身(《御览》引云一名芒硝,《大观本》作黑字)。生山谷。

【考据】

1. 《吴普》曰:消石,神农苦,扁鹊甘(凡出掌禹锡所引,亦见《御览》者,不箸所出)。

2. 《名医》曰:一名芒硝,生益州,及五都,陇西,西羌,采无时。

3. 案《范子计然》云:硝石出陇道,据《名医》,一名芒硝,又别出芒消条,非;北山经云:京山,其阴处有元(石肃),疑(石肃),即硝异文。

【今译】

味苦,性寒。

6. Xiaoshi（消石，niter，Sal Nitri）[1]

[Original Text]

[Xiaoshi（消石，niter，Sal Nitri），] bitter in taste and cold [in property], [is mainly used] to treat accumulation of heat in the five Zang-organs，[to relieve] distension and obstruction of the stomach，to clear away accumulation of undigested food [in the stomach and intestines], to promote discharge of waste and to eliminate evil-Qi[2]. [It can be] refined as paste and frequent taking will relax the body. [It] grows in mountains and valleys.

[Textual Research]

[In the book entitled] *Wu Pu Ben Cao*（《吴普本草》，*Wu Pu's Studies of Materia Medica*），[it says that according to] Agriculture God（神农），Xiaoshi（消石，niter，Sal Nitri）[is] bitter [in taste]；[according to] Qianque（扁鹊），[it is] sweet [in taste].

[In the book entitled] *Ming Yi Bie Lu*（《名医别录》，*Special Record of Great Doctors*），[it] says [that Xiaoshi（消石，niter，Sal Nitri) is also] called Mangxiao（芒硝），growing in Yizhou（益州），Wudu（五都），Longxi（陇西）and Xiqiang（西羌）. [It can be] collected at any time.

Notes

1. Xiaoshi（消石，niter，Sal Nitri），also called Mangxiao（芒

　　主治热邪聚集在五脏之中，胃胀满不通，能清除聚集在肠胃中未消化的食物，能清除人体中的糟粕，能纳入新的营养之物，能清除邪气。将其烧炼成膏状物，长期服用能使身体轻盈。该物生长在山谷之中。

硝），is a mineral medicinal，salty and bitter in taste，cold in property，entering the stomach meridian and the large intestine meridian，effective in reducing heat，promoting defecation，moistening dryness and softening hardness. Clinically it is used to treat accumulation and stagnation of excess-heat and dry feces. External application can treat redness，swelling and pain of the eyes；washing with it can treat erysipelas and abscess；dissolving in the mouth can treat swelling and pain of the throat and sore in the mouth；fumigating and washing with it can treat hemorrhoids and genital ulcer.

2. Evil-Qi refers to pathogenic factors.

7. 朴消

【原文】

味苦,寒。

主百病,除寒热邪气,逐六府积聚,结固,留癖,能化七十二种石。炼饵服之,轻身神仙。生山谷。

【考据】

1.《吴普》曰:朴硝石,神农岐伯雷公无毒,生益州,或山阴,入土,千岁不变,炼之不成,不可服(《御览》)。

2.《名医》曰:一名消石朴,生益州,有盐水之阳,采无时。

3. 案《说文》云:朴,木皮也,此盖消石外裹如玉璞耳,旧作硝,俗字。

【今译】

味苦,性寒。

主治各种疾病,能清除寒热性疾病和邪气,能清理六腑之中积聚

7. Puxiao（朴消，niter，Sal Nitri）[1]

[Original Text]

[Puxiao（朴消，niter，Sal Nitri），] bitter in taste and cold [in property，is used] to treat all diseases，to eliminate evil-Qi [that causes] cold and heat[2]，to expel accumulation [of pathogenic factors in] the six Fu-organs and fixed lump[3]，and to resolve seventy-two kinds of stones [in the body] [4]. To take refined [Puxiao（朴消，niter，Sal Nitri）will] relax the body like immortals. [It] exists in mountains and valleys.

[Textual Research]

[In the book entitled] *Wu Pu Ben Cao*（《吴普本草》，*Wu Pu's Studies of Materia Medica*），[it says that Puxiao（朴消，niter，Sal Nitri）is made of] natural Mangxiao（芒硝，mirabilite，Natrii Sulfas）. [According to] Agriculture God（神农），Qibo（岐伯）and Leigong（雷公），[it is] non-toxic，existing in soil in Yichou（益州）or Shanyin（山阴）. [It] never changes in thousands of years. [If] not refined，[it] cannot be taken.

[In the book entitled] *Ming Yi Bie Lu*（《名医别录》，*Special Record of Great Doctors*），[it] says [that Puxiao（朴消，niter，Sal Nitri）is also] called Xiaoshipu（消石朴），existing in Yizhou（益州）and containing salty element. [It can be] collected at any time.

[In] case [analysis in the book entitled] *Shuo Wen*（《说文》，

的邪物,能治疗难以治愈的痞块和癖气,能化解人体中七十二种结石之症。烧炼后服用,能使身体轻盈,像神仙一样。该物生长在山谷之中。

On Culture), [it] says [that the Chinese character] Pu (朴) [refers to] bark of wood that covers Xiaoshi (消石, niter, Sal Nitri), making it look like jade.

Notes

1. Puxiao (朴消, niter, Sal Nitri), also called Pixiao (皮硝), is a mineral medicinal made of Mangxiao (芒硝, mirabilite, Natrii Sulfas), bitter and salty in taste and cold in property, entering the stomach meridian and the large intestine meridian, effective in relieving heat, promoting defecation, moistening dryness and softening hardness. Clinically it is used to treat accumulation and stagnation of excess-heat, abdominal distension and constipation due to intestinal dryness.

2. This expression is also explained as pathogenic cold, pathogenic heat and pathogenic Qi.

3. Fixed lump refers to lump that exists for a long time and is difficult to resolve.

4. Seventy-two actually refers to all kinds of stones in the body. Stone here means calculosis.

8. 滑石

【原文】

味甘,寒。

主身热泄澼,女子乳难,癃闭。利小便,荡胃中积聚寒热,益精气。久服,轻身,耐饥,长年。生山谷。

【考据】

1.《名医》曰:一名液石,一名共石,一名脱石,一名番石,生赭阳,及太山之阴,或掖北,白山,或卷山,采无时。

2. 案《范子计然》云:滑石,白滑者善;南越志云:膋城县出膋石,即滑石也。

【今译】

味甘,性寒。

主治身体发热、泄泻,女子分娩艰难,小便困难。能使小便通畅,能治疗胃中积聚,寒热性疾病,能补益精气。长期服用,能使人身体轻盈,减退饥饿之感,寿命增加。该物生长在山谷之中。

8. Huashi（滑石，talcum，Talcum）[1]

[Original Text]

[Huashi（滑石，talcum，Talcum），] sweet in taste and cold [in property], [is mainly used] to treat fever，diarrhea，difficulty in delivering [baby] and anuresis. [It is quite effective in] promoting urination，dispelling accumulation in the stomach[2] and cold-heat [disease]，and replenishing essential Qi. Long-term taking [of it will enable people to] relax the body，tolerate hunger and prolong life. [It] exists in mountains and valleys.

[Textual Research]

[In the book entitled] *Ming Yi Bie Lu*（《名医别录》，*Special Record of Great Doctors*），[it] says [that Huashi（滑石，talcum，Talcum）is also] called Yeshi（液石），Gongshi（共石），Tuoshi（脱石）and Fanshi（番石），existing in Zheyang（赭阳），the back of Taishan（太山）or Yebei（掖北），Baishan（白山）or Juanshan（卷山）. [It can be] collected at any time.

[In the book entitled] *Fan Zi Ji Ran*（《范子计然》，*Studies About Fan Li's Teacher*），[it] says [that] Huashi（滑石，talcum，Talcum）is more effective [if it is] white and smooth. [In] *Nanyue's Annals*（南越志），[it says that] Huashi（滑石，talcum，Talcum）also exists in Liaocheng County（眷城县）[where it is called] Liaoshi（眷石）.

Notes

1. Huashi（滑石，talcum，Talcum），sweet and bland in taste，cold in property，entering the stomach meridian and bladder meridian，effective in clearing away heat，resolving toxin，promoting urination and excreting dampness. Clinically it is used to treat summer-heat attack，thirst，difficulty in urination，stranguria，edema，diarrhea due to dampness-heat，dysentery and jaundice.

2. Accumulation in the stomach refers to undigested food in the stomach.

9. 石胆

【原文】

味酸,寒。

主明目,目痛,金创,诸痫痉,女子阴蚀痛,石淋,寒热,崩中下血,诸邪毒气,令人有子。炼饵服之,不老,久服,增寿神仙。能化铁为铜,成金银(《御览》引作合成)。一名毕石,生山谷。

【考据】

1.《吴普》曰:石胆神农酸,小寒;李氏,大寒;桐君辛有毒;扁鹊苦无毒(《御览》引云,一名黑石,一名铜勒,生羌道或句青山,二月庚子辛丑采)。

2.《名医》曰:一名黑石,一名碁石,一名铜勒,生羌道,羌里,句青山,二月庚子辛丑日采。

3. 案《范子计然》云:石胆出陇西羌道;陶宏景云:仙经一名立制石,《周礼》疡医,凡疗疡以五毒攻之;郑云:今医方有五毒之药,作之合黄堥,置石胆,丹沙,雄黄,矾石,慈石,其中,烧之三日三夜,其烟上著,以鸡羽扫取之,以注创,恶肉破骨则尽出;图经曰:故翰林学士杨亿尝笔

9. Shidan（石胆，chalcanthite，Chalcanthitum）[1]

[Original Text]

[Shidan（石胆，chalcanthite，Chalcanthitum），] sour in taste and cold [in property]，[is mainly used] to improve vision and treat pain of the eyes，metal injury，convulsion due to epilepsy，genital ulceration and pain in women，stony stranguria，cold-heat [disease]，hemorrhage due to blood flooding and [diseases caused by] various pathogenic and toxic Qi. [It] enables people to conceive baby. Taking refined [Shidan（石胆，chalcanthite，Chalcanthitum）will make people] healthy and energetic. Frequent taking [of it will enable people] to live a life [as long as that of] immortals. [It] can melt iron into copper and become golden silver. [It is also] called Bishi（毕石），existing in mountains and valleys.

[Textual Research]

[In the book entitled] *Wu Pu Ben Cao*（《吴普本草》，*Wu Pu's Studies of Materia Medica*），[it says that according to] Agriculture God（神农），Shidan（石胆，chalcanthite，Chalcanthitum）[is] sour [in taste] and slightly cold [in property]；[according to] Li's（李氏），[it is] very cold [in property]；[according to] Tongjun（桐君），[it is] pungent [in taste] and toxic [in property]；[according to] Bianque（扁鹊），[it is] bitter [in taste] and non-toxic [in property].

记直史馆杨嵋,有疡生于颊,人语之,依郑法合烧,药成。注之疮中,遂愈。信古方攻病之速也。

【今译】

味酸,性寒。

能使眼睛明亮,能治疗眼睛肿痛,因金属创伤而导致的痈疮,各种癫痫病症,女子阴部溃疡疼痛,石淋病症,寒热性疾病,因崩漏而出血,各种邪气和毒气。使人能生育孩子。烧炼后服用,能使人长寿不老。长期服用,可增加寿命,使人像神仙一样长寿。能够将铁化为铜,含有金、含有银的又称为毕石,该物生长在山谷之中。

[In the book entitled] *Ming Yi Bie Lu* (《名医别录》, *Special Record of Great Doctors*), [it] says [that Shidan (石胆, chalcanthite, Chalcanthitum) is also] called Heishi (黑石), Qishi (碁石) and Tonglei (铜勒), existing in Qiangdao (羌道), Qiangli (羌里) and Juqingshan (句青山). [It can be] collected in February on the day of Xinchou (辛丑) in the year of Gengzi (庚子).

[In the book entitled] *Fan Zi Ji Ran* (《范子计然》, *Studies About Fan Li's Teacher*), [it] says [that] Shidan (石胆, chalcanthite, Chalcanthitum) exists in Qiangdao (羌道) in Longxi (陇西). Tao Hongjing (陶宏景) said [that it was also] called Lizhishi (立制石). [In the book entitled] *Zhou Li* (《周礼》, *Canon of Rites*), [it says that] ulcer can be treated with five medicinals. Zheng's (郑) [said that] the five medicinals used now include Shidan (石胆, chalcanthite, Chalcanthitum), Dansha (丹沙), Xionghuang (雄黄, realgar; Realgar), Fanshi (矾石, chalcanthite, Chalcanthitum) and Cishi (慈石, magnet), [which should be] heated for three days and three nights, the soot [of which] can be cleaned by besom made of chicken feathers.

Notes

1. Shidan (石胆) is another name of Danfan (胆矾, chalcanthite, Chalcanthitum), which is also called Lanfan (蓝矾). It is sour and pungent in taste, cold and toxic in property, effective in ceasing vomiting and wind-phlegm, drying dampness and removing toxin. Clinically it is used to treat congestion of wind-phlegm, sore-throat and epilepsy. External application can treat aphtha, ulcerative gingivitis and hemorrhoids.

10. 空青

【原文】

味甘,寒。

主青盲,耳聋。明目,利九窍,通血脉,养精神。久服,轻身延年不老。能化铜铁铅锡作金。生山谷。

【考据】

1.《吴普》曰:空青,神农甘,一经酸,久服,有神仙玉女来时,使人志高(《御览》)。

2.《名医》曰:生益州及越嶲山有铜处,铜精熏则生空青,其腹中空,三月中旬,采,亦无时。

3. 案《西山经》云:皇人之山,其下多青;郭璞云:空青曾青之属;《范子计然》云:空青出巴郡;《司马相如赋》云:丹青,张揖云青,青也;颜师古云:青,今之丹青也。

【今译】

味甘,性寒。

10.　Kongqing（空青，globular azurite，Azurite）[1]

〔Original Text〕

〔Kongqing（空青，globular azurite，Azurite），〕 sweet 〔in taste〕
and cold 〔in property，is used〕 to treat optic atrophy and deafness，
to improve vision，to disinhibit the nine orifices，to promote blood
circulation and to cultivate essence and spirit. Frequent taking 〔of it
will〕 relax the body and prolong life. 〔It〕 can transform copper，
iron，lead and tin into alloy. 〔It〕 exists in mountains and valleys.

〔Textual Research〕

〔In the book entitled〕 *Wu Pu Ben Cao* （《吴普本草》，*Wu Pu's
Studies of Materia Medica*），〔it〕 says 〔that according to〕 Agriculture
God（神农），Kongqing（空青，globular azurite，Azurite）〔is〕 sweet
〔in taste and may become〕 sour after application. Long-term taking
〔of it will create an ideal condition〕 for people to well cultivate
their health and mind，just like 〔being supported by〕 immortals and
jade maiden[2].

〔In the book entitled〕 *Ming Yi Bie Lu* （《名医别录》，*Special
Record of Great Doctors*），〔it〕 says 〔that Kongqing（空青，globular
azurite，Azurite）〕 exists in Yizhou（益州）and regions with caves in
Yuejuan（越巂）mountain. 〔It can be〕 collected in March or at any
time.

Guo Pu（郭璞）said 〔that〕 Kongqing（空青，globular azurite，

主治青盲症和耳聋。能使眼睛明亮，九窍通畅，血脉畅通。能滋养精神。长期服用，能使人身体轻盈，延年益寿，长寿不老。能把铜、铁、铅、锡化作合金。该物生长在山谷之中。

Azurite) belongs to Cengqing (曾青, azurite ore, Azuritum). [In the book entitled] *Fan Zi Ji Ran* (《范子计然》, *Studies About Fan Li's Teacher*), [it] says [that Kongqing (空青, globular azurite, Azurite) is] produced in Bajun (巴郡).

Notes

1. Kongqing (空青, globular azurite, Azurite) is a mineral medicinal, sweet and sour in taste, cold and slightly toxic in property, entering the liver meridian. It is effective in improving vision, resolving nebula, dispelling pathogenic wind and harmonizing the collaterals. Clinically it is used to treat blue blindness, night blindness, nebula and glaucoma as well as redness, swelling and pain of the eyes.

2. Jade maiden is a metaphor about the attendants of the Taoist immortals.

11. 曾青

【原文】

味酸,小寒。

主目痛止泪,出风痹,利关节,通九窍,破症坚积聚。久服轻身不老。能化金铜,生山谷。

【考据】

1.《名医》曰:生蜀中及越嶲,采无时。

2. 案管子揆度篇云:秦明山之曾青;《荀子》云:南海则有曾青,杨倞注,曾青,铜之精;《范子计然》云:曾青山宏农豫章,白青出新涂,青色者善;《淮南子》地形训云:青天八百岁生青曾;高诱云:青曾,青石也。

【今译】

味酸,性小寒。

主治眼睛肿痛,能止泪,消除风痹证。能使关节通畅,九窍畅通。能消散坚硬痞块和体内积聚。长期服用能使人身体轻盈,长寿不老。能将其化为金铜。该物生长在山谷之中。

11. Cengqing（曾青，azurite ore，Azuritum）[1]

[Original Text]

[Cengqing（曾青，azurite ore，Azuritum），] sour in taste and slightly cold [in property], [is mainly used] to treat pain of the eyes, to cease tearing, to resolve wind impediment, to disinhibit the nine orifices and to disperse hard lump and fixed accumulation. Long-term taking [of it will] relax the body and prolong life. [It] can transform into golden copper and exists in mountains and valleys.

[Textual Research]

[In the book entitled] *Ming Yi Bie Lu*（《名医别录》，*Special Record of Great Doctors*），[it] says [that Cengqing（曾青，azurite ore，Azuritum）] exists in Shuzhong（蜀中）and Yuejuan（越嶲）[and can be] collected at any time.

[According to] the analysis made by Yang Jing（杨倞），Cengqing（曾青，azurite ore，Azuritum）is the gist of copper.[In the book entitled] *Fan Zi Ji Ran*（《范子计然》，*Studies About Fan Li's Teacher*），[it] says [that] Cengqing（曾青，azurite ore，Azuritum）exists in Hongnong（宏农）and Yuzhang（豫章）.[If it is] white and blue，[it is] covered by something；[if it is just] blue，[it is natural and] excellent [in function].

Notes

1. Cengqing（曾青，azurite ore，Azuritum）is a mineral medicinal，sour in taste and cold in property，entering the liver meridian，effective in improving vision，clearing away heat，pacifying the liver and dispelling wind. Clinically it is used to treat wind-heat disease，redness，swelling and pain of the eyes，astringent itching，uncontrollable tearing，redness and ulceration of the eyelids.

神农本草经

12. 禹余粮

【原文】

味甘,寒。

主咳逆寒热,烦满(《御览》有瘕字),下赤白,血闭,症瘕,大热。炼饵服之,不饥,轻身延年。生池泽及山岛中。

【考据】

1.《名医》曰:一名白余粮,生东海及池泽中。

2. 案《范子计然》云:禹余粮出河东;《列仙传》云:赤斧,上华山取禹余粮;《博物志》云:世传昔禹治水,弃其所余食于江中,而为药也,按此出神农经,则禹非夏禹之禹,或本名白余粮,《名医》等移其名耳。

【今译】

味甘,性寒。

12. Yuyuliang（禹余粮，limonite，Limonitum）[1]

[Original Text]

[Yuyuliang（禹余粮，limonite，Limonitum），] sweet in taste and cold [in property], [is mainly used] to treat cough with dyspnea，cold-heat [disease], vexation and fullness[2]，red and white dysentery，amenorrhea，abdominal mass and severe heat[3] [disease]. Taking refined [Yuyuliang（禹余粮，limonite，Limonitum) will enable people] to tolerate hunger，relax the body and prolong life. [It] exists in lakes and swamps as well as mountains and islands.

[Textual Research]

[In the book entitled] *Ming Yi Bie Lu*（《名医别录》，*Special Record of Great Doctors*），[it] says [that Yuyuliang（禹余粮，limonite，Limonitum) is also] called Baiyuliang（白余粮），produced in Donghai（东海，East Sea) and Chize（池泽）.

[In the book entitled] *Fan Zi Ji Ran*（《范子计然》，*Studies About Fan Li's Teacher*），[it] says [that] Yuyuliang（禹余粮，limonite，Limonitum) is produced in Hedong（河东）. [In the book entitled] *Lie Xian Zhuan*（《列仙传》，*Story About Immortals*），[it] says [that] Yuyuliang（禹余粮，limonite，Limonitum) can be collected from Huashan（华山) with red axe.

主治咳嗽气逆,寒热性疾病,烦躁,郁闷,痢疾,赤白带下,经闭,症瘕,身体高热。烧炼后服用,能使人减少饥饿之感,身体轻盈,延年益寿。该物生长在池泽及山岛之中。

Notes

1. Yuyuliang （禹余粮，limonite，Limonitum） is a mineral medicinal，also called Yuliangshi （禹粮石） and Taiyi Yuyuliang （太乙禹余粮），sweet in taste and astringent in property，entering the meridians of the spleen，stomach and large intestine，effective in ceasing diarrhea，hemorrhage and leucorrhea. Clinically it is used to treat chronic diarrhea due to deficiency-cold，chronic dysentery，bloody stool，uterine flooding and spotting as well as leucorrhea.

2. Fullness refers to discomfort and restlessness in the chest and heart.

3. Severe heat refers to excess-heat syndrome/pattern caused by exuberance of Yang.

13. 太一余粮

【原文】

味甘,平。

主咳逆上气,症瘕,血闭,漏下。除邪气。久服耐寒暑,不饥,轻身,飞行千里,神仙。一名石脑,生山谷。

【考据】

1.《吴普》曰:太一禹余粮,一名禹哀,神农岐伯雷公甘平,李氏小寒,扁鹊甘无毒,生太山上,有甲,甲中有白,白中有黄,如鸡子黄色,九月采,或无时。

2.《名医》曰:生太白,九月采。

3. 案《抱朴子》金丹篇云:灵丹经,用丹沙,雄黄,雌黄,石硫黄,曾青,矾石,磁石,戎盐,太一禹余粮,亦用六一泥,及神室祭醮,合之,三十六日成。

【今译】

味甘,性平。

13. Taiyi Yuliang（太一余粮，limonite，Limonitum）[1]

[Original Text]

[Taiyi Yuliang（太一余粮，limonite，Limonitum），] sweet in taste and mild [in property], [is mainly used] to treat cough with dyspnea，abdominal mass，amenorrhea and dripping bleeding from vagina. [It also can be used] to eliminate evil-Qi. Long-term taking [of it will enable people] to tolerate cold，summer-heat and hunger，relaxing the body，walking for thousands of *li*[2] like immortals flying in the sky. [It is also] called Shinao（石脑）[and can be] found in mountains and valleys.

[Textual Research]

[In the book entitled] *Wu Pu Ben Cao*（《吴普本草》，*Wu Pu's Studies of Materia Medica*）says [that] Taiyi Yuliang（太一余粮，limonite，Limonitum）[is also] called Yu'ai（禹哀）[and that according to] Agriculture God（神农），Qibo（岐伯）and Leigong（雷公），[it is] sweet [in taste] and mild [in property]；[according to] Li's（李氏），[it is] slightly cold [in property]；[according to] Bianque（扁鹊），[it is] sweet [in taste] and non-toxic [in property]. [It] exists in Taishan（太山）like yellow egg [and can be] collected in September or at any time.

[In the book entitled] *Ming Yi Bie Lu*（《名医别录》，*Special Record of Great Doctors*），[it] says [that Taiyi Yuliang（太一余粮，

主治咳嗽并伴有气逆上行，症瘕，经闭，漏下出血淋漓不断。能清除邪气。长期服用能耐受寒冷和暑热之气，能使人减少饥饿之感，能使身体轻盈，能飞行千里，像神仙一样。又称为石脑，该物生长在山谷之中。

limonite, Limonitum)] exists in Taibai (太白) [and can be] collected in September.

[In the book entitled] *Bao Pu Zi* (《抱朴子》, *Primitive and Natural View*), [it] says [that] in the Chapter of Golden Bolus, Lingdanjing (灵丹经), [a magic bolus,] is made of Dansha (丹砂, cinnabar, Cinnabaris), Xionghuang (雄黄, realgar; Realgar), Cihuang (雌黄, orpiment ore, Orpimentum), 石硫黄, Cengqing (曾青, azurite ore, Azuritum), Fanshi (矾石, chalcanthite, Chalcanthitum), Cishi (磁石, magnetite ore, Magnetitum), Rongyan (戎盐, halite, Halitum) and Taiyi Yuliang (太一余粮, limonite, Limonitum) [which are] mixed up and cultivated for thirty-six days.

Notes

1. Taiyi Yuliang (太一余粮, limonite, Limonitum) is a mineral medicinal. It is also called Taiyi Yuyuliang (太一禹余粮) in some classics.

2. Li (里), a traditional unit of length used from antiquity to the present, is about 500m in length.

神农本草经

14. 白石英

【原文】

味甘，微温。

主消渴，阴痿不足，咳逆(《御览》引作呕)，胸膈间久寒，益气，除风湿痹(《御览》引作阴淫痹)。久服，轻身(《御览》引作身轻健)，长年。生山谷。

【考据】

1.《吴普》曰：白石英，神农甘，岐伯黄帝雷公扁鹊无毒，生太山，形如紫石英，白泽，长者二三寸，采无时(《御览》引云，久服，通日月光)。

2.《名医》曰：生华阴及太山。

3. 案《司马相如赋》，有白附，苏林云白附，白石英也，司马山云，出鲁阳山。

【今译】

味甘，性微温。

14. Baishiying（白石英，crystobalite，Quartz album）[1]

[Original Text]

[Baishiying（白石英，crystobalite，Quartz album），] sweet in taste and slightly warm [in property]，[is mainly used] to treat wasting-thirst，impotence，cough with dyspnea and frequent cold in the chest and diaphragm. [It can] replenish Qi and eliminate wind-dampness impediment. Long-term taking [of it will] relax the body and prolong life. [It] exists in mountains and valleys.

[Textual Research]

[In the book entitled] *Wu Pu Ben Cao*（《吴普本草》，*Wu Pu's Studies of Materia Medica*），[it] says [that according to] Agriculture God（神农），Baishiying（白石英，crystobalite，Quartz album）[is] sweet [in taste]；[according to] Qibo（岐伯），Yellow Emperor（黄帝）and Leigong（雷公），[it is] non-toxic. [It] exists in Taishan（太山），looking like Zishiying（紫石英，fluorite，Fluoritum），white and bright [in color]，about 2 or 3 *Cun*（寸）[in length]. [It can be] collected at any time.

[In the book entitled] *Ming Yi Bie Lu*（《名医别录》，*Special Record of Great Doctors*），[it] says [that Baishiying（白石英，crystobalite，Quartz album）can be] found in Huayin（华阴）and Taishan（太山）.

[In the book entitled] *Si Ma Xiang Ru Fu*（《司马相如赋》*Sima*

主治消渴症,因阳痿而阴茎不能勃起,咳嗽气逆,胸膈间长期有寒冷之感,能补益精气,能消除风湿邪所致痹证。长期服用,能使人身体轻盈,能使寿命增加。该物生长在山谷之中。

Xiangru Prose), ［it mentions］ Baifu（白附）. Su Lin（苏林）said ［that］ Baifu（白附）was Baishiying（白石英，crystobalite，Quartz album）and Sima Shan（司马山）said ［that it was］ found in Luyang （鲁阳）mountain.

Notes

1. Baishiying（白石英，crystobalite，Quartz album）is a mineral medicinal，sweet in taste and warm in property，entering the lung meridian， kidney meridian and heart meridian， effective in warming the kidney and lung，calming the heart and spirit and promoting urination. Clinically it is used to treat cough due to lung cold，panting，impotence，wasting-thirst，palpitation and difficulty in urination.

15. 紫石英

【原文】

味甘,温。

主心腹咳逆(《御览》引作呕逆),邪气,补不足,女子风寒在子宫,绝孕,十年无子。久服,温中,轻身延年。生山谷。

【考据】

1.《吴普》曰:紫石英,神农扁鹊味甘平,李氏大寒,雷公大温,岐伯甘无毒,生太山,或会稽,采无时,欲令如削,紫色达头如樗蒲者。

2. 又曰青石英,形如白石英,青端赤后者是,赤石英形如白石英,赤端白后者是,赤泽有光,味苦,补心气;黄石英形如白石英,黄色如金,赤端者是;黑石英,形如白石英,黑泽有光(《御览》掌禹锡引此节文)。

3.《名医》曰:生太山,采无时。

【今译】

味甘,性温。

15. Zishiying（紫石英，fluorite，Fluoritum）[1]

［Original Text］

［Zishiying（紫石英，fluorite，Fluoritum），］ sweet ［in］ taste ［and］ warm ［in property］，［is mainly used］ to treat ［disease in］ the heart and abdomen and cough with dyspnea，to supplement ［healthy Qi which is］ insufficient and to resolve wind-cold in the uterus ［that causes］ infertility for ten years. Long-term taking ［of it will］ warm the middle (internal organs)，relax the body and prolong life. ［It］ exists in mountains and valleys.

［Textual Research］

［In the book entitled］ *Wu Pu Ben Cao* （《吴普本草》，*Wu Pu's Studies of Materia Medica*），［it］ says ［that according to］ Agriculture God（神农）and Bianque（扁鹊），Zishiying（紫石英，fluorite，Fluoritum）［is］ sweet ［in］ taste ［and］ mild ［in property］；［according to］ Li's（李氏），［it is］ very cold ［in property］；［according to］ Leigong（雷公），［it is］ very warm ［in property］；［according to］ Qibo（岐伯），［it is］ non-toxic. ［It can be］ found in Taishan（太山）or Huiji（会稽）and collected at any time.

［It］ also says ［that among Zishiying（紫石英，fluorite，Fluoritum），］ the blue one（青石英）with blue tip and red back looks like Baishiying（白石英，crystobalite，Quartz album）；the red one （赤石英）with red tip and white back looks like Baishiying（白石英，

主治心腹有邪气，使人咳嗽气逆不已，能补充精气不足，能治疗女子子宫有风寒，不能怀孕，十年不能生子。长期服用，能温煦人体脏器，能使人身体轻盈，能延年益寿。该物生长在山谷之中。

crystobalite, Quartz album), red and bright [in color], bitter in taste and [effective in] tonifying heart-Qi; the yellow one (黄石英) as yellow as gold with red tip looks like Baishiying (白石英, crystobalite, Quartz album); the black one (黑石英) with black and bright [color] looks like Baishiying (白石英, crystobalite, Quartz album).

[In the book entitled] *Ming Yi Bie Lu* (《名医别录》, *Special Record of Great Doctors*), [it] says [that Zishiying (紫石英, fluorite, Fluoritum) can be] found in Taishan (太山) and collected at any time.

Notes

1. Zishiying (紫石英, fluorite, Fluoritum) is a mineral medicinal, sweet in taste and warm in property, entering the heart meridian and the liver meridian, effective in calming the heart, warming the lung and the uterus. Clinically it is used to treat palpitation, epilepsy, cough and panting due to lung cold.

16. 五色石脂

【原文】

味甘,平。

主黄疸,泄利,肠澼脓血,阴蚀,下血赤白,邪气痈肿,疽痔,恶疮,头疡,疥搔。久服,补髓益气,肥健,不饥,轻身延年。五石脂,各随五色补五脏。生山谷中。

【考据】

1.《吴普》曰:五色石脂,一名青、赤、黄、白、黑符。青符神农甘,雷公酸无毒,桐君辛无毒,李氏小寒,生南山,或海涯,采无时。赤符,神农雷公甘,黄帝扁鹊无毒,李氏小寒,或生少室,或生太山,色绛,滑如脂。黄符,李氏小寒,雷公苦,或生嵩山,色如钝脑,雁雏,采无时。白符,一名随髓,岐伯雷公酸无毒,李氏小寒,桐君甘无毒,扁鹊辛,或生少室天娄山,或太山。黑符,一名石泥,桐君甘无毒,生洛西山空地。

2.《名医》曰:生南山之阳,一本作南阳,又云黑石脂,一名石涅,一名石墨。

3. 案《吴普》引神农甘云云:五石脂各有条,后世合为一条也;《范

16. Five Colors of Shizhi （石脂，halloysite，Halloysitum）[1]

[Original Text]

[Five Colors of Shizhi （石脂，halloysite，Halloysitum） include] the blue one，the red one，the yellow one，the white one and the black one，sweet in taste [and] mild [in property]. [It is mainly used] to treat jaundice，diarrhea，stool with pus and blood，pudendal erosion，bloody stool with red and white elements，abscess and swelling [due to] evil-Qi，carbuncle，hemorrhoids，severe sore[2] ，head ulcer and scabies. Long-term taking [of it will] tonify marrow，replenish Qi，strengthen the body，tolerate hunger[3] ，relax the body and prolong life. Five Colors of Shizhi （石脂，halloysite，Halloysitum），existing in mountains，can tonify the five Zang-organs according to different colors. [It] exists in mountains and valleys.

[Textual Research]

[In the book entitled] *Wu Pu Ben Cao* （《吴普本草》，*Wu Pu's Studies of Materia Medica*），[it] says [that] Five Colors of Shizhi （石脂，halloysite，Halloysitum） are blue，red，yellow，white and black. [In terms of] the blue one，[according to] Agriculture God （神农），[it is] sweet [in taste]；[according to] Leigong （雷公），[it is] sour [in taste] and non-toxic；[according to] Tongjun （桐君），[it is] pungent [in taste] and non-toxic [in property]；[according to] Li's （李氏），[it is] slightly cold [in property]. [It] exists in Nanshan （南山） or Haiya （海涯），[and can be] collected at any time. [In terms of] the red one，[according to] Agriculture God （神农） and Leigong （雷公），[it is] sweet [in taste]；[according to] Yellow Emperor （黄帝） and Bianque （扁鹊），[it is] non-toxic [in property]；[according to] Li's （李氏），[it is] slightly cold [in

子计然》云：赤石脂出河东，色赤者善，《列仙传》云，赤须子好食石脂。

【今译】

味甘，性平。

主治黄疸，泄泻和痢疾，肠癖脓血，阴部溃疡，女子阴部出血，赤白带下，邪气痈肿，疽痛，痔疮，恶性痈疮，头部溃疡，疥疮瘙痒。长期服用，能补充骨髓，能补益精气，能使人身体康健，能减少饥饿之感，能使身体轻盈，能延年益寿。这五种石脂，各随其五色以补益五脏。该物生长在山谷之中。

property], existing in Shaoshi (少室) or Taishan (太山), appearing crimson and as slippery as lipid. [In terms of] the yellow one, [according to] Li's (李氏), [it is] slightly cold [in property]; [according to] Leigong (雷公), [it is] bitter [in taste], or existing in Songshan (嵩山), appearing like blunt brain and young geese, to be collected at any time. [In terms of] the white one, [according to] Qibo (岐伯) and Leigong (雷公), [it is] sour [in taste] and non-toxic [in property]; [according to] Li's (李氏), [it is] slightly cold [in property]; [according to] Tongjun (桐君), [it is] non-toxic [in property]; [according to] Bianque (扁鹊), [it is] pungent [in taste], existing in Tianlushan (天娄山) in Shaoshi (少室) or in Taishan (太山). [In terms of] the black one, also called Shini (石泥), [according to] Tongjun (桐君), [it is] non-toxic [in property], existing in vacant lands in Xishan (西山).

[In the book entitled] *Ming Yi Bie Lu* (《名医别录》, *Special Record of Great Doctors*), [it] says [that Five Colors of Shizhi (石脂, halloysite, Halloysitum)] exist in the adret of Nanshan (南山) or Nanyang (南阳), and the black one [is also] called Shinie (石涅) and Shimo (石墨).

[In the book entitled] *Wu Pu Ben Cao* (《吴普本草》, *Wu Pu's Studies of Materia Medica*), [it] says [that Five Colors of Shizhi (石脂, halloysite, Halloysitum)] were actually five independent medicinals in the times of Agriculture God (神农), but later on [they were] combined to form into one.

[In the book entitled] *Fan Zi Ji Ran* (《范子计然》, *Studies About Fan Li's Teacher*), [it] says [that] the red one exists in Hedong (河东) and [only when it is] red [can it be] excellent [in function].

Notes

1. Five Colors of Shizhi (石脂, halloysite, Halloysitum) actually refer to five kinds of mineral medicinals traditionally used to treat abscess, swelling, carbuncle and severe sore, especially the red one.

2. Severe sore refers to sudden occurrence of ulcer with local swelling and scorching pain, difficult to heal.

3. To tolerate hunger actually means no feeling of hunger.

17. 白青

【原文】

味甘,平。

主明目,利九窍,耳聋,心下邪气,令人吐,杀诸毒,三虫。久服通神明,轻身,延年不老。生山谷。

【考据】

1.《吴普》曰:神农甘平,雷公酸无毒,生豫章,可消而为铜(《御览》)。

2.《名医》曰:生豫章,采无时。

3. 案《范子计然》云:白青,出巴郡。

【今译】

味甘,性平。

能使眼睛明亮,九窍通畅,能治疗耳聋,能消除心下邪气,能令人

17. Baiqing（白青，azurite，Azurite）[1]

[Original Text]

［Baiqing（白青，azurite，Azurite），］sweet in taste ［and］ mild ［in property］, ［is mainly used］ to improve vision, to disinhibit the nine orifices, to cure deafness, to eliminate evil-Qi in the heart[2] through vomiting, ［to remove］ various toxin and to kill three kinds of worms. Long-term taking ［of it will］ improve the spirit, broaden the mind, relax the body, prolong life and prevent aging. ［It］ exists in mountains and valleys.

[Textual Research]

［In the book entitled］ *Wu Pu Ben Cao*（《吴普本草》, *Wu Pu's Studies of Materia Medica*）, ［it］ says ［that according to］ Agriculture God（神农）, ［Baiqing（白青，azurite，Azurite) is］ sweet ［in taste］ and mild ［in property］; ［according to］ Leigong（雷公）, ［it is］ sour ［in taste］ and non-toxic ［in property］. ［It］ exists in Yuzhang（豫章）and can transform into copper.

［In the book entitled］ *Ming Yi Bie Lu*（《名医别录》, *Special Record of Great Doctors*）, ［it］ says ［that it］ exists in Yuzhang（豫章）and can be collected at any time.

［In the book entitled］ *Fan Zi Ji Ran*（《范子计然》, *Studies About Fan Li's Teacher*）, ［it］ says ［that］ Baiqing（白青，azurite，Azurite）exists in Bajun（巴郡）.

呕吐,能消解各种毒素,能清除三种虫子。长期服用能使神志清晰,精神旺盛,身体轻盈,能延年益寿,长寿不老。该物生长在山谷之中。

Notes

1. Baiqing（白青，azurite，Azurite）was the ancient name of Bianqing（扁青，azurite，Azurite），also called Biqing（碧青）and Shiqing（石青），sour and salty in taste，mild and slightly toxic in property，entering the liver meridian，effective in removing phlegm and breaking bending，harmonizing the liver and ceasing fright，improving vision and expelling nebula. When made into pills and powder，it can treat wind-phlegm，epilepsy，coma and infantile convulsion.

2. Heart here refers to the chest，especially the stomach.

神农本草经

18. 扁青

【原文】

味甘,平。

主目痛,明目,折跌,痈肿,金疮不瘳,破积聚,解毒气(《御览》引作辟毒),利精神。久服,轻身不老。生山谷。

【考据】

1.《吴普》曰:扁青,神农雷公小寒无毒,生蜀郡,治丈夫内绝,令人有子(《御览》引云,治痈脾风痹,久服轻身)。

2.《名医》曰:生朱崖武都朱提,采无时。

3. 案《范子计然》云:扁青出宏农豫章。

4. 上,玉、石,上品一十八种,旧同。

【今译】

味甘,性平。

18. Bianqing（扁青，azurite，Azurite）[1]

[Original Text]

[Bianqing（扁青，azurite，Azurite），] sweet in taste [and] mild [in property], [is mainly used] to improve vision, to treat traumatic injury, abscess, swelling, injury [caused by] metal and difficult to heal, to resolve accumulation, to remove toxic Qi and to harmonize essence and spirit. Long-term taking [of it will] relax the body and prolong life. [It] exists in mountains and valleys.

[Textual Research]

[In the book entitled] *Wu Pu Ben Cao* (《吴普本草》, *Wu Pu's Studies of Materia Medica*), [it] says [that according to] Agriculture God（神农）and Leigong（雷公）, Bianqing（扁青，azurite，Azurite）[is] slightly cold and toxic [in property], existing in Shujun（蜀郡）, improving male sexual function and enabling people to conceive baby.

[In the book entitled] *Tai Ping Yu Lan* (《太平御览》, *Imperial Studies in Taiping Times*), [it] says [that Bianqing（扁青，azurite，Azurite）can] treat abscess of the spleen and wind impediment. Long-term taking [of it can] relax the body.

[In the book entitled] *Ming Yi Bie Lu* (《名医别录》, *Special Record of Great Doctors*), [it] says [that Bianqing（扁青，azurite，Azurite）] exists in Zhuya（朱崖）, Wudu（武都）and Zhuti（朱提）

主治眼睛肿痛,能使眼睛明亮,能治疗跌打损伤,痈肿,金属损伤所致的难以治愈的痈疮,能破解积聚,能解除毒气,有利于精神和顺。长期服用,能使人身体轻盈,长寿不老。该物生长在山谷之中。

and can be collected at any time.

［In the book entitled］ *Fan Zi Ji Ran* （《范子计然》, *Studies About Fan Li's Teacher*）, ［it］ says ［that］ Bianqing（扁青, azurite, Azurite）exists in Hongnong（宏农）and Yuzhang（豫章）.

Notes

1. As explained in ［1］ in number 17, Bianqing（扁青, azurite, Azurite）and Baiqing（白青, azurite, Azurite）are actually of the same thing.

19. 菖蒲

【原文】

味辛,温。

主风寒湿痹,咳逆上气,开心孔,补五脏,通九窍,明耳目,出声音。久服轻身,不忘,不迷惑,延年。一名昌阳(《御览》引云,生石上,一寸九节者,久服轻身云云,《大观本》,无生石上三字,有云一寸九节者良,作黑字),生池泽。

【考据】

1.《吴普》曰:菖蒲一名尧韭(艺文类聚引云,一名昌阳)。

2.《名医》曰:生上洛,及蜀郡严道,五月十二日采根,阴干。

3. 案《说文》云茚,菖蒲也,益州生,菥茚茚也,《广雅》云,邛昌阳,菖蒲也,《周礼》醢人云,菖本,郑云菖本,菖蒲根,切之四寸为菹,春秋左《传》云,食以菖歜;杜预云:菖歜,菖蒲菹;吕氏春秋云:冬至后五旬七日,菖始生,菖者百草之先,于是始耕;《淮南子》说山训云:菖羊去蚤虱而来蛉穷;高诱云:菖羊,菖蒲;《列仙传》云:商邱子胥食菖蒲根,务光服蒲韭根,《离骚》草木疏云,沈存中云:所谓兰荪,即今菖蒲是也。

19. Changpu（菖蒲，acorus，Acorus Calamus）[1]

［Changpu（菖蒲，acorus，Acorus Calamus），］pungent in taste and warm［in property］，［is mainly used］to treat impediment of wind，cold and dampness［as well as］cough with dyspnea，to open the heart orifice，to tonify the five Zang-organs，to improve hearing，vision and voice. Long-term taking［of it can］relax the body，preventing amnesia，avoiding confusion and prolonging life.［It］，also known as Changyang（昌阳），grows in lakes and swamps.

［Textual Research］

［In the book entitled］*Wu Pu Ben Cao*（《吴普本草》，*Wu Pu's Studies of Materia Medica*），［it］says［that］Changpu（菖蒲，acorus，Acorus Calamus）is also called Yaojiu（尧韭）

［In the book entitled］*Ming Yi Bie Lu*（《名医别录》，*Special Record of Great Doctors*），［it］says［that Changpu（菖蒲，acorus，Acorus Calamus）］grows in Shangluo（上洛）and Yandao（严道）in Shujun（蜀郡）. The root［should be］collected on May 12，and dried in the shade.

［In］case［analysis in the book entitled］*Shuo Wen*（《说文》，*On Culture*），［it］says［that］Changpu（菖蒲，acorus，Acorus Calamus）grows in Yizhou（益州）.［In the book entitled］*Guang Ya*（《广雅》，*The First Chinese Encyclopedic Dictionary*），［it］says［that］Changpu（菖蒲，acorus，Acorus Calamus）grows in

【今译】

味辛,性温。

主治风寒湿邪所致痹证,咳嗽并伴有气逆上行,能开通心窍,能补益五脏,能使九窍畅通,能使听力清楚,能清晰视力,能发出声音。长期服用能使人身体轻盈,能消除健忘症,能使人不迷惑,能延年益寿。又称为昌阳,该物生长在池泽中。

Changyang（昌阳）. [In the book entitled] *Zhou Li*（《周礼》, *Canon of Rites*）, [it says that] the root of Changpu（菖蒲, acorus, Acorus Calamus) can be cut into 4 *Cun*（寸）to produce into sauerkraut. [In the book entitled] *Lǚ Shi Chun Qiu*（《吕氏春秋》, *Lǚ's History About Spring and Autumn Period*）, [it] says [that] Changpu（菖蒲, acorus, Acorus Calamus）begins to grow after Winter Solstice [which is] the first grass to grow after winter.

Notes

1. Changpu（菖蒲, acorus, Acorus Calamus）, also known as Shichangpu（石菖蒲）, is a herbal medicinal, pungent in taste and warm in property, entering the heart meridian, liver meridian and spleen meridian, effective in opening orifices, dispelling phlegm, resolving dampness and harmonizing the middle（internal organs）. Clinically it is used to treat coma due to heat disease, epilepsy, phlegm syncope, amnesia, deafness, chest distress, abdominal distension and pain, lockjaw and dysentery. It is also called Changyang（昌阳）, Yaojiu（尧韭）, Shuijiancao（水剑草）and Yaochangpu（药菖蒲）.

73

20. 菊花

【原文】

味苦,平。

主诸风头眩,肿痛,目欲脱,泪出,皮肤死肌,恶风湿痹。久服,利血气,轻身,耐老延年。一名节华,生川泽及田野。

【考据】

1.《吴普》曰:菊华一名白华(初学记),一名女华,一名女茎。

3.《名医》曰:一名日精,一名女节,一名女华,一名女茎,一名更生,一名周盈,一名傅延年,一名阴成,生雍州。正月采根,三月采叶,五月采茎,九月采花,十一月采实,皆阴干。

3. 案《说文》云:蘜治墙也,蘜日精也,似秋华,或省作蘜,《尔雅》云,蘜治墙;郭璞云:今之秋华菊,则蘜、蘜、蘜、皆秋华,字、惟今作菊,《说文》以为大菊瞿麦,假音用之也。

【今译】

味苦,性平。

20. Juhua（菊花，flower of florists chrysanthemum，Flos Chrysanthemi）[1]

[Original Text]

[Juhua （菊花，flower of florists chrysanthemum，Flos Chrysanthemi），] bitter in taste and mild [in property]，[is mainly used] to treat dizziness of head with swelling and pain，eyes tending to prolapse [due to distending pain]，tearing，numbness of skin like withered muscle，aversion to wind and dampness impediment. Long-term taking [of it will] promote circulation of blood and flow of Qi，relaxing the body，preventing aging and prolonging life. [It is also] called Jiehua （节华），growing in valleys，swamps and fields.

[Textual Research]

[In the book entitled] *Wu Pu Ben Cao* （《吴普本草》，*Wu Pu's Studies of Materia Medica*），[it] says [that] Juhua（菊花，flower of florists chrysanthemum，Flos Chrysanthemi）is also known as Baihua（白华），Nǔhua（女华）and Nǔjing（女茎）.

[In the book entitled] *Ming Yi Bie Lu* （《名医别录》，*Special Record of Great Doctors*），[it] says [that Juhua（菊花，flower of florists chrysanthemum，Flos Chrysanthemi）is also] called Rijing （日精），Nǔjie（女节），Nǔhua（女华），Nǔjing（女茎），Gengsheng （更生），Zhouying（周盈），Fuyannian（傅延年）and Yincheng（阴

主治各种风邪所致的头目眩晕,眼睛肿痛欲脱,泪流不止,皮肤因失去知觉而出现的类似死亡的肌肉,麻风病,湿邪所致痹证。长期服用,有利于血气的运行,能使人身体轻盈,不易衰老,能延年益寿。又称为节华,该物生长在山川和平泽之中及田野。

成），growing in Yongzhou(雍州)．［Its］root ［should be］collected in January，［its］leaves ［should be］collected in March，［its］stalks ［should be］collected in May，［its］flowers ［should be］collected in September and ［its］fruits ［should be］collected in November，all ［of which should be］dried in the shade.

Notes

1. Juhua （菊 花，flower of florists chrysanthemum，Flos Chrysanthemi) is a herbal medicinal，sweet and bitter in taste，cool in property，entering the liver meridian and lung meridian，effective in dispersing wind，pacifying the liver，improving vision and removing toxin. Clinically it is used to treat exogenous wind-heat disease，headache，dizziness，redness of the eyes，furuncle and swelling.

21. 人参

【原文】

味甘,微寒。

主补五脏,安精神,定魂魄,止惊悸,除邪气,明目,开心益智。久服,轻身延年。一名人衔,一名鬼盖。生山谷。

【考据】

1.《吴普》曰:人参一名土精,一名神草,一名黄参,一名血参,一名人微,一名玉精,神农甘小寒,桐君雷公苦,岐伯黄帝甘无毒,扁鹊有毒,生邯郸,三月生叶,小兑,核黑,茎有毛,三月九月采根,根有头足手面目如人(《御览》)。

2.《名医》曰:一名神草,一名人微,一名土精,一名血参,如人形者有神,生上党及辽东,二月四月八月上旬采根,竹刀刮,暴干,无令见风。

3. 案《说文》云:参,人参,药草,出上党;《广雅》云:地精,人参也;《范子计然》云:人参出上党,状类人者善。刘敬叔异苑云:人参一名土精,生上党者佳,人形皆具,能作儿啼。

21. Renshen（人参，ginseng，Radix Ginseng） [1]

［Original Text］

［Renshen（人参，ginseng，Radix Ginseng），］ sweet ［in］ taste and mild and cold ［in property］，［is mainly used］ to tonify the five Zang-organs，to calm essence and spirit，to tranquilize the ethereal soul and corporeal soul，to cease fright and palpitation，to improve vision，to soothe the heart and to promote wisdom. Long-term taking ［of it will］ strengthen the body and prolong life. ［It is］ either called Renxian（人衔）or Guigai（鬼盖）. ［It］ grows in mountains and valleys.

［Textual Research］

［In the book entitled］ *Wu Pu* Ben cao（《吴普本草》，*Wu Pu's Studies of Materia Medica*），［it］ says ［that］ Renshen（人参，ginseng，Radix Ginseng）［is also］ called either Tujing（土精，earth essence），or Huangshen（黄参，yellow ginseng），or Huangcao（神草，god herb），or Xueshen（血参，red ginseng），or Renwei（人微，human subtlety），or Yujing（玉精，jade essence）. ［According to］ Agriculture God（神农），［it is］ sweet ［in taste］ and mild cold ［in property］；［according to］ Tongjun（桐君）and Leigong（雷公），［it is］ bitter ［in taste］；［according to］ Qibo（岐伯）and Yellow Emperor（黄帝），［it is］ sweet ［in taste］ and non-toxic ［in property］；［according to］ Bianque（扁鹊），［it is］ sweet ［in taste］

【今译】

味甘,性微寒。

能补益五脏,能安静精神,能安定魂魄,能制止惊风和心悸,能清除邪气,能使眼睛明亮,能开启心灵,能增加智慧。长期服用,能使人身体轻盈,能延年益寿。又称为人衔,又称为鬼盖。该物生长在山谷之中。

and toxic [in property], growing in Handan（邯郸）[in the Hebei Province]. [It begins] to grow leaves in March. [Its] root, looking like a man with head, feet, hands, face and eyes, [should be] collected in May and September.

[In] case [analysis in the book entitled] *Shuo Wen*（《说文》, *On Culture*）, [it] says [that] Renshen（人参, ginseng, Radix Ginseng）is a medicinal and grows in Shangdang（上党）. [In the book entitled] *Guang Ya*（《广雅》, *The First Chinese Encyclopedic Dictionary*）, [it] says [that the so-called] Dijing（地精, earth essence）refers to Renshen（人参, ginseng, Radix Ginseng）. [In the book entitled] *Fan Zi Ji Ran*（《范子计然》, *Studies About Fan Li's Teacher*）, [it] says [that] Renshen（人参, ginseng, Radix Ginseng）grows in Shangdang（上党）and looks like a good person.

Notes

1. Renshen（人参, ginseng, Radix Ginseng）is a herbal medicinal. Its stalks, leaves, flowers and roots all can be used as medicinals. It is sweet and slightly bitter in taste, warm in property, entering the spleen meridian and lung meridian, effective in supplementing Qi, preventing prolapse, tonifying the spleen, replenishing the lung, producing fluid and calming spirit. Clinically it is used to treat severe disease, chronic disease and massive hemorrhage.

22. 天门冬

【原文】

味苦,平。

主诸暴风湿偏痹,强骨髓,杀三虫,去伏尸。久服轻身,益气延年。一名颠勒(《尔雅》注引云,门冬一名满冬,今无文)。生山谷。

【考据】

1.《名医》曰:生奉高山,二月七月八月采根,暴干。

2. 案《说文》云墙,墙蘼,满冬也;《中山经》云:条谷之山,其草多宜冬;《尔雅》云:墙蘼,满冬;《列仙传》云:赤须子食天门冬;《抱朴子·仙药》云:天门冬,或名地门冬,或名筵门冬,或名颠棘,或名淫羊食,或名管松。

【今译】

味苦,性平。

22. Tianmendong（天门冬，asparagus，Radix Asparagi）[1]

[Original Text]

［Tianmendong（天门冬，asparagus，Radix Asparagi），］bitter in taste and mild ［in property］，［is mainly used］to treat wind-dampness ［that causes］paralysis，to strengthen bones and marrow，to kill three kinds of worms and to eliminate Fushi（伏尸，serious disease caused by overstrain）[2]．Long-term taking ［of it will］relax the body，replenish Qi and prolong life．［It］，also called Dianlei（颠勒），grows in mountains and valleys．

[Textual Research]

［In the book entitled］*Ming Yi Bie Lu*（《名医别录》，*Special Record of Great Doctors*），［it］says ［that Tianmendong（天门冬，asparagus，Radix Asparagi）］grows in Fenggaoshan（奉高山），the root ［of which should be］collected in February，July and August and dried in the sun．

［In］case ［analysis in the book entitled］*Shuo Wen*（《说文》，*On Culture*），［it］says ［that the herb called］Qiang（墙）or Qiangmi（墙蘼）is also Tianmendong（天门冬，asparagus，Radix Asparagi）．［The same idea is also mentioned in the book entitled *Er Ya*（《尔雅》，*Elegance Canon*）］．

［In the book entitled］*Bao Pu Zi*（《抱朴子》，*Primitive and*

　　主治各种暴风暴湿所致之半生不随、疼痛萎弱，能强壮骨髓，能杀死多种寄生虫，能消除形若死尸之病。长期服用能使人身体轻盈，能补益精气，能延年益寿。又称为颠勒。该物生长在山谷之中。

Natural View）about magic medicinals（仙药），［it］says［that］ Tianmendong（天门冬，asparagus，Radix Asparagi）［is］also called Dimendong（地门冬），Yanmendong（筵门冬），Dianci（颠棘），Yinyangshi（淫羊食）or Guansong（管松）.

Notes

1. Tianmendong（天门冬，asparagus，Radix Asparagi）is a herbal medicinal，sweet and slightly bitter in taste，cold in property，entering the lung meridian and kidney meridian，effective in nourishing Yin to replenish the lung，clearing the lung to stop cough and moistening dryness. Clinically it is used to treat fever due to Yin deficiency，dry cough，hemoptysis and panting.

2. Fushi（伏尸，serious disease caused by overstrain）is the name of a disease characterized by aversion to cold，tidal fever，cough，panting，hemoptysis，insufficiency of Qi，emaciation，weakness and night sweating.

23. 甘草

【原文】

味甘,平。

主五脏六府寒热邪气,坚筋骨,长肌肉,倍力,金疮,尰,解毒。久服轻身延年(《御览》引云一名美草,一名密甘,《大观本》,作黑字)。生川谷。

【考据】

1.《名医》曰:一名密甘,一名美草,一名密草,一名蕗(当作藞)草,生河西积沙山,及上郡,二月八日除日,采根暴干,十日成。

2. 案《说文》云:苷,甘草也,藞,大苦也,苦,大苦苓也;《广雅》云:美草,甘草也,《毛诗》云隰有苓,《传》云,苓,大苦;《尔雅》云:藞,大苦;郭璞云:今甘草,蔓延生,叶似荷,青黄,茎赤黄,有节,节有枝相当,或云藞似地黄,此作甘,省字,藞,苓通。

【今译】

味甘,性平。

23. Gancao（甘草，licorice，
Radix Glycyrrhea Praeparata）[1]

[Original Text]

[Gancao（甘草，licorice，Radix Glycyrrhea Praeparata），] sweet in taste [and] mild [in property]，[is mainly used] to treat [diseases caused by] pathogenic cold and heat in the five Zang-organs and six Fu-organs，to strengthen sinews and bones，to promote muscles，to increase strength，to cure traumatic injury and swollen foot，and to resolve toxin. Long-term taking [of it will] relax the body and prolong life. [It] grows in mountain valleys and river valleys.

[Textual Research]

[In the book entitled] *Ming Yi Bie Lu*（《名医别录》，*Special Record of Great Doctors*），[it] says [that Gancao（甘草，licorice，Radix Glycyrrhea Praeparata）is also] called Migan（密甘），Meicao（美草），Micao（密草）and Lucao（蕗草），growing in a mountain with sand in Hexi（河西）and Shangjun（上郡）. [Its] root [should be] collected on February 8，and dried in the sun for 10 days.

[In] case [analysis in the book entitled] *Shuo Wen*（《说文》，*On Culture*），[it] says [that the so-called] Gan（苷）refers to Gancao（甘草，licorice，Radix Glycyrrhea Praeparata）. [In the book entitled] *Guang Ya*（《广雅》，*The First Chinese Encyclopedic Dictionary*），[it] says [that] Meicao（美草）actually refers to

主治五脏六腑中的寒热性疾病和邪气,能使筋骨强壮,能增长肌肉,能增强力气,能治疗因金属疮伤而导致的痈疮,能消除脚肿,能解除毒气。长期服用能使人身体轻盈,能延年益寿。该物生长在山川河谷之中。

Gancao（甘草，licorice，Radix Glycyrrhea Praeparata）.

[According to] Guo Pu（郭璞），Gancao（甘草，licorice，Radix Glycyrrhea Praeparata）grows for a long time. [Its] leaves look like that of lotus; [its] stalks are red and yellow; [its] joints bear twigs.

Notes

1. Gancao（甘草，licorice，Radix Glycyrrhea Praeparata）is a herbal medicinal, sweet in taste and mild in property, entering the spleen meridians and the lung meridian, effective in tonifying the spleen and stomach, resolving urgency, ceasing pain, dispelling phlegm, stopping cough, removing toxin and regulating all medicinals. Clinically it is used to treat deficiency of the spleen and kidney, abdominal and thoracic pain, cough, palpitation, swelling and pain of the throat, ulcer and poisoning.

24. 干地黄

【原文】

味甘,寒。

主折跌绝筋,伤中,逐血痹,填骨髓,长肌肉,作汤,除寒热积聚,除痹,生者尤良。久服,轻身不老。一名地髓,生川泽。

【考据】

1.《名医》曰:一名芐,一名芑,生咸阳,黄土地者佳,二月八日采根阴干。

2. 案《说文》云:芐,地黄也,礼曰钘毛牛藿,羊芐,豕薇;《广雅》云:地髓,地黄也;《尔雅》云:芐,地黄;郭璞云:一名地髓,江东呼芐;《列仙传》云:吕尚服地髓。

【今译】

味甘,性寒。

主治跌打损伤,内脏损伤,能治疗因血虚所致痹证,能使骨髓充实,

24. Gandihuang（干地黄，dried rehmannia，Radix Rehmanniae）[1]

[Original Text]

[Gandihuang（干地黄，dried rehmannia，Radix Rehmanniae），] sweet in taste and cold [in property]，[is mainly used] to treat fracture of bones and sinews due to falling and visceral injury，to expel blood impediment，to enrich marrow，and to promote growth of muscles. [When] made into decoction，[it can] eliminate accumulation of cold and heat and impediment [syndrome/pattern]. [The therapeutic effect of] raw [Dihuang（地黄，rehmannia，Radix Rehmanniae)] is better [than that of the processed one]. Long-term taking [of it will] relax the body and prevent aging. [It is] also known as Disui（地髓）and grows in valleys and swamps.

[Original Research]

[In the book entitled] *Ming Yi Bie Lu*（《名医别录》，*Special Record of Great Doctors*），[it] says [that Gandihuang（干地黄，dried rehmannia，Radix Rehmanniae）is also] called Bian（芐）and Qi（芑），growing in Xianyang（咸阳）. [The one that grows] in yellow soil is better [than those that grow in other areas]. [Its] root [should be collected on February 8，and dried in the shade.

[In] case [analysis in the book entitled] *Shuo Wen*（《说文》，*On Culture*），[it] says [that] Bian（芐）refers to Dihuang（地黄，

能增长肌肉。煎煮成汤剂,能消除寒热性疾病,能解除积聚,能祛除痹证。生地黄疗效更好。长期服用,能使人身体轻盈,长寿不老。又称为地髓,该物生长在山川和平泽之中。

rehmannia，Radix Rehmanniae). [In the book entitled] *Guang Ya* (《广雅》, *The First Chinese Encyclopedic Dictionary*), [it] says [that] Disui（地髓）is actually Dihuang（地黄，rehmannia，Radix Rehmanniae). [In the book entitled] *Lie Xian Zhuan*（《列仙传》, *Story about Immortals*), [it] says [that] Lǚ Shang（吕尚）[2][liked] to take Disui（地髓）.

Notes

1. Gandihuang（干地黄，dried rehmannia，Radix Rehmanniae)，also called Ganshengdi（干生地），or abbreviated as Shengdi （生地），is a dried herbal medicinal，sweet and bitter in taste，cool in property，entering the heart meridian，liver meridian and kidney meridian，effective in clearing away heat，nourishing Yin，cooling the blood and moistening dryness. Clinically it is used to treat fever due to Yin deficiency，wasting-thirst，epistaxis，vaginal flooding and spotting（metrostaxis and metrorrhagia），irregular menstruation，genital injury and constipation.

2. Lǚ Shang（吕尚）was another name of Jiang Ziya（姜子牙，about 1156 BC‑1017 BC) who was a great scholar in the late of the Shang Dynasty（商朝，from about 1600 BC to 1046 BC) and helped the first king of the Zhou Dynasty（周朝，from 1046 BC to 256 BC) to overthrow the Shang Dynasty.

25. 术

【原文】

味苦,温。

主风寒湿痹,死肌,痉疸,止汗,除热,消食,作煎饵。久服,轻身延年,不饥。一名山蓟(艺文类聚引作山筋),生山谷。

【考据】

1.《吴普》曰:术,一名山连,一名山芥,一名天苏,一名山姜(艺文类聚)。

2.《名医》曰:一名山姜,一名山连,生郑山,汉中,南郑,二月三月八月九月,采根暴干。

3. 案《说文》云:术,山蓟也;《广雅》云:山姜,术也,白术,牡丹也;《中山经》云:首山草多术;郭璞云:术,山蓟也;《尔雅》云:术,山蓟;郭璞云:今术似蓟,而生山中;《范子计然》云:术出三辅,黄白色者善;《列仙传》云:涓子好饵术;《抱朴子·仙药》云:术一名山蓟,一名山精,故神药经曰:必欲长生,长服山精。

25. Zhu（术，rhizome or herb of Japanese galangal Rhizoma seu Herba Alpiniae Japonicae）[1]

［Original Text］

［Zhu（术，rhizome or herb of Japanese galangal Rhizoma seu Herba Alpiniae Japonicae），］bitter in taste and warm in property］，［is mainly used］to treat impediment［due to］wind，cold and dampness，numbness of muscles，convulsion and jaundice，to eliminate heat and to promote digestion.［It should be］made into decoction［for treating disease］. Long-term taking［of it will］relax the body，prolong life and expel［the sense of］hunger.［It is］also called Shanji（山蓟），growing in mountains and valleys.

［Textual Research］

［In the book entitled］*Wu Pu Ben Cao*（《吴普本草》，*Wu Pu's Studies of Materia Medica*），［it］says［that Zhu（术，rhizome or herb of Japanese galangal Rhizoma seu Herba Alpiniae Japonicae）is］also called Shanlian（山连），Shanjie（山芥），Tiansu（天苏）and Shanjiang（山姜）.

［In the book entitled］*Ming Yi Bie Lu*（《名医别录》，*Special Record of Great Doctors*），［it］says［that Zhu（术，rhizome or herb of Japanese galangal Rhizoma seu Herba Alpiniae Japonicae），］also called Shanjiang（山姜）and Shanlian（山连），grows in Zhengshan（郑山），Hanzhong（汉中）and Nanzheng（南郑）.［From］February and March to August and September，its root［can be］collected and dried in the sun.

［In］case［analysis in the book entitled］*Shuo Wen*（《说文》，

【今译】

味苦,性温。

主治风寒湿邪所致之痹证,能消除肌肉坏死,能祛除痉挛和黄疸,能止汗,能消除热邪所致之病,能使食物消化。能作煎剂服用。长期服用,能使人身体轻盈,能延年益寿,能减少饥饿之感。又称为山蓟,该物生长在山谷之中。

神农本草经

On Culture）, ［it］ says ［that］ Zhu （术，rhizome or herb of Japanese galangal Rhizoma seu Herba Alpiniae Japonicae） is also called Shanji （山蓟）. ［In the book entitled］ *Guang Ya* （《广雅》，*The First Chinese Encyclopedic Dictionary*）, Zhu （术，rhizome or herb of Japanese galangal Rhizoma seu Herba Alpiniae Japonicae） is also called Shanjiang （山姜） while Baizhu （白术） refers to Mudan （牡丹，moutan，Cortex Moutan Radicis）. ［In］ case ［analysis in the book entitled］ *Zhong Shan Jing* （《中山经》，*Central Mountain Canon*）, ［it］ says ［that］ most of the grasses in mountains are Zhu （术，rhizome or herb of Japanese galangal Rhizoma seu Herba Alpiniae Japonicae）. ［In the book entitled］ *Fan Zi Ji Ran* （《范子计然》，*Studies About Fan Li's Teacher*）, ［it］ says ［that］ Zhu （术，rhizome or herb of Japanese galangal Rhizoma seu Herba Alpiniae Japonicae） grows in three regions and the yellow and white ones are better ［than any others］.

Notes

1. Zhu （术，rhizome or herb of Japanese galangal Rhizoma seu Herba Alpiniae Japonicae）, a combined term of Baizhu （白术，rhizome of largehead atractyloes，Rhizoma Atractylodis Macrocephalae） and Cangzhu （苍术，rhizome of swordlike atractylodes，rhizome of Chinese atractylodes，Rhizoma Atractylodis）, sweet and bitter in taste and astringent in property, entering the spleen meridian and stomach meridian, effective in fortifying the spleen, harmonizing the middle (internal organs), drying dampness and promoting discharge of water. Clinically it is used to treat spleen deficiency, poor appetite, weakness, indigestion, abdominal and thoracic deficiency and distension, diarrhea, phlegm with retained fluid, edema and threatened abortion.

26. 菟丝子

【原文】

味辛,平。

主续绝伤,补不足,益气力,肥健人。汁去面䵟。久服明目,轻身延年。一名菟芦,生川泽。

【考据】

1.《吴普》曰:菟丝,一名玉女,一名松萝,一名鸟萝,一名鸭萝,一名复实,一名赤网,生山谷(《御览》)。

2.《名医》曰:一名菟缕,一名唐蒙,一名玉女,一名赤网,一名菟累,生朝鲜田野,蔓延草木之上,色黄而细为赤网,色浅而大为菟累,九月,采实暴干。

3. 案《说文》云:蒙,玉女也;《广雅》云:菟邱,菟丝也,女萝,松萝也;《尔雅》云:唐蒙,女萝,女萝,菟丝,又云蒙,玉女;《毛诗》云:爰采唐矣,《传》云唐蒙,菜名,又茑与女萝,《传》云,女萝,菟丝松萝也;陆玑云:今菟丝蔓连草上生,黄赤如金,今合药,菟丝子是也,非松萝,松萝自蔓松上,枝正青,与菟丝异;《楚词》云:被薜荔兮带女萝;王逸云:女萝,菟

26. Tusizi（菟丝子，seed of Chinese dodder，Semen Cuscutae）[1]

[Original Text]

[Tusizi（菟丝子，seed of Chinese dodder，Semen Cuscutae），] pungent in taste and mild [in property]，[is mainly used] to treat fracture of bones and sinews，to improve insufficiency，to increase energy and to strengthen the body. Juice [of Tusizi（菟丝子，seed of Chinese dodder，Semen Cuscutae）can] resolve facial blackspot. Long-term taking [of it can] improve vision，relax the body and prolong life. [It is also] called Tulu（菟芦），growing in valleys and swamps.

[Textual Research]

[In the book entitled] *Wu Pu Ben Cao*（《吴普本草》，*Wu Pu's Studies of Materia Medica*），[it] says [that Tusizi（菟丝子，seed of Chinese dodder，Semen Cuscutae）is also] called Yunǔ（玉女），Songluo（松萝），Niaoluo（鸟萝），Yaluo（鸭萝），Fushi（复实）and Chiwang（赤网），growing in mountains and valleys.

[In the book entitled] *Ming Yi Bie Lu*（《名医别录》，*Special Record of Great Doctors*），[it] says [that Tusizi（菟丝子，seed of Chinese dodder，Semen Cuscutae）is also] called Tulǔ（菟缕），Tangmeng（唐蒙），Yunǔ（玉女），Tulei（菟累）and Tulei（菟累），growing in the fields of Chaoxian（朝鲜）and over the branches of grasses and trees. [If it is] yellow and thin，[it] is Chiwang（赤网）；[if it is] tint and large，[it] is Tulei（菟累）. [It should be] collected in September and dried in the sun.

丝也；《淮南子》云：千秋之松，下有茯苓，上有菟丝，高诱注云，茯苓，千岁松脂也，菟丝生其上，而无根，旧作菟，非。

【今译】

味辛，性平。

能通过补益主治外伤所致之筋伤骨折，能补充精气不足，能补益气力，能使人身体康健。其汁能祛除面部黑斑。长期服用能使眼睛明亮，身体轻盈，能延年益寿。又称为菟芦，该物生长在山川和平泽之中。

[In] case [analysis in the book entitled] *Shuo Wen* (《说文》, *On Culture*), [it] says [that the so-called] Meng (蒙) [actually refers to] Yunǔ (玉女). [In the book entitled] *Guang Ya* (《广雅》, *The First Chinese Encyclopedic Dictionary*), [it] says [that the so-called] Tuqiu (菟邱) [refers to] Tusi (菟丝, Chinese dodder, Semen Cuscutae) [and the so-called] Nǔluo (女萝) [refers to] Songluo (松萝).

Lu Ji (陆玑) said, "Now Tusi (菟丝, seed of Chinese dodder, Semen Cuscutae) extends to the branches of grasses and trees in growing. [It looks] yellow and red, like gold. [The so-called] Tusizi (菟丝子, seed of Chinese dodder, Semen Cuscutae) is [actually] a combined medicinal, different from Songluo (松萝, long usnea filament, Filum Usneae). Songluo (松萝, long usnea filament, Filum Usneae) grows over the pine tree with blue branches.

[In the book entitled] *Huai Nan Zi* (《淮南子》, *A Philosophy Book*) Compiled by Liu An, King in Huainan, [it] says [that], over a thousand years old spine tree, Fuling (茯苓, poria, Poria) grows in the lower and Tusi (菟丝, Chinese dodder, Semen Cuscutae) grows in the upper.

Gao Xiuzhu (高诱注) said [that] Fuling (茯苓, poria, Poria) is the turpentine of a spine tree growing for a thousand years and Tusi (菟丝, Chinese dodder, Semen Cuscutae) grows over it without any root.

Notes

1. Tusizi (菟丝子, seed of Chinese dodder, Semen Cuscutae) is pungent and sweet in taste, mild in property, entering the liver meridian and the kidney meridian, effective in tonifying kidney essence, nourishing the liver, improving vision and protecting fetus. Clinically it is used to treat ache of the waist and knees, impotence, seminal emission, enuresis, frequent urination, dizziness and poor eyesight.

27. 牛膝

【原文】

味苦酸(《御览》作辛)。

主寒(《御览》作伤寒),湿痿痹,四肢拘挛,膝痛不可屈伸,逐血气伤,热,火烂,堕胎。久服轻身耐老(《御览》作能老)。一名百倍,生川谷。

【考据】

1.《吴普》曰:牛膝,神农甘,一经酸,黄帝扁鹊甘,李氏温,雷公酸无毒,生河内,或临邛,叶如夏蓝,茎,本赤,二月八月采(《御览》)。

2.《名医》曰:生河内及临朐,二月八月十月,采根,阴干。

3.案《广雅》云:牛茎牛膝也;陶宏景云:其茎有节似膝,故以为名也,膝当为膝。

【今译】

味苦,性酸。

主治寒湿之邪所引起的痿证和痹证,能消解四肢拘挛,能缓解因膝

27. Niuxi（牛膝，root of twotooth achyranthes, Radix Achyranthis Bidentatae）[1]

［Original Text］

［Niuxi（牛膝，root of twotooth achyranthes, Radix Achyranthis Bidentatae），］bitter and sour in taste，［is mainly used］to treat cold ［damage］，wilting and impediment［due to］dampness，spasm of the four limbs，inability of the knee to extend and bend［due to］pain，［disease caused by］Qi［stagnation］and blood［stasis］，canker ［caused by］fire and abortion. Long-term taking［of it will］relax the body and prevent aging.［It is also］called Baibei（百倍），growing in mountain valleys and river valleys.

［Textual Research］

［In the book entitled］*Wu Pu Ben Cao*（《吴普本草》，*Wu Pu's Studies of Materia Medica*），［it］says［that according to］Agriculture God（神农），Yellow Emperor（黄帝）and Bianque（扁鹊），［Niuxi （牛膝，root of twotooth achyranthes，Radix Achyranthis Bidentatae）is］sweet［in taste］；［according to］Li's（李氏），［it is］warm［in property］；［according to］Leigong（雷公），［it is］sour［in taste］and non-toxic［in property］.［It］grows in Henei（河内）or Linqiong（临邛）with green leaves，stalks and red trunks.［It can be］collected in February and August.

［In the book entitled］*Ming Yi Bie Lu*（《名医别录》，*Special*

部疼痛而不能弯曲直伸,能祛除气滞血瘀所致的病症,能治疗因火热所致的溃疮,能堕胎。长期服用能使人身体轻盈,不易衰老。又称为百倍,该物生长在山川河谷之中。

Record of Great Doctors），［it］says［that it］grows in Henei（河内）and Linqu（临朐）.［Its］root［can be］collected in February, August and October, and dried in the shade.

［In the book entitled］ *Guang Ya*（《广雅》，*The First Chinese Encyclopedic Dictionary*），［it］says［that the so-called］Niujing（牛茎）is actually Niuxi（牛膝, root of twotooth achyranthes, Radix Achyranthis Bidentatae）. Tao Hongjing（陶宏景）said［that there are some］joints in its stalks,［looking］like knees. That is why it is so named.

Notes

1. Niuxi（牛膝, root of twotooth achyranthes, Radix Achyranthis Bidentatae）is a herbal medicinal, bitter and sour in taste, mild in property, entering the liver meridian and kidney meridian, effective in activating the blood, dispersing stasis and resolving swelling. Clinically it can be used to treat amenorrhea, abdominal mass, aching pain of the waist and spine, stranguria, bloody urine, throat impediment, abscess and swelling.

28. 茺蔚子

【原文】

味辛,微温。

主明目益精,除水气。久服轻身,茎主瘾疹痒,可作浴汤。一名益母,一名益明,一名大札。生池泽。

【考据】

1.《名医》曰:一名贞蔚,生海滨,五月采。

2.案《说文》云:萑,蓷也,《广雅》云:益母,茺蔚也,《尔雅》云:萑,蓷;郭璞云:今茺蔚也;《毛诗》云:中谷有蓷,《传》云,蓷;鵻也;陆玑云:旧说及魏博士济阴周元明,皆云庵闾,是也,韩诗及三苍说,悉云益母,故曾子见益母而感;刘歆曰蓷,臭秽,臭秽即茺蔚也,旧作茺,非。

【今译】

味辛,性微温。

28. Chongweizi（茺蔚子，wormwoodlike motherwort herb，Herba Leonuri）[1]

[Original Text]

［Chongweizi（茺蔚子，wormwoodlike motherwort herb，Herba Leonuri），］pungent in taste and slightly warm［in property］，［is mainly used］to improve vision，to replenish essence and to eliminate water-Qi[2]．Long-term taking［of it will］relax the body．［Its］stalks［can］treat urticaria with itching．［It can be］decocted to wash［the body of the patient for treatment］．［It is also］called Yimu（益母），Yiming（益明）and Dazha（大札），growing in lakes and swamps.

[Textual Research]

［In the book entitled］*Ming Yi Bie Lu*（《名医别录》，*Special Record of Great Doctors*），［it］says［that Chongweizi（茺蔚子，wormwoodlike motherwort herb，Herba Leonuri）is also］named Zhenwei（贞蔚），growing in Haibin（海滨），［and can be］collected in May.

［In］case［analysis in the book entitled］*Shuo Wen*（《说文》，*On Culture*），［it］says［that the so-called］Tui（萑）[3] refers to Huan（萑）[4]．［In the book entitled］*Guang Ya*（《广雅》，*The First Chinese Encyclopedic Dictionary*），［it］says［that］Yimu（益母）refers to Chongweizi（茺蔚子，wormwoodlike motherwort herb，

能使眼睛明亮，能补益精气，能消除水气。长期服用能使人身体轻盈。其茎能主治癥疹所致之剧痒，可煎煮成洗浴用的汤剂。又称为益母，又称为益明，又称为大札。该物生长在池泽中。

Herba Leonuri).

Notes

1. Chongweizi（茺蔚子，wormwoodlike motherwort herb，Herba Leonuri），also called Yimu Caozi（益母草子）and Xiaohuma（小胡麻），is a herbal medicinal，pungent and sweet in taste，slightly cold and toxic in property，entering the liver meridian and the spleen meridian，effective in activating the blood，regulating menstruation，clearing the liver and improving vision. Clinically it is used to treat irregular menstruation，dysmenorrhea，morbid leucorrhea，blood stasis and abdominal pain after delivery of baby and hypertension as well as swelling and pain of the eyes.

2. The so-called water-Qi（水气）actually refers to edema.

3. Tui（蓷）is another name of Chongweizi（茺蔚子，wormwoodlike motherwort herb，Herba Leonuri）.

4. Huan（萑）is another name of Chongweizi（茺蔚子，wormwoodlike motherwort herb，Herba Leonuri），but also refers to Luwei（芦苇，reed，Phragmites Communis）.

29.　女萎

【原文】

味甘,平。

主中风暴热,不能动摇,跌筋结肉,诸不足。久服,去面黑皯,好颜色,润泽,轻身不老。生山谷。

【考据】

1.《吴普》曰:女萎一名葳蕤,一名玉马,一名地节,一名虫蝉,一名乌萎,一名荧,一名玉竹,神农苦,一经甘,桐君雷公扁鹊甘无毒,黄帝辛,生太山山谷,叶青黄相值如姜,二月七月采,治中风暴热,久服轻身(《御览》),一名左眄,久服轻身耐老(同上)。

2.《名医》曰:一名荧,一名地节,一名玉竹,一名马熏,生太山及邱陵,立春后采,阴干。

3. 案《尔雅》云:荧委萎;郭璞云:药草也,叶似竹,大者如箭,竿,有节,叶狭而长,表白裹青,根大如指,长一二尺,可啖;陶宏景云:按本经有女萎,无萎蕤,别录有萎蕤,而为用正同,疑女萎即萎蕤也,惟名异耳;陈藏器云:魏志樊阿传,青粘,一名黄芝,一名地节,此即萎蕤。

29. Nǚwei（女萎，stem of October clematis，Caulis Clematidis Apiifoliae）[1]

[Original Text]

[Nǚwei（女萎，stem of October clematis，Caulis Clematidis Apiifoliae），] sweet in taste [and] mild [in property]，[is mainly used] to treat wind attack with sudden high fever，difficulty to move，convulsion and tension of sinews and muscles [as well as syndromes/patterns of] various deficiency. Long-term taking [of it can] remove facial blackspots，lustering facial expression，moistening [superficies]，relaxing the body and preventing aging. [It] grows in mountains and valleys.

[Textual Research]

[In the book entitled] *Wu Pu Ben Cao*（《吴普本草》，*Wu Pu's Studies of Materia Medica*），[it] says [that] Nǚwei（女萎，stem of October clematis，Caulis Clematidis Apiifoliae）[is also] called Weirui（葳蕤），Yuma（玉马），Dijie（地节），Chongchan（虫蝉），Wuwei（乌萎），Ying（荧）and Yuzhu（玉竹）. [According to] Agriculture God（神农）[it is] bitter [in taste and] sweet [after] processing. [According to] Tongjun（桐君），Leigong（雷公）and Bianque（扁鹊），[it is] sweet [in taste] and non-toxic [in property]；[according to] Yellow Emperor（黄帝），[it is] pungent [in taste]. [It] grows in the valleys in Taishan（太山）. [Its] leaves

【今译】

味甘,性平。

主治因中风所致的暴热,身体不能正常活动,筋骨肌肉凝聚而挛急,能治疗各种不足之症。长期服用,能消除面部黑斑,能使面部色彩美丽,能滋润面部光泽,能使人身体轻盈,长寿不老。该物生长在山谷之中。

are green and yellow like ginger. ［It should be］ collected in February and July ［and can be used］ to treat wind attack with high fever. Long-term taking ［of it will］ relax the body.

［In the book entitled］ *Ming Yi Bie Lu* (《名医别录》, *Special Record of Great Doctors*)，［it］ says ［that Nǔwei (女萎, stem of October clematis, Caulis Clematidis Apiifoliae) is also］ called Ying (荧)，Dijie (地节)，Yuzhu (玉竹) and Maxun (马熏)，growing in Taishan (太山) and Qiuling (邱陵). ［It should be］ collected in the Beginning of Spring and dried in the shade.

Guo Pu said (郭璞)，"［Nǔ wei (女萎, stem of October clematis, Caulis Clematidis Apiifoliae) is］ a medicinal herb. ［Its］ leaves look like bamboo or like arrow ［if it is］ large and long. There are joints in its stalks，externally white and internally green. The root is big and long，about one or two *Chi* (尺) ［in length］.

Notes

1. Nǔwei (女萎, stem of October clematis, Caulis Clematidis Apiifoliae) is a medicinal herb，also known as Yuzhu (玉竹)，Weirui (葳蕤) and Lingdangcai (铃铛菜)，sweet in taste and mild in property，entering the lung meridian and the stomach meridian，effective in enriching Yin，moistening dryness，eliminating vexation，ceasing thirst，softening sinews and strengthening the heart. Clinically it is used to treat heat disease with fluid damage，Yin deficiency with dryness and heat，dry cough without sputum，vexation with thirst and polyorexia.

30. 防葵

【原文】

味辛,寒。

主疝瘕,肠泄,膀胱热结,溺不下,咳逆,温疟,癫痫,惊邪狂走。久服,坚骨髓,益气轻身。一名梨盖。生川谷。

【考据】

1.《吴普》曰:房葵一名梨盖,一名爵离,一名房苑,一名晨草,一名利如,一名方盖,神农辛,小寒,桐君扁鹊无毒,岐伯雷公黄帝苦,无毒,茎叶如葵,上黑黄,二月生根,根大如桔梗,根中红白,六月花白,七月八月实白,三月三日采根(《御览》)。

2.《名医》曰:一名房慈,一名爵离,一名农果,一名利茹,一名方盖,生临淄,及嵩高太山少室,三月三日,采根暴干。

3. 案《博物志》云:防葵与狼毒相似。

【今译】

味辛,性寒。

30. Fangkui（防葵，oreoselinum，Radix Peucedani Praeruptori）[1]

[Original Text]

[Fangkui（防葵，oreoselinum，Radix Peucedani Praeruptori），] pungent in taste and cold [in property]，[is mainly used] to treat hernia and abdominal lump[2]，diarrhea，heat accumulation in the bladder，anuria，cough with dyspnea，warm malaria，epilepsy and running wildly [due to] fright. Long-term taking [of it will] strengthen bone marrow，replenish Qi and relax the body. [It is also] called Ligai（梨盖），growing in mountain valleys and river valleys.

[Textual Research]

[In the book entitled] *Wu Pu Ben Cao*（《吴普本草》，*Wu Pu's Studies of Materia Medica*），[it] says [that Fangkui（防葵，oreoselinum，Radix Peucedani Praeruptori) is also] called Ligai（梨盖），Jueli（爵离），Fangyuan（房苑），Chencao（晨草），Liru（利如）and Fanggai（方盖），etc. [According to] Agriculture God（神农），[it is] pungent [in taste] and slightly cold [in property]；[according to] Tongjun（桐君）and Bianque（扁鹊），[it is] non-toxic [in property]；[according to] Qibo（岐伯），Leigong（雷公）and Yellow Emperor（黄帝），[it is] bitter [in taste] and non-toxic [in property]. [Its] stalks and leaves look like sunflower with black and yellow color in the upper. [Its] root begins to grow in February，as

主治疝瘕，泄泻，膀胱热结，小便不通，咳嗽气逆，暑热之邪所致的疟疾，癫痫，受惊而狂奔。长期服用，能使骨髓强健，能补益精气，能使人身体轻盈。又称为梨盖。该物生长在山川河谷之中。

large as that of Jiegeng （桔梗，platycodon grandiflorum，Radix Platycodi）. The root is red and white, the flower turns white in June and the fruit becomes white in July and August. The root [should be] collected on March 3.

[In the book entitled] *Ming Yi Bie Lu* （《名医别录》，*Special Record of Great Doctors*）, [it] says [that Fangkui （防葵，oreoselinum，Radix Peucedani Praeruptori）, also] called Fangci （房慈）, Jueli （爵离）, Nongguo （农果）, Liru （利茹） and Fanggai （方盖）, grows in Linzi （临淄）, Songgao （嵩高）, Taishan （太山） and Shaoshi （少室）. The root [should be] collected on March 3 and dried in the sun.

[In the book entitled] *Bo Wu Zhi* （《博物志》，*History of All Plants*）, [it] says [that] Fangkui （防葵，oreoselinum，Radix Peucedani Praeruptori） is similar to Langdu （狼毒，Chinese stellera root, fischer euphorbia root, Radix Stellerae Chamaejasmis seu Euphorbiae Fischerianae）.

Notes

1. Fangkui （防葵，oreoselinum，Radix Peucedani Praeruptori） is a herbal medicinal, pungent and bitter in taste, cold and non-toxic in property, effective in treating hernia and abdominal lump, diarrhea, heat accumulation in the bladder, anuria, cough with dyspnea, epilepsy, deficiency and weakness of the five Zang-organs, lower abdominal mass, oral dryness and amassment of water in the bladder.

2. Hernia and abdominal lump refer to pathological conditions. One is transformation of pathogenic wind into heat that transmits to the lower energizer and mixes with dampness, characterized by lower abdominal heat and pain, difficulty in urination and turbid urine. The other is wind-cold mixed with the blood in the abdomen, characterized by protrusion of the abdomen and pain involving the waist.

31. 柴胡

【原文】

味苦,平。

主心腹,去肠胃中结气,饮食积聚,寒热邪气,推陈致新。久服,轻身明目益精。一名地熏。

【考据】

1.《吴普》曰:茈葫,一名山菜,一名茹草,神农岐伯雷公苦无毒,生冤句,二月八月采根(《御览》)。

2.《名医》曰:一名山菜,一名茹草,叶一名芸蒿,辛香可食,生宏农及冤句,二月八月采根暴干。

3. 案《博物志》云:芸蒿叶似邪蒿,春秋有白蒻,长四五寸,香美可食,长安及河内并有之;《夏小正》云:正月采芸,月令云仲春芸始生;吕氏春秋云:菜之美者,华阳之芸,皆即此也,急就篇有芸;颜师古注云:即今芸蒿也,然则是此茈胡叶矣,茈柴前声相转,《名医》别录,前胡条,非;陶宏景云:本经上品,有茈胡而无此,晚来医乃用之。

31. Chaihu（柴胡，bupleurum，Radix Bupleuri）[1]

[Original Text]

［Chaihu（柴胡，bupleurum，Radix Bupleuri），］bitter in taste and mild ［in property］, ［is mainly used］ to treat ［disorders of］ the heart and abdomen，to eliminate binding of Qi in the intestines and stomach ［as well as］ accumulation of ［undigested］ food ［in the stomach］，to remove evil-Qi in cold and heat，and to get rid of the stale to bring forth the fresh. Long-term taking ［of it will］ relax the body，improve vision and replenish essence. ［It is also］ called Dixun（地熏）.

[Textual Research]

［In the book entitled］ *Wu Pu Ben Cao*（《吴普本草》，*Wu Pu's Studies of Materia Medica* ），［it］ says ［that］ Chaihu（柴胡，bupleurum，Radix Bupleuri) is also called Shancai（山菜）and Rucao（茹草）.［According to］ Agriculture God（神农），Qibo（岐伯）and Leigong（雷公），［it is］ bitter ［in taste］ and non-toxic ［in property］.［Its］ root ［should be］ collected in February and August.

［In the book entitled］ *Ming Yi Bie Lu*（《名医别录》，*Special Record of Great Doctors* ），［it］ says ［that Chaihu（柴胡，bupleurum，Radix Bupleuri) is also］ called Shancai（山菜），Rucao（茹草）and Yunhao（芸蒿）.［It is］ pungent，sweet and edible.［It］ grows in Hongnong（宏农）and Yuanju（冤句）.［Its］ root ［can be］ collected

【今译】

　　味苦,性平。

　　主治心腹疾患,能解除肠胃气结,能消除积聚于肠胃中的未消化饮食,能治疗寒热性疾病,能祛除邪气,能清除人体中的糟粕,能纳入新的营养之物。长期服用,能使人身体轻盈,能使眼睛明亮,能补益精气。又称为地熏。

in February and August, and dried in the sun.

[In the book entitled] *Bo Wu Zhi* (《博物志》, *History of All Plants*), [it] says [that] the leaves of Chaihu (柴胡, bupleurum, Radix Bupleuri) are similar to those of Xiehao (邪蒿, common seseli herb, Herba Seselis Seseloidis) and Bairuo (白翡, large rhizome of hindu lotus, Rhizoma Nelumbinis) in spring and autumn, about four to five *Cun* (寸), fragrant and edible. [It] grows in Chang'an (长安) and Henei (河内).

[In the book entitled] *Lǚ Shi Chun Qiu* (《吕氏春秋》, *Lǚ's History of Spring and Autumn Period*) says [that Chaihu (柴胡, bupleurum, Radix Bupleuri) is like] a fragrant vegetable, like cole in Huayang (华阳).

Notes

1. Chaihu (柴胡, bupleurum, Radix Bupleuri) is a herbal medicinal, also known as Dixun (地熏), Shancai (山菜), Gucao (菇草) and Chaicao (柴草), bitter in taste and slightly cold in property, entering the liver meridian and gallbladder meridian, effective in harmonizing the external and internal, soothing the liver and promoting Yang. Clinically it is used to treat common cold, fever, alternate cold and heat, malaria, liver depression and Qi stagnation, distension and pain of the chest and rib-side, anal prolapse, uterine prolapse and irregular menstruation.

32. 麦门冬

【原文】

味甘,平。

主心腹,结气伤中伤饱,胃络脉绝,羸瘦短气。久服轻身,不老不饥。生川谷及堤阪。

【考据】

1.《吴普》曰:一名马韭,一名衅冬,一名忍冬,一名忍陵,一名不死药,一名仆垒,一名随脂(太平《御览》引云,一名羊韭,秦,一名马韭,一名禹韭,韭,越一名羊齐,一名麦韭,一名禹韭,一名衅韭,一名禹余粮),神农岐伯甘平,黄帝桐君雷公甘无毒,李氏甘小温,扁鹊无毒,生山谷肥地,叶如韭,肥泽丛生,采无时,实青黄。

2.《名医》曰:秦名羊韭,齐名麦韭,楚名马韭,越名羊蓍,一名禹葭,一名禹余粮,叶如韭,冬夏长生,生函谷肥土,石间久废处,二月三月八月十月采,阴干。

3. 案《说文》云:荵,荵冬草;《中山经》云:青要之山,是多仆累,据《吴普》说,即麦门冬也,忍,荵,垒,累,音同;陶宏景云:实如青珠,根似

32. Maimendong（麦门冬，ophiopogon，Radix Ophiopogonis）[1]

[Original Text]

[Maimendong（麦门冬，ophiopogon，Radix Ophiopogonis），] sweet [in] taste [and] mild [in property]，[is mainly used] to treat [disorders of] the heart and abdomen，damage caused by stagnation of Qi，exhaustion of the collaterals of the stomach meridian，emaciation and shortness of breath. Long-term taking [of it will] relax the body，prevent aging and hunger. [It] grows in mountain valleys，river valleys and Tiban（堤阪，a rugged and uneven area）.

[Textual Research]

[In the book entitled] *Wu Pu Ben Cao*（《吴普本草》，*Wu Pu's Studies of Materia Medica*），[it] says [that Maimendong（麦门冬，ophiopogon，Radix Ophiopogonis）is also] called Majiu（马韭），Xidong（羊冬），Rendong（忍冬），Renling（忍陵），Busiyao（不死药），Pulei（仆垒），Suizhi（随脂）. [According to] Agriculture God（神农）and Qibo（岐伯），[it is] sweet [in taste] and mild in [proptery；[according to] Yellow Emperor（黄帝），Tongjun（桐君）and Leigong（雷公），[it is] sweet [in taste] and non-toxic [in property]；[according to] Li's（李氏），[it is] sweet [in taste] and slightly warm [in property]；[according to] Bianque（扁鹊），[it is] non-toxic [in property]. [It] grows in valleys and fertile land. [Its]

穬麦,故谓麦门冬。

【今译】

味甘,性平。

主治心腹气结,内脏损伤,伤食,因胃络损伤而跳动停止,能治疗身体瘦弱,呼吸气短。长期服用能使人身体轻盈,长寿不老,能减少饥饿之感。该物生长在山川河谷之中以及河堤与崎岖之地中。

leaves look like Chinese chives [and its] fruits are yellow. [It can be] collected at any time.

[In the book entitled] *Ming Yi Bie Lu* (《名医别录》, *Special Record of Great Doctors*), [it] says [that Maimendong (麦门冬, ophiopogon, Radix Ophiopogonis) is named differently in different regions, such as] Yangjiu (羊韭) in Qin (秦) [area], Maijiu (麦韭) in Qi (齐) [area], Majiu (马韭) in Chu (楚) [area] and Yangqi (羊蓍) in Yue (越) [area], etc. [Its] leaves look like Chinese chives. [It] grows in valleys and fertile land, developing prosperously in winter and summer. [It can be] collected in February, March, August and October, and dried in the shade.

Notes

1. Maimendong (麦门冬, ophiopogon, Radix Ophiopogonis) is a herbal medicinal, sweet and slightly bitter in taste, cold in property, entering the heart meridian, the lung meridian and the stomach meridian, effective in clearing the heart, moistening the lung, nourishing the stomach and producing fluid. Clinically it is used to treat vexation due to heat pain, thirst due to fluid damage, dry cough due to dryness of the lung, hemoptysis, nosebleed, lung abscess, wasting-thirst and constipation due to intestinal dryness.

33. 独活

【原文】

味苦,平。

主风寒所击,金疮止痛,贲豚,痫痓,女子疝瘕。久服,轻身耐老。一名羌活,一名羌青,一名护羌使者。生川谷。

【考据】

1.《吴普》曰:独活一名胡王使者,神农黄帝苦无毒,八月采,此药有风花不动,无风独摇(《御览》)。

2.《名医》曰:一名胡王使者,一名独摇草,此草得风不摇,无风自动,生雍州,或陇西南安,二月八月采根暴干。

3. 案《列仙传》云:山图服羌活独活,则似二名,护羌胡王皆羌字缓声,犹专诸为专设诸,庚公差为瘐公之斯,非有义也。

【今译】

味苦,性平。

主治因风寒损伤所致的疾患,因金属创伤,能消除疼痛,能治疗贲

33. Duhuo（独活，pubescent angelica，Radix Angelicae Pubescentis）[1]

［**Original Text**］

［Duhuo （独活，pubescent angelica，Radix Angelicae Pubescentis），］bitter in taste and mild ［in property］，［is mainly used］to treat wind-cold attack，relieving pain ［caused by］metal injury，running piglet，epilepsy and hernia-conglomeration in woman[2]．［It is also］called Qianghuo（羌活），Qiangqing（羌青）and Huqiang Shizhe（护羌使者），growing in mountain valleys and river valleys.

［**Textual Research**］

［In the book entitled］*Wu Pu Ben Cao*（《吴普本草》，*Wu Pu's Studies of Materia Medica*），［it］says ［that］Duhuo（独活，pubescent angelica，Radix Angelicae Pubescentis）［is also］called Huwang Shizhe（胡王使者）．［According to］Agriculture God（神农）and Yellow Emperor（黄帝），［it is］bitter ［in taste］and non-toxic ［in property］．［It can be］collected in August. The flowers in this herb never move ［when］wind is blowing．［but always］move ［when there is］no wind.

［In the book entitled］*Ming Yi Bie Lu*（《名医别录》，*Special Record of Great Doctors*），［it］says ［that Duhuo（独活，pubescent angelica，Radix Angelicae Pubescentis）is also］called Huwang

豚，癫痫，抽搐以及女子疝瘕。长期服用，能使人身体轻盈，不易衰老。又称为羌活，又称为羌青，又称为护羌使者。该物生长在山川河谷之中。

Shizhe（胡王使者）and Duyaocao（独摇草）. This herb never moves [when] wind is blowing, but spontaneously move [when there is] no wind. [It] grows in Yongzhou（雍州）or Nan'an（南安）in Longxi（陇西）. [Its] root [should be] collected in February and August, and dried in the sun.

Notes

1. Duhuo （独活, pubescent angelica, Radix Angelicae Pubescentis) is a herbal medicinal, also known as Rouduhuo（肉独活）and Chuanduhuo（川独活）, pungent and bitter in taste and warm in property, entering the kidney meridian and bladder meridian, effective in dispelling pathogenic wind, dispersing pathogenic cold and relieving pain. Clinically it is used to treat wind, cold and dampness impediment, aching pain of the knees and waist, convulsion and pain of hands and feet, common cold and headache.

2. The so-called hernia-conglomeration in woman is a disease characterized by pain and heat in the lower abdomen, difficulty in urination, turbid urine and pain involving the waist and back caused by accumulation of wind-heat in the lower abdomen and its mixture with pathogenic dampness.

34. 车前子

【原文】

味甘,寒,无毒。

主气癃,止痛,利水道小便,除湿痹。久服轻身耐老。一名当道,生平泽。

【考据】

1.《名医》曰:一名芣苢,一名虾蟆衣,一名牛遗,一名胜舄,生真定邱陵阪道中,五月五日采,阴干。

2. 案《说文》云:芣一曰芣苢,苢,芣苢,一名马舄,其实如李,令人宜子,周书所说,《广雅》云当道马舄也;《尔雅》云:舄苢马,舄,马舄车前;郭璞云:今车前草,大叶长穗,好生道边,江东呼为虾蟆衣,又蕵,牛蕵;孙炎云:车前一名牛蕵,《毛诗》云采采芣苢,《传》云芣苢,马舄,马舄,车前也;陆玑云:马舄一名车前,一名当道,喜在牛迹中生,故曰车前当道也,今药中车前子,是也,幽州人谓之牛舌草。

34. Cheqianzi（车前子，seed of Asiatic plantain，Semen Plantaginis）[1]

[Original Text]

［Cheqianzi（车前子，seed of Asiatic plantain，Semen Plantaginis），］sweet in taste，cold and non-toxic［in property］，［is mainly used］to treat Qi block，relieving pain，to disinhibit waterway［in the body］and urination，and to eliminate dampness impediment. Long-term taking［of it can］relax the body and prevent aging.［It is also］called Dangdao（当道）and grows in［the areas with］plains and swamps.

[Textual Research]

［In the book entitled］*Ming Yi Bie Lu*（《名医别录》，*Special Record of Great Doctors*），［it］says［that Cheqianzi（车前子，seed of Asiatic plantain，Semen Plantaginis），is also］called Fuyi（苤苢），Xiamoyi（虾蟆衣），Niuyi（牛遗）and Shengxi（胜舄），growing in mountains in Zhending（真定）and Qiuling（邱陵）.［It can be］collected on May 5 and dried in the shade.

Guo Pu（郭璞）said，"Now Cheqianzi（车前子，seed of Asiatic plantain，Semen Plantaginis）bears large leaves and long tassels，often growing in the sides of roads."

【今译】

味甘,性寒,无毒。

主治气癃,能消除疼痛,能通利水道,能疏通小便,能祛除湿邪所致痹证。长期服用能使人身体轻盈,不易衰老。又称为当道,该物生长在平川水泽之中。

Notes

1. Cheqianzi（车前子，seed of Asiatic plantain，Semen Plantaginis）is a herbal medicinal，also known as Cheqianshi（车前实），Fengyan Qianren（凤眼前仁）and Qianren（前仁），sweet in taste and cold in property，entering the kidney meridian and the bladder meridian，effective in disinhibiting water，clearing heat，improving vision and eliminating phlegm. Clinically it is used to treat dysuria，stranguria，morbid leucorrhea，diarrhea and dysentery due to summer-heat and dampness.

35. 木香

【原文】

味辛,温。

主邪气,辟毒疫,温鬼,强志,主淋露。久服,不梦寤魇寐。生山谷。

【考据】

1.《名医》曰:一名蜜香,生永昌。

【今译】

味辛,温。

主治邪气所致之症,能解除毒邪传染,能祛除温热性疾患,能增强记忆力,能治疗因淋雨雾气所致之疾患。长期服用,不会使人睡眠中因噩梦而惊醒。该物生长在山谷之中。

35. Muxiang（木香，root of common aucklandia，Radix Aucklandiae）[1]

[Original Text]

［Muxiang （木香，root of common aucklandia，Radix Aucklandiae），］ pungent in taste and warm ［in property］，［is mainly used］ to eliminate evil-Qi，to prevent ［invasion of］ toxin and pestilence，to strengthen memory，and to treat severe heat ［disease］ and ［disease caused by］ rain，fog and dew. Long-term taking ［of it will］ avoid nightmare and sudden waking up ［due to fright］．［It］ grows in mountains and valleys.

[Textual Research]

［In the book entitled］ *Ming Yi Bie Lu*（《名医别录》，*Special Record of Great Doctors*），［it］ says ［that Muxiang（木香，root of common aucklandia，Radix Aucklandiae）is also］ called Mixiang（蜜香）and grows in Yongchang（永昌）.

Notes

1. Muxiang（木香，root of common aucklandia，Radix Aucklandiae）is a herbal medicinal，bitter and pungent in taste，warm in property，entering the liver meridian，the spleen meridian and the kidney meridian，effective in promoting Qi to flow，relieving pain，warming the middle（the internal organs）and harmonizing the stomach. Clinically it is used to treat cold attack，Qi stagnation，epigastric and abdominal distension and pain，vomiting，diarrhea and dysentery.

36. 薯蓣

【原文】

味甘,温。

主伤中,补虚羸,除寒热邪气,补中益气力,长肌肉。久服耳目聪明,轻身不饥,延年。一名山芋,生山谷。

【考据】

1.《吴普》曰:薯蓣,一名诸署(《御览》作署豫,作诸署,艺文类聚,亦作诸),齐越名山芋,一名修脆,一名儿草(《御览》引云,秦楚名玉延,齐越名山芋,郑赵名山芋,一名玉延)神农甘小温,桐君雷公甘(御引作苦),无毒,或生临朐钟山,始生,赤茎细蔓,五月华白,七月实青黄,八月熟落,根中白,皮黄,类芋(《御览》引云,二月八月采根,恶甘遂)。

2.《名医》曰:秦楚名玉延,郑越名土诸,生嵩高,二月八月采根,暴干。

3. 案《广雅》云:玉延,薯豫,薯蓣也;北山经云:景山草多薯豫;郭璞云:根似羊蹄可食,今江南单呼为薯,语有轻重耳;《范子计然》云:薯豫本出三辅,白色者善;本章衍义云:山药上一字犯宋英庙讳,下一字曰

36. Shuyu（薯蓣，dioscorea，Rhizoma Dioscoreae）[1]

[Original Text]

[Shuyu（薯蓣，dioscorea，Rhizoma Dioscoreae），] sweet [in] taste [and] warm [in property]，[is mainly used] to treat middle damage[2]，to improve deficiency and emaciation，to eliminate evil-Qi in cold and heat，to tonify the middle（internal organs），to increase energy and to promote [growth of] muscles. Long-term taking [of it can] improve hearing and vision，relaxing the body，relieving hunger and prolonging life. [It is also] called Shanyu（山芋），growing in mountains and valleys.

[Textual Research]

[In the book entitled] *Wu Pu Ben Cao*（《吴普本草》，*Wu Pu's Studies of Materia Medica*），[it] says [that Shuyu（薯蓣，dioscorea，Rhizoma Dioscoreae）is also] called Zhushu（诸署），Shanyu（山芋），Xiucui（修脆）and Ercao（儿草）. [According to] Agriculture God（神农），[it is] sweet [in taste] and slightly warm [in property]；[according to] Tongjun（桐君）and Leigong（雷公），[it is] sweet [in taste] and non-toxic [in property]，growing in Zhongshan（钟山）in Linqu（临朐）. [When it] begins to grow，the stalks are red and thin. [In] May，[its] flowers are white；[in] July，[its] fruits are green and yellow and become ripe [in] August. [Its] root is white and [its] peel is yellow.

蓣,唐代宗名豫,故改下一字为药。

【今译】

味甘,性温。

主治内脏损伤,能补益虚弱消瘦,能消除寒热性疾病和邪气,能补充人体内脏,能增强气力,能增长肌肉。长期服用能使人听力增强,视力清明,身体轻盈,能减少饥饿之感,能延年益寿。又称为山芋,该物生长在山谷之中。

［In the book entitled］ *Ming Yi Bie Lu* （《名医别录》，*Special Record of Great Doctors*），［it］ says ［that Shuyu （薯蓣，dioscorea，Rhizoma Dioscoreae) is also］ called Yuyan （玉延） in Qin （秦） and Chu （楚）［areas］，and Tuzhu （土诸） in Zheng （郑） and Yue （越）［areas］．［It］ grows in Songgao （嵩高）．［Its］ root ［can be］ collected in February and August，and dried in the sun．

Notes

1. Shuyu （薯蓣，dioscorea，Rhizoma Dioscoreae)］ is a herbal medicinal，sweet in taste and mild in property，entering the spleen meridian and the kidney meridian，effective in treating diarrhea due to spleen deficiency，chronic dysentery，overstrain，cough，seminal emission，leucorrhea，frequent urination and diabetes．

2. The so-called middle damage means deficiency disease caused by injury of the internal organs．

37. 薏苡仁

【原文】

味甘,微寒。

主筋急拘挛,不可屈伸,风湿痹,下气。久服轻身,益气。

其根下三虫,一名解蠡。生平泽及田野。

【考据】

1.《名医》曰:一名屋菼,一名起实,一名赣,生真定,八月采实,采根无时。

2. 案《说文》云:蔇,蔇苢,一曰蔇英,赣,一曰薏蔇;《广雅》云:赣,起实,蔇目也,吴越春秋,鲧娶于有莘氏之女,名曰女嬉,年壮未孳,嬉于砥山,得薏苡而吞之,意若为人所感,因而妊孕,后汉书马援传,援在交趾,常饵薏苡实,用能轻身省欲以胜瘴,蔇,俗作薏,非。

【今译】

味甘,性微寒。

主治筋急紧而拘挛,不能弯曲直伸,风湿邪所致痹证,能使气下行

37. Yiyiren（薏苡仁，coix，Semen Coicis）[1]

[Original Text]

[Yiyiren（薏苡仁，coix，Semen Coicis），] sweet in taste and slightly cold [in property], [is mainly used] to treat spasm and tension of sinews, inability to bend and stretch, wind-dampness impediment and [cough and panting through] descending Qi. Long-term taking [of it can] relax the body and replenish Qi.

[Its] root [can be used to] eliminate three worms[2]. [It is also] called Xieli（解蠡），growing in plains，swamps and fields.

[Textual Research]

[In the book entitled] *Ming Yi Bie Lu*（《名医别录》，*Special Record of Great Doctors*），[it] says [that Yiyiren（薏苡仁，coix，Semen Coicis) is also] called Wutan（屋菼），Qishi（起实）and Gan（赣），growing in Zhending（真定）. [It can be] collected in August and [its] root [can be] collected at any time.

Notes

1. Yiyiren（薏苡仁，coix，Semen Coicis) is a herbal medicinal，sweet and bland in taste，cool in property，entering the spleen meridian，the lung meridian and the kidney meridian，effective in fortifying the spleen，tonifying the lung，clearing heat and resolving dampness. Clinically it is used to treat diarrhea，edema，lung

以降逆。长期服用,能使人身体轻盈,能补益精气。

其根能祛除三种虫子,又称为解蠹。该物生长在平川水泽之中及田野之上。

abscess, stranguria, leucorrhea, flat wart, stomach cancer and uterine cancer.

2. The three worms refer to three kinds of worms in the intestines, i.e. long worm, red worm and short worm.

Agriculture
God's Canon of
Materia Medica

38. 泽泻

【原文】

味甘,寒。

主风寒湿痹,乳难,消水,养五脏,益气力,肥健。久服耳目聪明,不饥,延年,轻身,面生光,能行水上。一名水泻,一名芒芋,一名鹄泻。生池泽。

【考据】

1.《名医》曰:生汝南,五六八月采根,阴干。

2. 案《说文》云:藚水写也;《尔雅》云:蕍蕮;郭璞云:今泽蕮,又藚,牛脣;郭璞云,《毛诗》《传》云:水舄也,如续断,寸寸有节,拔之可复,《毛诗》云,言采其藚,《传》云,藚,水舄也;陆玑云:今泽舄也,其叶如车前草大,其味亦相似,徐州广陵人食之。

【今译】

味甘,性寒。

主治风寒湿邪所致痹证,分娩困难,能消除水液,能滋养五脏,能补

38. Zexie（泽泻，alsma，Rhizoma Alismatis）[1]

[Original Text]

[Zexie（泽泻，alsma，Rhizoma Alismatis），] sweet in taste and cold [in property], [is mainly used] to treat wind，cold and dampness impediment and difficulty in delivering baby，to eliminate water，to nourish the five Zang-organs，to increase energy and to strengthen the body. Long-term taking [of it can] improve hearing and vision，relieve hunger，prolong life，relax the body，luster the facial expression，just like walking over river. [It is also] called Shuixie（水泻），Mangyu（芒芋）and Huxie（鹄泻），growing in lakes and swamps.

[Textual Research]

[In the book entitled] *Ming Yi Bie Lu*（《名医别录》，*Special Record of Great Doctors*），[it] says [that Zexie（泽泻，alsma，Rhizoma Alismatis）] grows in Runan（汝南）. [Its] root [can be] collected in May，June and August，and dried in the shade.

Luji（陆玑）said，"The leaves of Zexie（泽泻，alsma，Rhizoma Alismatis）are as large as those of Cheqianzi（车前子，seed of Asiatic plantain，Semen Plantaginis），its taste is also similar [to that of Cheqianzi（车前子，seed of Asiatic plantain，Semen Plantaginis）]. People from Guangling（广陵）in Xuzhou（徐州）like to take it."

益气力,能使人身体康健。长期服用能使人听力增强,视力清明,能减少饥饿之感,能延年益寿,能身体轻盈,能使面部光彩,如同行走在水上一样。又称为水泻,又称为芒芋,又称为鹄泻。该物生长在池泽中。

Notes

1. Zexie （泽泻，alsma，Rhizoma Alismatis） is a herbal medicinal, sweet in taste and cold in property, entering the kidney meridian and bladder meridian, effective in promoting urination, eliminating dampness and resolving heat. Clinically it is used to treat dysuria, edema, beriberi, diarrhea, stranguria and leucorrhea.

39. 远志

【原文】

味苦,温。

主咳逆,伤中,补不足,除邪气,利九窍,益智慧,耳目聪明,不忘,强志倍力。久服,轻身不老。叶名小草,一名棘菀(陆德明《尔雅》音义引作䒶),一名棘绕(《御览》作要绕),一名细草。生川谷。

【考据】

1.《名医》曰:生太山及冤句,四月采根叶,阴干。

2.案《说文》云:菀,棘菀也;《广雅》云:蕀苑,远志也,其上谓之小草;《尔雅》云:葽绕,蕀菀;郭璞云:今远志也,似麻黄,赤华,叶锐而黄。

【今译】

味苦,性温。

主治咳嗽气逆,内脏损伤,能补充精气不足,能清除邪气,能使九窍通畅,能增加智慧,能使人听力增强,视力清明,能消除健忘症,能提高

39. Yuanzhi（远志，polygala root，
Radix Polygalae）[1]

[Original Text]

[Yuanzhi（远志，polygala root，Radix Polygalae），] bitter in taste and warm [in property], [is mainly used] to treat cough with dyspnea and internal damage, to improve insufficiency, to eliminate evil-Qi, to disinhibit nine orifices, to replenish wisdom and to ensure hearing, vision, memory, energy and strength. Long-term taking [of it will] relax the body and prevent aging. [Its] leaves are called small grass. [It is also] called Ciyuan（棘菀），Cirao（棘绕）and Xicao（细草），growing in mountain valleys and river valleys.

[Textual Research]

[In the book entitled] *Ming Yi Bie Lu*（《名医别录》，*Special Record of Great Doctors*），[it] says [that Yuanzhi（远志，polygala root，Radix Polygalae）] grows in Taishan（太山）and Yuanju（冤句）. [Its] root and leaves [can be] collected in April and dried in the shade.

[In the book entitled] *Guang Ya*（《广雅》，*The First Chinese Encyclopedic Dictionary*），[it] says [that] Ciyuan（蒬菀）refers to Yuanzhi（远志，polygala root，Radix Polygalae），the tip of which looks like a small grass.

Guo Pu（郭璞）said，"Now Yuanzhi（远志，polygala root，

记忆力，能增强气力。长期服用，能使人身体轻盈，长寿不老。其叶之名为小草，又称为棘菀，又称为棘绕，又称为细草。该物生长在山川河谷之中。

Radix Polygalae) looks like Mahuang （麻黄，ephedra，Herba Ephedrae）[because it bears] red flowers and sharp yellow leaves. "

Notes

1. Yuanzhi（远志，polygala root，Radix Polygalae）is a herbal medicinal，bitter and pungent in taste，warm in property，entering the heart meridian，the lung meridian and the kidney meridian，effective in tranquilizing the mind，strengthening the will，dispelling phlegm and ceasing cough. Clinically it is used to treat palpitation，amnesia and seminal emission.

40. 龙胆

【原文】

味苦,涩。

主骨间寒热,惊痫邪气。续绝伤,定五脏,杀蛊毒。久服益智,不忘,轻身,耐老。一名陵游,生山谷。

【考据】

1.《名医》曰:生齐朐及冤句,二月八月十一月十二月,采根,阴干。

【今译】

味苦,性涩。

主治骨间寒热性疾病,惊风,癫痫及邪气侵袭。能通过补益治疗外伤所致之筋伤骨折,能安静五脏,能消杀虫毒。长期服用能增强智慧,能消除健忘,能使人身体轻盈,不易衰老。又称为陵游,该物生长在山谷之中。

40. Longdan（龙胆，root of rough gentian，Radix Gentianae）[1]

［Original Text］

［Longdan（龙胆，root of rough gentian，Radix Gentianae），］bitter in taste and astringent［in property］，［is mainly used］to resolve cold-heat in the bones and evil-Qi in fright and epilepsy，continuously to repair severe injury，to strengthen the five Zang-organs and to kill mysterious toxin[2]．Long-term taking［of it will］enrich wisdom，avoid amnesia，relax the body and prevent aging．［It is also］called Lingyou（陵游），growing in mountains and valleys．

［Textual Research］

［In the book entitled］*Ming Yi Bie Lu*（《名医别录》，*Special Record of Great Doctors*），［it］says［that Longdan（龙胆，root of rough gentian，Radix Gentianae）］grows in Qiqu（齐朐）and Yuanju（冤句）．［Its］root［can be］collected in February，August，November and December，and dried in the shade．

Notes

1．Longdan（龙胆，root of rough gentian，Radix Gentianae）is a herbal medicinal，bitter in taste and cold in property，entering the liver meridian and the gallbladder meridian，effective in purging excess-fire in the liver and gallbladder，eliminating dampness-heat in the lower energizer．Clinically it is used to treat headache，swollen eyes，swelling and pain of the throat，swelling and pain of the ears with sores，jaundice，epilepsy，infantile convulsive epilepsy，infection of urethra，swelling and pain of testicles，genital itching and eczema in the genitals and lower legs．

153

41. 细辛

【原文】

味辛,温。

主咳逆,头痛,脑动,百节拘挛,风湿痹痛,死肌。久服明目,利九窍,轻身长年。一名小辛,生山谷。

【考据】

1.《吴普》曰:细辛一名细草(《御览》引云,一名小辛),神农黄帝雷公桐君辛小温,岐伯元毒,李氏小寒,如葵叶,色赤黑,一根一叶相连(《御览》引云,三月八月采根)。

2.《名医》曰:生华阴,二月八月采根,阴干。

3. 案《广雅》云:细条,少辛,细辛也;《中山经》云:浮戏之山,上多少辛;郭璞云:细辛也;《管子·地员篇》云:小辛大蒙;《范子计然》云:细辛出华阴,色白者善。

【今译】

味辛,温。

41. Xixin (细辛, as arum, Herba Asari) [1]

[Original Text]

[Xixin (细辛, as arum, Herba Asari),] pungent in taste and warm [in property], [is mainly used] to treat cough with dyspnea, headache, head shaking, spasm of joints, wind-dampness impediment and pain, and numbness of muscles. Long-term taking [of it can] improve vision, disinhibit nine orifices, relax the body and prolong life. [It is also] called Xiaoxin (小辛), growing in mountains and valleys.

[Textual Research]

[In the book entitled] *Wu Pu Ben Cao* (《吴普本草》, *Wu Pu's Studies of Materia Medica*), [it] says [that] Xixin (细辛, as arum, Herba Asari) is also called Xicao (细草). [According to] Agriculture God (神农), Yellow Emperor (黄帝), Leigong (雷公) and Tongjun (桐均), [it is] pungent [in taste] and slightly warm [in property]; [according to] Qibo (岐伯), [it is] quite toxic; [according to] Li's (李氏), [it is] slightly cold [in property]. [It is just] like the leaves of sunflower, red and black in color, one root connected with one leaf. [According to the book entitled] *Tai Ping Yu Lan* (《太平御览》, *Imperial Studies in Taiping Times*), [it can be] collected in March and August.

[In the book entitled] *Ming Yi Bie Lu* (《名医别录》, *Special*

主治咳嗽气逆,头痛,头颅颤动,关节拘急挛缩,风湿邪所致痹证,疼痛,肌肉坏死。长期服用能使眼睛明亮,九窍通畅,身体轻盈,寿命延长。又称为小辛,该物生长在山谷之中。

Record of Great Doctors), [it] says [that Xixin（细辛, as arum, Herba Asari)] grows in Huayin（华阴). [Its] root [can be] collected in February and August and dried in the shade.

[In the book entitled] *Guang Ya* (《广雅》, *The First Chinese Encyclopedic Dictionary*), [it] says [that the so-called] Xitiao（细条) and Shaoxin（少辛) actually refer to Xixin（细辛, as arum, Herba Asari). [In] case [analysis in the book entitled] *Zhong Shan Jing* (《中山经》, *Central Mountain Canon*), [it] says [that] Shaoyin（少辛) usually grows in Fuxi（浮戏) mountain. [In the book entitled] *Fan Zi Ji Ran* (《范子计然》, *Studies About Fan Li's Teacher*), [it] says [that] Xixin（细辛, as arum, Herba Asari) grows in Huayin（华阴) and the best one is white in color.

Notes

1. Xixin（细辛, as arum, Herba Asari) is a herbal medicinal, pungent in taste and warm in property, entering the lung meridian and the kidney meridian, effective in expelling wind and dispersing cold, relieving pain, warming the lung to resolve phlegm and unobstructing nostrils. Clinically it is used to treat common cold, wind-cold disease, headache, wind-cold and dampness impediment, cough and panting due to drinking cold water and nasal sinusitis.

42. 石斛

【原文】

味甘,平。

主伤中,除痹,下气,补五脏虚劳,羸瘦,强阴。久服厚肠胃,轻身,

延年。一名林兰(御览引云,一名禁生,观本,作黑字),生山谷。

【考据】

1.《吴普》曰:石斛,神农甘平,扁鹊酸,李氏寒(《御览》)。

2.《名医》曰:一名禁生,一名杜兰,一名石蓬,生六安水傍石上,七

月八月,采茎,阴干。

3. 案《范子计然》云:石斛,出六安。

【今译】

味甘,性平。

42. Shihu（石斛，dendrobe，Herba Dendrobii）[1]

［Original Text］

［Shihu（石斛，dendrobe，Herba Dendrobii），］sweet in taste and mild ［in property］，［is mainly used］to treat internal damage[2]，to eliminate impediment，［promote］Qi to descend，to tonify the five Zang-organs ［to treat］ deficiency ［due to］ overstrain and emaciation，and to strengthen Yin. Long-term taking ［of it will］ invigorate the intestines and stomach，relax the body and prolong life. ［It is also］ called Linlan（林兰），growing in mountains and valleys.

［Textual Research］

［In the book entitled］ *Wu Pu Ben Cao*（《吴普本草》，*Wu Pu's Studies of Materia Medica*），［it］says［that according to］Agriculture God（神农），［Shihu（石斛，dendrobe，Herba Dendrobii）is］sweet ［in taste］and mild［in property］；［according to］Bianque（扁鹊），［it is］sour［in taste］；［according to］Li's（李氏），［it is］cold［in property］.

［In the book entitled］ *Ming Yi Bie Lu*（《名医别录》，*Special Record of Great Doctors*），［it］says［that Shihu（石斛，dendrobe，Herba Dendrobii）is also］called Jinsheng（禁生），Dulan（杜兰）and Shizhu（石蓫），growing over stones beside the river in Liu'an（六安）. ［Its］stalks［can be］collected in July and August and dried in

主治内脏损伤，能祛除痹证，能使气下行以降逆，能补益五脏虚劳，能治疗身体瘦弱，能增强阴液。长期服用能使肠胃厚实，能使人身体轻盈，能延年益寿。又称为林兰，该物生长在山谷之中。

the shade.

［In the book entitled］ *Fan Zi Ji Ran* （《范子计然》，*Studies About Fan Li's Teacher*），［it］ says ［that］ Shihu （石斛，dendrobe，Herba Dendrobii) grows in Liu'an （六安）.

Notes

1. Shihu （石斛，dendrobe，Herba Dendrobii） is a herbal medicinal，sweet and bland in taste，slightly cold in property，entering the lung meridian，the stomach meridian and the kidney meridian，effective in enriching Yin，nourishing the stomach，clearing heat and producing fluid. Clinically it is used to treat heat disease with Yin damage，dryness of the mouth and tongue，and deficiency-heat after illness.

2. The so-called internal damage refers to damage of the internal organs.

43. 巴戟天

【原文】

味辛,微温。

主大风邪气,阴痿不起。强筋骨,安五脏,补中,增志,益气。生山谷。

【考据】

1.《名医》曰:生巴郡及下邳,二月八月,采根,阴干。

【今译】

味辛,性微温。

主治大风邪气所致之症,因阳痿而阴茎不能勃起。能强健筋骨,能安静五脏,能补益人体内脏,能增强记忆力,能补益精气。该物生长在山谷之中。

43. Bajitian（巴戟天，root of medicinal indianmulberry，Radix Morindae Officinalis）[1]

［Original Text］

［Bajitian （巴戟天，root of medicinal indianmulberry，Radix Morindae Officinalis），］ pungent in taste and slightly warm ［in property］，［is mainly used］ to treat leprosy ［caused by］ evil-Qi and impotence，to strengthen sinews and bones，to pacify the five Zang-organs，to tonify the middle （internal organs），to increase intelligence and to replenish Qi. ［It］ grows in mountains and valleys.

［Textual Research］

［In the book entitled］ *Ming Yi Bie Lu* （《名医别录》，*Special Record of Great Doctors*），［it］ says ［that Bajitian （巴戟天，root of medicinal indianmulberry，Radix Morindae Officinalis）］ grows in Bajun （巴郡） and Xiapi （下邳）．［Its］ root ［can be］ collected in February and August and dried in the shade.

163

Notes

1. Bajitian （巴戟天，root of medicinal indianmulberry，Radix Morindae Officinalis） is a herbal medicinal，pungent and sweet in taste，slightly warm in property，entering the liver meridian and the kidney meridian，effective in tonifying kidney-Yang，strengthening the sinews and bones，expelling wind-warm pathogenic factors. Clinically it is used to treat impotence due to insufficiency of kidney-Yang，seminal emission，premature ejaculation，spermatorrhea and pain of the waist and knees.

44. 白英

【原文】

味甘,寒。

主寒热,八疸,消渴,补中益气。久服,轻身延年。一名谷菜(元本误作黑字),生山谷。

【考据】

1.《名医》曰:一名白草,生益州,春采叶,夏采茎,秋采花,冬采根。

2. 案《尔雅》云:苻,鬼目;郭璞云:今江东有鬼目草茎似葛,叶圆而毛,子如耳珰也,赤色丛生,《唐本》注;白英云,此鬼目草也。

【今译】

味甘,性寒。

44. Baiying（白英，bittersweet herb，bitter nightshade herb，Herba Solani）[1]

[Original Text]

[Baiying（白英，bittersweet herb，bitter nightshade herb，Herba Solani），] sweet in taste and cold [in property]，[is mainly used] to treat cold-heat [disease]，eight kinds of jaundice and wasting-thirst，to tonify the middle（the internal organs）and to replenish Qi. Long-term taking [of it will] relax the body and prolong life. [It] grows in mountains and valleys.

[Textual Research]

[In the book entitled] *Ming Yi Bie Lu*（《名医别录》，*Special Record of Great Doctors*），[it] says [that Baiying（白英，bittersweet herb，bitter nightshade herb，Herba Solani）is also] called Baicao（白草），growing in Yizhou（益州）. [In] the spring，[its] leaves [can be] collected；[in] the summer，[its] stalks [can be] collected；[in] the autumn，[its] flowers [can be] collected；[in] the winter，[its] root [can be] collected.

Guo Pu（郭璞）said，"Now in the east of Changjiang River，there is a herb [called] Guimucao（鬼目草），the stalks look like Ge（葛，lobed kudzuvine，Puerariae），the leaves are round and hairy，the seeds are like earbob，red in color and growing in great variety. [In] an edition [of canon published in] the Tang [Dynasty，it]

主治寒热性疾病，八种黄疸和消渴，能充实人体内脏，能补益精气。长期服用，能使人身体轻盈，能延年益寿。又称为谷菜，该物生长在山谷之中。

explains [that] Guimucao (鬼目草) actually refers to Baiying (白英, bittersweet herb, bitter nightshade herb, Herba Solani)."

Notes

1. Baiying （白英, bittersweet herb, bitter nightshade herb, Herba Solani) is a herbal medicinal, sweet in taste, cold and non-toxic in property, entering the liver meridian and the stomach meridian, effective in clearing heat, expelling dampness, resolving toxin and dispersing swelling. Clinically it is used to treat jaundice, edema, stranguria, cholecystitis, gallstone and rheumatoid arthritis.

45. 白蒿

【原文】

味甘,平。

主五脏邪气,风寒湿痹,补中益气,长毛发,令黑,疗心悬,少食,常饥。久服,轻身,耳目聪明,不老。生川泽。

【考据】

1.《名医》曰:生中山,二月采。

2. 案《说文》云:蘩,白蒿也,艾,冰台也;《广雅》云:蘩,母,旁勃也;《尔雅》云:艾,冰台;郭璞云:今艾,白蒿;《夏小正》云:二月采蘩;《传》云:蘩,由胡,由胡者,繁母也,繁母者,旁勃也;《尔雅》云:蘩,皤蒿;郭璞云:白蒿,又蘩,由胡;郭璞云:未详;《毛诗》云:于以采蘩,《传》云蘩,皤蒿也,又采蘩祁祁;《传》云:蘩,白蒿也;陆玑云:凡艾,白色者为皤蒿;《楚词》王逸注云:艾,白蒿也,按皤白,音义皆相近,艾,是药名,《本草经》无者,即白蒿是也,《名医》别出艾条,非。

45. Baihao（白蒿，sievers wormwood herb，Herba Artemisiae Sieversianae）[1]

[Original Text]

[Baihao（白蒿，sievers wormwood herb，Herba Artemisiae Sieversianae），] sweet [in] taste and mild [in property]，[is mainly used] to treat evil-Qi in the five Zang-organs，wind-cold and dampness impediment，to tonify the middle（the internal organs）and to replenish Qi，to promote growth of hair，to blacken [hair]，to relieve suspension of the stomach[3]，to increase appetite and [to make people] frequently [feel] hungry[4]. Long-term taking [of it will] relax the body，improve hearing and vision，and prevent aging. [It] grows in valleys and swamps.

[Textual Research]

[In the book entitled] *Ming Yi Bie Lu*（《名医别录》，*Special Record of Great Doctors*），[it] says [that Baihao（白蒿，sievers wormwood herb，Herba Artemisiae Sieversianae）] grows in Zhongshan（中山）and [can be] collected in February.

Notes

1. Baihao（白蒿，sievers wormwood herb，Herba Artemisiae Sieversianae）is herbal medicinal，sweet in taste，mild and non-toxic in property，effective in clearing heat and expelling dampness，

【今译】

味甘,性平。

主治五脏中的邪气,风寒湿邪所致痹证,能充实人体内脏,能补益精气,能使毛发增长、变黑,能消解胃中的空悬之感,能治疗食欲不足,能增强食欲。长期服用,能使身体轻盈,听力增强,视力清明,长寿不老。该物生长在山川和平泽之中。

cooling the blood and ceasing bleeding, replenishing Qi and preventing aging. Clinically it can be used to treat wind-dampness and cold-heat, jaundice with heat bind, generalized yellowing, dysuria, mass in the large intestine, heat stagnation and cold damage.

2. Suspension of the stomach means deficiency of the stomach.

3. To make people frequently feel hungry means to treat poor appetite.

46. 赤箭

【原文】

味辛,温。

主杀鬼精物,蛊毒恶气。久服益气力,长阴,肥健,轻身,增年。一名离母,一名鬼督邮。生川谷。

【考据】

1.《吴普》曰:鬼督邮,一名神草,一名阎狗,或生太山,或少室,茎箭赤无叶,根如芋子,三月四月八月,采根,日干,治痈肿(《御览》)。

2.《名医》曰:生陈仓雍州,及太山少室,三月四月八月采根,暴干。

3. 案《抱朴子》云:按仙方中,有合离草,一名独摇,一名离母,所以谓之合离,离母者,此草为物,下根如芋魁,有游子十二枚,周环之,去大魁数尺,虽相须,而实不相连,但以气相属耳,别说云,今医家见用天麻,即是此赤箭根。

【今译】

味辛,性温。

46. Chijian（赤箭，rhizome of tall gastrodia，Rhizoma Gastrodiae）[1]

[Original Text]

[Chijian （赤箭，rhizome of tall gastrodia，Rhizoma Gastrodiae），] pungent in taste and warm [in property]，[is mainly used] to kill ghost-like strange things[2]，[and to resolve] worm toxin and vicious Qi[3]. Long-term taking [of it will] replenish energy，nourish Yin，cultivate health，relax the body，and prolong life. [It is also] called Limu（离母）and Guiduyou（鬼督邮），growing in mountain valleys and river valleys.

[Textual Research]

[In the book entitled] *Wu Pu Ben Cao*（《吴普本草》，*Wu Pu's Studies of Materia Medica*），[it] says [that Chijian（赤箭，rhizome of tall gastrodia，Rhizoma Gastrodiae）is also] called Guiduyou（鬼督邮），Shencao（神草）and Yangou（阎狗），growing in Taishan（太山）or Shaoshi（少室）. [Its] stalks are red without leaves and [its] root looks like Yuzi（芋子，dasheen seed，Semen Colocasiae Esculentae）. [Its] root [can be] collected in March，April and August，and dried in the sun. [According to the book entitled] *Tai Ping Yu Lan*（《太平御览》，*Imperial Studies in Taiping Times*），[it can be used] to treat abscess and swelling.

[In the book entitled] *Ming Yi Bie Lu*（《名医别录》，*Special Record*

能杀除鬼怪邪气,能治疗虫毒恶气所致之病患。长期服用能补益气力,能增强阴液,能使人身心康健,身体轻盈,能延长寿命。又称为离母,又称为鬼督邮。该物生长在山川河谷之中。

of Great Doctors），［it］says［that Chijian（赤箭，rhizome of tall gastrodia，Rhizoma Gastrodiae）］grows in Yongzhou（雍州）in Chencang（陈仓）and Shaoshi（少室）in Taishan（太山）.［Its］root［can be collected］in March，April and August，and dried in the sun.

［In the book entitled］*Bao Pu Zi*（《抱朴子》，*Primitive and Natural View*），［it］says［that］in Miraculous Formulae there is［a herbal medicinal called］Lihecao（合离草），［which refers to Chijian（赤箭，rhizome of tall gastrodia，Rhizoma Gastrodiae），also］called Duyao（独摇）and Limu（离母）.［Its］root looks like Yukui（芋魁，dasheen tuber，Tuber Colocasiae Esculentae）.［The so-called］Tianma（天麻）used now in medicine is actually the root of Chijian（赤箭，rhizome of tall gastrodia，Rhizoma Gastrodiae）.

Notes

1. Chijian（赤箭，rhizome of tall gastrodia，Rhizoma Gastrodiae）is a herbal medicinal，sweet and pungent in taste，mild in property，entering the liver meridian. Effective in relieving wind and fright. Clinically it is used to treat vertigo due to deficiency-wind，headache due to wind attack，numbness of limbs，paralysis，epilepsy and infantile convulsion.

2. The so-called ghost-like strange things refer to the causes of strange diseases that are difficult to be diagnosed.

3. The so-called worm toxin and vicious Qi refer to complicated and severe disease caused by strange elements or vicious toxin，such as serious hepatitis，paroxysmal dysentery and schistosomiasis.

47. 奄闾子

【原文】

味苦,微寒。

主五脏瘀血,腹中水气,胪张留热,风寒湿痹,身体诸痛。久服,轻身延年不老。生川谷。

【考据】

1.《吴普》曰:奄闾,神农雷公桐君岐伯苦小温无毒,李氏温,或生上党,叶青厚两相当,七月花曰,九月实黑,七月九月十月采,驴马食仙去(《御览》)。

2.《名医》曰:䮫驴食之神仙,生雍州,亦生上党,及道边,十月采实,阴干。

3. 案《司马相如赋》,有奄闾,张揖云奄闾,蒿也,子可治疾。

【今译】

味苦,性微寒。

主治五脏瘀血之症,能消除腹中水气积聚,能消解腹中胀满,体内

47. Yanlǔzi（奄闾子，Herb of ghostplant wormwood，Artemisia Lactiflora）[1]

[Original Text]

[Yanlǔzi（奄闾子，Herb of ghostplant wormwood，Artemisia Lactiflora），] bitter in taste and slightly cold [in property], [is mainly used] to treat blood stasis in the five Zang-organs, abdominal edema，abdominal distension，heat accumulation，wind-cold and dampness impediment and various pain in the body. Long-term taking [of it will] relax the body，prolong life and prevent aging. [It] grows in mountain valleys and river valleys.

[Textual Research]

[In the book entitled] *Wu Pu Ben Cao*（《吴普本草》，*Wu Pu's Studies of Materia Medica*），[it] says [that according to] Agriculture God（神农），Leigong（雷公），Tongjun（桐均）and Qibo（岐伯），Yanlǔzi（奄闾子，Herb of ghostplant wormwood，Artemisia Lactiflora) is slightly warm and non-toxic [in property]；[according to] Li's（李氏），[it is] warm [in property]. [It] may grow in Shangdang（上党）and [its] leaves are green and thick. [According to the book entitled] *Tai Ping Yu Lan*（《太平御览》，*Imperial Studies in Taiping Times*），[its] flowers blossom in July and [it] turns black in September. [In] July and September，[it can be] collected.

郁热,能治疗风寒湿邪所致痹证以及身体中的各种疼痛之患。长期服用,能使人身体轻盈,能延年益寿,能长寿不老。该物生长在山川河谷之中。

[In the book entitled] *Ming Yi Bie Lu* (《名医别录》, *Special Record of Great Doctors*), [it] says [that when] mule has grazed Yanlǔzi（奄闾子, Herb of ghostplant wormwood，Artemisia Lactiflora)], [it will become] immortal. Yanlǔzi（奄闾子, Herb of ghostplant wormwood，Artemisia Lactiflora）grows in Yongzhou（雍州）and Shangdang（上党）in roadsides. [It can be] collected in October and dried in the shade.

Notes

1. Yanlǔzi（奄闾子, Herb of ghostplant wormwood，Artemisia Lactiflora）is a herbal medicinal，bitter in taste and slightly cold in property，entering the liver meridian of foot-Jueyin，effective in expelling blood stasis and dampness. Clinically it is used to treat blood stasis in the five Zang-organs，abdominal edema，abdominal distension，amenorrhea due to blood stasis，blood stagnation and abdominal pain after delivery of baby，traumatic injury and wind-dampness impediment and pain.

48. 析蓂子

【原文】

味辛,微湿。

主明目,目痛泪出,除痹,补五脏,益精光。久服,轻身不老。一名蔑析,一名大蕺,一名马辛。生川泽及道旁。

【考据】

1.《吴普》曰:析蓂一名析目,一名荣冥,一名马骍,雷公神农扁鹊辛,李氏小温,四月采干,二十日生道旁,得细辛良,畏干姜,苦参荠实,神农无毒,生野田,五月五日采阴干,治腹胀(《御览》)。

2.《名医》曰:一名大荠,生咸阳,四月五月采,暴干。

3. 案《说文》云:蓂,析蓂,大荠也;《广雅》云:析蓂,马辛也;《尔雅》云:析蓂大荠;郭璞云:荠叶细,俗呼之曰老荠,旧作蒺,非。

【今译】

味辛,性微湿。

能使眼睛明亮,能消解因眼睛肿痛而泪流不止,能祛除痹证,能充

48. Ximingzi（析蓂子，pennycress seed，Semen Thlaspi Arvensa）[1]

[Original Text]

[Ximingzi（析蓂子，pennycress seed，Thlaspi Arvensa），] pungent in taste and slightly damp [in property]，[is mainly used] to improve vision，treat pain of the eyes with spontaneous tearing，to eliminate impediment，to tonify the five Zang-organs and to replenish eyesight. Long-term taking [of it will] relax the body and prevent aging. [It is also] called Miexi（蔑析），Daji（大蕺）and Maxin（马辛），growing in valleys，swamps and roadsides.

[Textual Research]

[In the book entitled] *Wu Pu Ben Cao*（《吴普本草》，*Wu Pu's Studies of Materia Medica*），[it] says [that] Ximingzi（析蓂子，pennycress seed，Thlaspi Arvensa）is also called Ximu（析目），Rongmin（荣冥）and Maxing（马骍）. [According to] Leigong（雷公），Agriculture God（神农）and Bianque（扁鹊），[it is] pungent [in taste]；[according to] Li's（李氏），[it is] slightly warm [in property]，[and can be] collected and dried in April. [According to] Agriculture God（神农），[it is] non-toxic，grows in wild land and [can be] collected and dried in the shade on May 5. [According to the book entitled] *Tai Ping Yu Lan*（《太平御览》，*Imperial Studies in Taiping Times*），[it can be used] to treat abdominal

实五脏,能补益精气光。长期服用,能使人身体轻盈,能长寿不老。又称为蒇析,又称为大戟,又称为马辛。该物生长在山川和平泽之中及道路旁边。

distension.

[In the book entitled] *Ming Yi Bie Lu* (《名医别录》, *Special Record of Great Doctors*), [it] says [that Ximingzi (析蓂子, pennycress seed, Thlaspi Arvensa) is also] called Daji (大荠), grows in Xianyang (咸阳) and [can be] collected and dried in the sun in April and May.

Notes

1. Ximingzi (析蓂子, pennycress seed, Thlaspi Arvense), also similar to seed of boor's mustard, seed of dish mustard, seed of field pennycress, seed of wild cress in English, is a herbal medicinal, bitter and sweet in taste, mild in property, effective in harmonizing the middle (the internal organs) and resolving dampness, clearing heat and removing toxin, soothing the sinews and activating the collaterals, improving vision and disinhibiting water. Clinically it is used to treat indigestion, nephritis, endometritis, ulcer, abscess, swelling and pain.

49. 蓍实

【原文】

味苦,平。

主益气,充肌肤,明目,聪慧先知。久服,不饥不老,轻身。生山谷。

【考据】

1.《吴普》曰:蓍实味苦酸平无毒,主益气,充肌肤,明目聪慧,先知,久服,不饥不老,轻身,生少室山谷,八月九月采实暴干(《御览》)。

2.《名医》曰:生少室,八月九月采实,日干。

3. 案《说文》云:蓍,蒿属,生千岁,三百茎;《史记》龟策《传》云:蓍,百茎共一根。

【今译】

味苦,性平。

49. Shishi（菩实，alpine yarrow fruit，Fructus Achilleae Alpinae）[1]

[Original Text]

[Shishi （菩 实，alpine yarrow fruit，Fructus Achilleae Alpinae），] bitter in taste and mild [in property]，[is mainly used] to replenish Qi，to enrich muscles，to improve vision，[to make people more] intelligent and know [the future] in advance. Long-term taking [of it can] relieve hunger，prevent aging and relax the body. [It] grows in mountains and valleys.

[Textual Research]

[In the book entitled] *Wu Pu Ben Cao* （《吴普本草》，*Wu Pu's Studies of Materia Medica* ），[it] says [that] Shishi（菩实，alpine yarrow fruit，Fructus Achilleae Alpinae），bitter and sour in taste，mild and non-toxic [in property]，[is mainly used] to replenish Qi，enrich muscles，improve vision，[make people more] intelligent and know [the future] in advance. Long-term taking [of it can] relieve hunger，prevent aging and relax the body. [It] grows in mountains and valleys in Shaoshi （少室）. [According to the book entitled] *Tai Ping Yu Lan* （《太平御览》，*Imperial Studies in Taiping Times* ），[it can be] collected and dried in the sun in August and September.

[In the book entitled] *Ming Yi Bie Lu* （《名医别录》，*Special Record of Great Doctors* ），[it] says [that Shishi（菩实，alpine yarrow

能补益精气，能充盈肌肤，能使眼睛明亮，能使人聪慧并能预知未来。长期服用，能使人减少饥饿之感，能长寿不老，能使身体轻盈。该物生长在山谷之中。

fruit，Fructus Achilleae Alpinae)] grows in Shaoshi（少室）and [can be] collected and dried in the sun in August and September.

[In] case [analysis in the book entitled] *Shuo Wen* （《说文》，*On Culture*）, [it] says [that] Shishi（蓍实，alpine yarrow fruit，Fructus Achilleae Alpinae) grows for thousands of years with three hundred stalks. [In the book entitled] *Shi Ji* （《史记》，*Records of History*）, [it] says [that] in Shishi（蓍实，alpine yarrow fruit，Fructus Achilleae Alpinae) there are a hundred stalks but just one root.

Notes

1. Shishi（蓍实，alpine yarrow fruit，Fructus Achilleae Alpinae) is a herbal medicinal，bitter and sour in taste，mild and non-toxic in property， effective in replenishing Qi， enriching muscles and improving vision. There is no information about which meridian it enters and what specific diseases it can be used to treat in clinical practice.

50. 六芝（赤芝、黑芝、青芝、白芝、黄芝、紫芝）

【原文】

赤芝，味苦，平。主胸中结，益心气，补中，增慧智，不忘。久食，轻身，不老，延年，神仙。一名丹芝。

黑芝，味咸，平。主癃，利水道，益肾气，通九窍，聪察。久食，轻身，不老，延年，神仙。一名元芝。

青芝，味酸，平。主明目，补肝气，安精魂，仁恕，久食，轻身，不老，延年，神仙。一名龙芝。

白芝，味辛，平。主咳逆上气，益肺气，通利口鼻，强志意，勇悍，安魄。久食，轻身，不老，延年，神仙。一名玉芝。

黄芝，味甘，平。主心腹五邪，益脾气，安神，忠信，和乐。久食，轻身，不老，延年，神仙。一名金芝。

紫芝，味甘，温。主耳聋，利关节，保神，益精气，坚筋骨，好颜色。久服，轻身，不老，延年。一名木芝。生山谷（旧作六种，今并）。

【考据】

1.《吴普》曰：紫之一名木芝。

50. Liuzhi（六芝，six fragrant herbs）

[Original Text]

Chizhi（赤芝，red fragrant herb），bitter in taste and mild [in property，[is mainly used] to resolve stagnation in the chest，to replenish heart-Qi，to tonify the middle（internal organs），to increase intelligence and to avoid amnesia. Long-term taking [of it can] relax the body，prevent aging and prolong life like immortals. [It is also] called Danzhi（丹芝）.

Heizhi（黑芝，black fragrant herb），salty in taste and mild [in property]，[is mainly used] to treat dysuria，to disinhibit water，to replenish kidney-Qi，to unobstruct nine orifices and to increase intelligence. Long-term taking [of it can] relax the body，prevent aging，prolong life like immortals. [It is also] called Yuanzhi（元芝）.

Qingzhi（青芝，green fragrant herb），sour in taste and mild [in property]，[is mainly used] to improve vision，to tonify liver-Qi，to pacify essence and ethereal soul and to cultivate morality. Long-term taking [of it can] relax the body，prevent aging，prolong life like immortals. [It is also] called Longzhi（龙芝）.

Baizhi（白芝，white fragrant herb），pungent in taste and mild [in property]，[is mainly used] to treat cough with dyspnea，to replenish lung-Qi，to disinhibit mouth and nose，to invigorate spirit，to strengthen body resistance and to pacify ethereal soul.

2.《名医》曰:赤芝生霍山,黑芝生恒山,青芝生太山,白芝生华山,黄芝生嵩山,紫芝生高夏地上,色紫,形如桑(《御览》),六芝皆无毒,六月八月采。

3.案《说文》云:芝,神草也;《尔雅》云:茵芝;郭璞云:芝一岁三华,瑞草;礼内则云:芝栭;卢植注云:芝,木芝也;《楚词》云:采三秀于山间;王逸云:三秀谓芝草;后汉书《华陀传》:有漆叶青面散;注引陀传曰:青面者,一名地节,一名黄芝,主理五脏,益精气,本字书无面字,相传音女廉反;《列仙传》云:吕尚服泽芝;《抱朴子·仙药》云:赤者如珊瑚,白者如截肪,黑者如泽漆,青者如翠羽,黄者如紫金,而皆光明洞彻如坚冰也。

【今译】

赤芝,味苦,性平。

主治胸中郁结不舒,能补益心气,能充实人体内脏,能增强智慧,能消除健忘之症。长期食用,能使人身体轻盈,能长寿不老,能延年益寿,像神仙一样。又称为丹芝。

黑芝,味咸,性平。

主治小便不利,能通利水道,能补益肾气,能使九窍畅通,能使人聪明而有才智。长期食用,能使人身体轻盈,能长寿不老,能延年益寿,像神仙一样。又称为元芝。

青芝,味酸,性平。

能使眼睛明亮,能滋补肝气,能安静精神和魂魄,能使人宽厚仁慈。

Long-term taking [of it can] relax the body, prevent aging, prolong life like immortals. [It is also] called Yuzhi（玉芝）.

Huangzhi（黄芝, yellow fragrant herb）, sweet [in] taste [and] mild [in property], [is mainly used] to resolve five kinds of evil in the heart and abdomen, to pacify the spirit and [to enable people to be] loyal and happy. Long-term taking [of it can] relax the body, prevent aging, prolong life like immortals. [It is also] called Jinzhi（金芝）.

Zizhi（紫芝, purple fragrant herb）, sweet [in] taste [and] warm [in property], [is mainly used] to treat deafness, soothe joints, to protect the spirit, to replenish essence and Qi, to strengthen sinews and bones and to luster facial expression. Long-term taking [of it can] relax the body, prevent aging, prolong life like immortals. [It is also] called Muzhi（木芝）, growing in mountains and valleys.

[Textual Research]

[In the book entitled] *Ming Yi Bie Lu*（《名医别录》, *Special Record of Great Doctors*）, [it] says [that] Chizhi（赤芝, red fragrant herb）grows in Huoshan（霍山）, Heizhi（黑芝, black fragrant herb）grows in Hengshan（恒山）, Qingzhi（青芝, green fragrant herb）grows in Taishan（太山）, Baizhi（白芝, white fragrant herb）grows in Huashan（华山）, Huangzhi（黄芝, yellow fragrant herb）grows in Songshan（嵩山）and Zizhi（紫芝, purple fragrant herb）grows in Gaoxia（高夏）. All these six fragrant herbs are non-toxic [and can be] collected in June and August.

[In] case [analysis in the book entitled] *Shuo Wen*（《说文》, *On*

长期食用,能使人身体轻盈,能长寿不老,能延年益寿,像神仙一样。又称为龙芝。

白芝,味辛,性平。

主治咳嗽及呼吸困难,能补益肺气,能通利口鼻,能增强记忆力,能使人勇猛强壮,能安静魂魄。长期食用,能使人身体轻盈,能长寿不老,能延年益寿,像神仙一样。又称为玉芝。

黄芝,味甘,性平。

主治心腹中的五种邪气,能补益脾气,能安静精神,能使人忠信诚实,和乐舒畅。长期食用,能使人身体轻盈,能长寿不老,能延年益寿,像神仙一样。又称为金芝。

紫芝,味甘,性温。

主治耳聋,能使关节通畅,能保全神气,能补益精气,能使筋骨强壮,能使面部色彩美丽。长期服用,能使人身体轻盈,能长寿不老,能延年益寿。又称为木芝。该物生长在山谷之中。

Culture），[it] says [that] fragrant herbs are magical herbs. Guo Pu
（郭璞）said, "Fragrant herb bears three flowers in a year and is
auspicious." 　[In the book entitled] *Bao Pu Zi* （《抱朴子》,
Primitive and Natural View），[it] says [that] Chizhi（赤芝, red
fragrant herb）is like coral，Baizhi（白芝, white fragrant herb）is
like cut lipid，Heizhi（黑芝, black fragrant herb）is like Ziqi（泽漆,
sun spurge，Herba Euphorbiae Helioscopiae），Qingzhi（青芝, green
fragrant herb）is like feathers of peacock，and Huangzhi（黄芝,
yellow fragrant herb）is like violet gold. All [of them are] bright
and icy.

51. 卷柏

【原文】

味辛,温。

主五脏邪气,女子阴中寒热痛,症瘕,血闭,绝子。久服轻身,和颜色。一名万岁。生山谷石间。

【考据】

1.《吴普》曰:卷柏,神农辛,桐君雷公甘(《御览》引云,一名豹足,一名求股,一名万岁,一名神枝,时,生山谷)。

2.《名医》曰:一名豹足,一名求股,一名交时,生常山,五月七月采,阴干。

3. 案《范子计然》云:卷柏,出三辅。

【今译】

味辛,性温。

51. Juanbai（卷柏，tamariskoid spikemoss herb；pulvinate spikemoss herb，Herba Selaginellae）[1]

[Original Text]

[Juanbai（卷柏，tamariskoid spikemoss herb；pulvinate spikemoss herb，Herba Selaginellae），] pungent in taste and warm [in property]，[is mainly used] to expel evil-Qi in the five Zang-organs and to treat cold-heat pain in the uterus，abdominal mass，amenorrhea and infertility. Long-term taking [of it will] relax the body and luster facial expression. [It is also] called Wansui（万岁）and grows in mountain valleys and stones.

[Textual Research]

[In the book entitled] *Wu Pu Ben Cao*（《吴普本草》，*Wu Pu's Studies of Materia Medica*），[it] says [that according to] Agriculture God（神农），Juanbai（卷柏，tamariskoid spikemoss herb；pulvinate spikemoss herb，Herba Selaginellae）is pungent [in taste]；[according to] Tongjun（桐均）and Leigong（雷公），[it is] sweet [in taste]. [According to the book entitled] *Tai Ping Yu Lan*（《太平御览》，*Imperial Studies in Taiping Times*），[it is also] called Baozu（豹足），Qiugu（求股），Wansui（万岁）and Shenji（神枝），usually growing in mountains and valleys.

[In the book entitled] *Ming Yi Bie Lu*（《名医别录》，*Special Record of Great Doctors*），[it] says [that Juanbai（卷柏，tamariskoid

主治五脏中的邪气,能治疗女子阴部的寒热性疾病和疼痛,症瘕,经闭,不孕之症。长期服用,能使人身体轻盈,能使面部色泽调和。又称为万岁。该物生长在山谷之中和石头之间。

spikemoss herb; pulvinate spikemoss herb, Herba Selaginellae) is also] called Baozu (豹足), Qiugu (求股), Jiaoshi (交时) and Changshan (常山). [It can be] collected in May and July and dried in the shade.

[In the book entitled] *Fan Zi Ji Ran* (《范子计然》, *Studies About Fan Li's Teacher*), [it] says [that] Juanbai (卷柏, tamariskoid spikemoss herb; pulvinate spikemoss herb, Herba Selaginellae) grows in Sanpu (三辅).

Notes

1. Juanbai (卷柏, tamariskoid spikemoss herb; pulvinate spikemoss herb, Herba Selaginellae) is a herbal medicinal, pungent in taste and mild in property, entering the liver meridian, effective in activating the blood. Clinically it is used to treat amenorrhea, abdominal mass, traumatic injury. When baked, it can be used to treat hematemesis, hematochezia, hematuria and uterine bleeding.

52. 蓝实

【原文】

味苦,寒。

主解诸毒,杀蛊蚑,注鬼,螫毒。久服,头不白,轻身。生平泽。

【考据】

1.《名医》曰:其茎叶可以染青,生河内。

2. 案《说文》云:葴马蓝也,蓝,染青草也;《尔雅》云:葴,马蓝;郭璞云:今大叶冬蓝也,《周礼》掌染草;郑注云:染草,蓝茜,象斗之属,《夏小正》五月启灌蓝;《毛诗》云:终朝采蓝,《笺》云,蓝,染草也。

【今译】

味苦,性寒。

能消解各种毒气,能杀除虫毒和蚂蟥毒,能消除引发传染病的怪异之邪,能祛除虫毒和蛇毒。长期服用,能使人头发不变白,能使人身体轻盈。该物生长在平川水泽之中。

52. Lanshi（蓝实，indigoplant fruitFructus Polygoni Tingtorii）[1]

[Original Text]

[Lanshi（蓝实，indigoplant fruitFructus Polygoni Tingtorii），] bitter in taste and cold [in property], [is mainly used] to resolve various toxin, to kill toxic worms, to remove ghost[2] and snake toxin. Long-term taking [of it can] prevent white hair and relax the body. [It] grows in plains and swamps.

[Textual Research]

[In the book entitled] *Ming Yi Bie Lu*（《名医别录》, *Special Record of Great Doctors*）, [it] says [that] the root and leaves [of Lanshi（蓝实，indigoplant fruitFructus Polygoni Tingtorii）] dye green. [It] grows in Henei（河内）.

Notes

1. Lanshi（蓝实，indigoplant fruitFructus Polygoni Tingtorii）is a herbal medicinal, bitter in taste, cold and non-toxic in property, effective in resolving various toxin, enriching marrow, improving vision and hearing, soothing the five Zang-organs, regulating the six Fu-organs, unobstructing joints, strengthening the body and replenishing the heart.

2. The so-called ghost here refers to unknown cause of infectious disease.

53. 芎䓖

【原文】

味辛,温。

主中风入脑,头痛,寒痹,筋挛,缓急,金疮,妇人血闭,无子。生川谷。

【考据】

1.《吴普》曰:芎䓖(《御览》引云一名香果),神农黄帝岐伯雷公辛无毒,扁鹊酸无毒,李氏生温熟寒,或生胡无桃山阴,或太山(《御览》作或斜谷西岭,或太山),叶香细青黑,文赤如藁本,冬夏丛生,五月华赤,七月实黑,茎端两叶,三月采,根有节,似马衔状。

2.《名医》曰:一名胡䓖,一名香果,其叶名蘼芜,生武功斜谷西岭,三月四月,采根暴干。

3. 案《说文》云:营,营䓖,香草也,芎,司马相如说或从弓;春秋《左传》云:有山鞠穷乎;杜预云:鞠穷所以御湿;《西山经》云:号山,其草多芎䓖;郭璞云:芎䓖一名江蓠;《范子计然》云:芎䓖生始无,祜者善(有脱字);《司马相如赋》:有芎䓖;司马贞引司马彪云:芎䓖似藁本;郭璞云:

53. Xiongqiong（芎䓖，xiongqiong rhizome，Rhizoma Chuanxiong）[1]

[Original Text]

[Xiongqiong（芎䓖，xiongqiong rhizome，Rhizoma Chuanxiong），] pungent in taste and warm [in property], [is mainly used] to treat headache [caused by] invasion of [pathogenic] wind into the brain, cold impediment, spasm of sinews, convulsion, trauma [caused by] metal, amenorrhea and infertility. [It] grows in mountain valleys and river valleys.

[Textual Research]

[In the book entitled] *Wu Pu Ben Cao*（《吴普本草》, *Wu Pu's Studies of Materia Medica*），[it] says [that] Xiongqiong（芎䓖, Xiongqiongherb， Rhizoma Chuanxiong ），[according to] Agriculture God（神农），Yellow Emperor（黄帝），Qibo（岐伯）and Leigong（雷公），[is] pungent [in taste] and non-toxic [in property]；[according to] Bianque（扁鹊），[it is] non-toxic [in property]；[according to] Li's（李氏），[it is] warm [in property if it is] raw and cold [in property if it is] processed. [It] grows in Shanyin（山阴）or Taishan（太山），or valleys in Xiling（西岭） [according to the book entitled] *Tai Ping Yu Lan*（《太平御览》, *Imperial Studies in Taiping Times*）. [Its] leaves are sweet [in taste], thin [in structure], green and black [in color with] the

今历阳呼为江离。

【今译】

味辛,性温。

主治因风邪入脑而头痛和因寒痹所致的筋脉挛拘,能使挛拘的筋脉舒畅正常,能治疗因金属损伤而导致的痈疮,女性因血脉闭塞所致的经闭以及不孕之症。该物生长在山川河谷之中。

神农本草经

texture like [that of] Gaoben (藁本, rhizome of Chinese ligusticum, rhizome of jehol ligusticum, Rhizoma Ligustici). [It] grows prosperously in winter and summer. [In] May, [its] flowers are red; [in] July, [its] fruits are black. [Its] stalks and leaves [can be] collected in March. There are joints [in its] root, like gag bit.

[In the book entitled] *Ming Yi Bie Lu* (《名医别录》, *Special Record of Great Doctors*), [it] says [that Xiongqiong (芎䓖, Xiongqiongherb, Rhizoma Chuanxiong) is also] called Huqiong (胡 䓖) and Xiangguo (香果), its leaves are called Miwu (蘼芜), growing in Wugong (武功) and valleys in Xiling (西岭). [Its] root [can be] collected in March and April and dried in the sun.

Notes

1. Xiongqiong (芎䓖, xiongqiong rhizome, Rhizoma Chuanxiong) is a herbal medicinal, pungent in taste and warm in property, entering the liver meridian and the heart meridian, effective in activating the blood and promoting flow of Qi, dispersing wind and ceasing pain. Clinically it is used to treat irregular menstruation, abdominal pain due to blood stasis and Qi stagnation, dysmenorrheal, amenorrhea, migraine, distension and pain of the chest and rib-side, coronary heart disease and angina.

54. 蘼芜

【原文】

味辛,温。

主咳逆,定惊气,辟邪恶,除蛊毒鬼注,去三虫,久服通神。一名薇芜。生川泽。

【考据】

1.《吴普》曰:蘼芜,一名芎䓖(《御览》)。

2.《名医》曰:一名茳蓠,芎䓖苗也,生雍州及冤句,四月五月,采叶暴干。

3. 案《说文》云:蘼,蘼芜也,蓠,茳蓠,蓠芜;《尔雅》云:靳茞蘼芜;郭璞云:香草,叶小如委状;《淮南子》云:似蛇床;《山海经》云:臭如蘼芜,《司马相如赋》,有江离蘼芜;司马贞引樊光云:藁本,一名蘼芜,根名勒芷。

【今译】

味辛,性温。

54. Miwu（蘼芜，javenile leaf of chuanxiong，Folium Chuanxiong Juvenile）[1]

[Original Text]

[Miwu（蘼芜，javenile leaf of chuanxiong，Folium Chuanxiong Juvenile），] pungent in taste and warm [in property]，[is mainly used] to treat cough with dyspnea，to relieve fright，to avoid [invasion of] evil[2]，to eliminate worm toxin and consumptive disease[3]，and to expel three worms[4]. Long-term taking [of it will] invigorate the spirit. [It is also] called Weiwu（薇芜），growing in valleys and swamps.

[Textual Research]

[In the book entitled] *Ming Yi Bie Lu*（《名医别录》，*Special Record of Great Doctors*），[it] says [that Miwu（蘼芜，javenile leaf of chuanxiong，Folium Chuanxiong Juvenile）is also] called Jiangli（茳蓠），growing in Yongzhou（雍州）and Yuanju（冤句）.[In] April and May，[its] leaves [can be] collected and dried in the sun.

Notes

1. Miwu（蘼芜，javenile leaf of chuanxiong，Folium Chuanxiong Juvenile）is a herbal medicinal，pungent in taste and warm in property，entering the heart meridian and the liver meridian，effective in expelling pathogenic wind and dispersing

205

　　主治咳嗽气逆,能安静惊恐状态,能消除邪恶之气,能治疗虫毒及鬼怪物所致病症,能祛除三种虫子。长期服用能使神气通畅。又称为蔷芜。该物生长在山川和平泽之中。

pathogenic cold. Clinically it is used to treat headache due to attack of pathogenic wind, vertigo, epiphora induced by wind and cough.

2. Evil here refers to severe pathogenic factors.

3. Consumptive disease refers to the disease caused by infection of worm toxin, characterized by cough, hemoptysis, chest pain, tidal fever, night sweating and steaming heat in the bones.

4. The so-called three worms actually refer to three kinds of diseases caused by worm toxin.

55. 黄连

【原文】

味苦,寒。

主热气目痛,眦伤泣出,明目(《御览》引云,主茎伤,《大观本》,无),肠澼,腹痛,下利,妇人阴中肿痛。久服,令人不忘。一名王连。生川谷。

【考据】

1.《吴普》曰:黄连,神农岐伯黄帝雷公苦无毒,李氏小寒,或生蜀郡,太山之阳(《御览》)。

2.《名医》曰:生巫阳及蜀郡,太山,二月八月采。

3.案《广雅》云:王连,黄连也;《范子计然》云:黄连出蜀郡,黄肥坚者善。

【今译】

味苦,性寒。

55. Huanglian（黄连，coptis，Rhizoma Coptidis）[1]

[Original Text]

[Huanglian（黄连，coptis，Rhizoma Coptidis），] bitter in taste and cold [in property], [is mainly used] to relieve pain of the eyes [due to] heat Qi and epiphora [due to] eyelid injury, to improve vision, to treat diarrhea, abdominal pain, dysentery, vulval swelling and pain. Long-term taking [of it will] invigorate memory. [It is also] called Wanglian（王连），growing in mountain valleys and river valleys.

[Textual Research]

[In the book entitled] *Wu Pu Ben Cao*（《吴普本草》，*Wu Pu's Studies of Materia Medica*），[it] says [that] Huanglian（黄连，coptis，Rhizoma Coptidis），[according to] Agriculture God（神农），Qibo（岐伯），Yellow Emperor（黄帝）and Leigong（雷公），[is] bitter [in taste] and non-toxic [in property]；[according to] Li's（李氏），[it is] slightly cold [in property].[According to the book entitled] *Tai Ping Yu Lan*（《太平御览》，*Imperial Studies in Taiping Times*），[it] grows in Shujun（蜀郡）and the sunny side of Taishan（太山）.

[In the book entitled] *Ming Yi Bie Lu*（《名医别录》，*Special Record of Great Doctors*），[it] says [that Huanglian（黄连，coptis，Rhizoma Coptidis）] grows in Wuyang（巫阳），Shujun（蜀郡）and

　　主治热邪之气所致的眼睛肿痛，因眼角损伤而泪流不止，能使眼睛明亮，能治疗泄泻，腹痛，痢疾，女性阴部肿痛。长期服用，令人能消除健忘之症。又称为王连。该物生长在山川河谷之中。

Taishan（太山）. [It can be] collected in February and August.

[In the book entitled] *Guang Ya*（《广雅》, *The First Chinese Encyclopedic Dictionary*）, [it] says [that the so-called] Wanglian （王连） actually refers to Huanglian （黄连, coptis, Rhizoma Coptidis）. [In the book entitled] *Fan Zi Ji Ran*（《范子计然》, *Studies About Fan Li's Teacher*）, [it] says [that] Huanglian（黄连, coptis, Rhizoma Coptidis）grows in Shujun （蜀郡）. [If it is] yellow, thick and hard, [it is] more effective.

Notes

1. Huanglian （黄连, coptis, Rhizoma Coptidis）is a herbal medicinal, bitter in taste and cold in property, entering the heart meridian, the stomach meridian and the large intestine meridian, effective in clearing heat and drying dampness, purging fire and resolving toxin. Clinically it is used to treat heat disease with vexation, unconsciousness and delirium, internal accumulation of dampness-heat, abdominal mass, vomiting, diarrhea and dysentery.

56. 络石

【原文】

味苦,温。

主风热,死肌,痈伤,口干舌焦,痈肿不消,喉舌肿,水浆不下。久服,轻身明目,润泽,好颜色,不老延年。一名百鲮。生川谷。

【考据】

1.《吴普》曰:落石,一名鳞石,一名明石,一名县石,一名云华,一名云珠,一名云英,一名云丹,神农苦小温,雷公苦无毒,扁鹊桐君甘无毒,李氏大寒,云药中君,采无时(《御览》)。

2.《名医》曰:一名石磋,一名略石,一名明石,一名领石,一名县石,生太山或石山之阴,或高山岩石上,或生人间,正月采。

3. 案《西山经》云:上申之山多硌石,疑即此;郭璞云:硌,磊硌大石儿,非也;《唐本》注云:俗名耐冬,山南人谓之石血,以其包络石木而生,故名络石,别录谓之石龙藤,以石上生者良。

56. Luoshi（络石，fruit of Chinese starjasmine，Fructus Trachelospermi）[1]

［Original Text］

［Luoshi （络石，fruit of Chinese starjasmine，Fructus Trachelospermi），］ bitter in taste and warm ［in property］, ［is mainly used］ to treat wind-heat ［disease］, numbness of muscles，abscess ［due to infection of traumatic］ injury，dryness of the mouth and tongue，abscess and swelling ［that is］ hard to resolve，swelling of the throat and tongue，difficulty in drinking water and taking porridge. Long-term taking ［of it will］ relax the body，improve vision，luster the facial expression，prevent aging and prolong life. ［It is also］ called Bailing （百鲮），growing in mountain valleys and river valleys.

［Textual Research］

［In the book entitled］ *Wu Pu Ben Cao* （《吴普本草》，*Wu Pu's Studies of Materia Medica* ），［it］ says ［that Luoshi （络石，fruit of Chinese starjasmine，Fructus Trachelospermi） is also］ called Luoshi （落石），Linshi （鳞石），Mingshi （明石），Xianshi （县石），Yunhua （云华），Yunzhu （云珠），Yunying （云英） and Yundan （云丹）. ［According to］ Agriculture God （神农），［it is］ bitter ［in taste］ and slightly warm ［in property］；［according to］ Leigong （雷公），［it is］ bitter ［in taste］ and non-toxic ［in property］；［according to］

【今译】

味苦,性温。

主治风热之症,肌肉坏死,因外部感染所致的痈疮,口干舌焦,痈肿不能消解,喉舌肿胀,水粥不能下咽。长期服用,能使人身体轻盈,能使眼睛明亮,能滋润面部光泽,能使面部色彩美丽,能长寿不老,能延年益寿。又称为百鲮。该物生长在山川河谷之中。

Bianque（扁鹊）and Tongjun（桐均），[it is] sweet [in taste] and non-toxic [in property]；[according to] Li's（李氏），[it is] serious cold [in property]. [According to the book entitled] *Tai Ping Yu Lan*（《太平御览》，*Imperial Studies in Taiping Times*），[it can be] collected at any time.

[In the book entitled] *Ming Yi Bie Lu*（《名医别录》，*Special Record of Great Doctors*），[it] says [that Luoshi（络石，fruit of Chinese starjasmine，Fructus Trachelospermi）is also] called Shicuo（石磋），Lüèshi（略石），Mingshi（明石），Lingshi（领石）and Xianshi（县石），growing in Taishan（太山），or the shady side of Shishan（石山），or over the stones in high mountains，or in farmland. [It can be] collected in January.

Notes

1. Luoshi（络石，fruit of Chinese starjasmine，Fructus Trachelospermi）is a herbal medicinal，bitter in taste，slightly cold in property，entering the heart meridian，the liver meridian and the kidney meridian，effective in expelling pathogenic wind，unobstructing the collaterals，resolving stasis and ceasing bleeding. Clinically it is used to treat wind-dampness impediment and pain，spasm of sinews and vessels，abscess，swelling and throat impediment.

57. 蒺藜子

【原文】

味苦,温。

主恶血,破癥结积聚,喉痹,乳难。久服,长肌肉,明目轻身。一名旁通,一名屈人,一名止行,一名豺羽,一名升推(《御览》引云,一名君水香,《大观本》,无文)。生平泽,或道旁。

【考据】

1.《名医》曰:一名即藜,一名茨,生冯翊,七月八月,采实,暴干。

2. 案《说文》云:茨,蒺藜也;诗曰:墙上有茨,以茨为茅苇,开屋字;《尔雅》云:茨,蒺藜;郭璞云:布地蔓生细叶,子有三角刺人;《毛诗》云:墙上有茨;《传》云:茨,蒺藜也,旧本作蒺藜,非。

【今译】

味苦,性温。

主治因瘀滞所致的死血之症,能破解癥结积聚之症,能治疗喉痹和

57. Jilizi (蒺藜子, fruit of puncturevine caltrap, Fructus Tribuli) [1]

[Original Text]

[Jilizi (蒺藜子, fruit of puncturevine caltrap, Fructus Tribuli),] bitter in taste and warm [in property], [is mainly used] to resolve seriously stagnated blood, to disperse accumulation of abdominal mass, and to treat throat impediment and difficulty in delivering baby. Long-term taking [of it will] promote growth of muscles, improve vision and relax the body. [It is also] called Pangtong (旁通), Quren (屈人), Zhixing (止行), Caiyu (豺羽) and Shengtui (升推), growing in plains, swamps or roadsides.

[Textual Research]

[According to the book entitled] *Tai Ping Yu Lan* (《太平御览》, *Imperial Studies in Taiping Times*), [it is also] called Junshuixiang (君水香), growing in pools or at roadsides. [In the book entitled] *Ming Yi Bie Lu* (《名医别录》, *Special Record of Great Doctors*), [it] says [that Jilizi (蒺藜子, fruit of puncturevine caltrap, Fructus Tribuli) can be] collected in July and August and dried in the sun.

Note

1. Jilizi (蒺藜子, fruit of puncturevine caltrap, Fructus Tribuli)

分娩困难。长期服用，能增长肌肉，能使眼睛明亮，能使人身体轻盈。又称为旁通，又称为屈人，又称为止行，又称为豺羽，又称为升推。该物生长在平川水泽之中，或道旁。

is a herbal medicinal, sometimes also referring to Ziyunyingzi (紫云英子, seed of Chinese milkvetch, Semen Astragali Sinici). It is bitter in taste, mild and slightly warm in property, entering the liver meridian and the lung meridian, effective in pacifying the liver, soothing the liver, expelling wind and improving vision. Clinically it is used to treat headache, vertigo, discomfort of the chest, distension and pain of the breast, measles and itching.

58. 黄耆

【原文】

味甘,微温。

主痈疽久败疮,排脓,止痛,大风癞疾,五痔,鼠瘘,补虚,小儿百病。一名戴糁。生山谷。

【考据】

1.《名医》曰:一名戴椹,一名独椹,一名芰草,一名蜀脂,一名百本,生蜀郡白水汉中,二月十月采,阴干。

【今译】

味甘,性微温。

主治痈疽以及久治不愈之疮,能排出脓肿,能消除疼痛,能治疗麻风,癫痫症,五种痔疮及瘰疬症,能补益虚弱症,能治疗各种小儿疾病。又称为戴糁。该物生长在山谷之中。

58. Huangqi (黄耆, root of membranous milkvetch; root of Mongolian milkvetch, Radix Astragali) [1]

[Original Text]

[Huangqi (黄耆, root of membranous milkvetch; root of Mongolian milkvetch, Radix Astragali),] sweet in taste and slightly warm [in property], [is mainly used] to treat injury [caused by] chronic carbuncle and ulcer, to resolve pus, to cease pain, [to treat] severe leprosy, five [kinds of] hemorrhoids and scrofula, to improve deficiency [and to treat] various infantile diseases. [It is also] called Daishen (戴糁), growing in mountains and valleys.

[Textual Research]

[In the book entitled] *Ming Yi Bie Lu* (《名医别录》, *Special Record of Great Doctors*), [it] says [that Huangqi (黄耆, root of membranous milkvetch; root of Mongolian milkvetch, Radix Astragali) is also] called Daishen (戴椹), Dushen (独椹), Jicao (芨草), Shuzhi (蜀脂) and Baiben (百本), growing in Baishui (白水) and Hanzhong (汉中) in Shujun (蜀郡). [It can be] collected in February and October and dried in the shade.

Notes

1. Huangqi (黄耆) is another name of Huangqi (黄芪, root of membranous milkvetch; root of Mongolian milkvetch, Radix Astragali), with the same pronunciation but different characters. It is a herbal medicinal, sweet in taste and slightly warm in property, entering the spleen meridian and the lung meridian, effective in tonifying the middle (the internal organs) and replenishing Qi, securing the superficies and promoting urination, resolving pus and enriching muscles. Clinically it is used to treat deficiency and weakness of the spleen and stomach, poor appetite and fatigue, Qi deficiency and spontaneous sweating, night sweating, Qi deficiency and edema, nephritis and edema.

59. 肉松蓉

【原文】

味甘,微温。

主五劳七伤,补中,除茎中寒热痛,养五脏,强阴,益精气,多子,妇
人症瘕。久服轻身。生山谷。

【考据】

1.《吴普》曰:肉苁蓉,一名肉松蓉,神农黄帝咸,雷公酸小温(《御
览》作李氏小温),生河西(《御览》作东),山阴,地,长三四寸丛生,或代
郡(览御下有雁门二字),二月至八月,采(《御览》引云,阴干用之)。

2.《名医》曰:生河西及代郡雁门,五月五日采,阴干。

3. 案《吴普》云:一名肉松蓉,当是古本,蓉即是容字,俗写苁蓉,非
正字也。

4. 陶宏景云:是野马精落地所生,生时似肉,旧作肉苁蓉,非。

【今译】

味甘,性微温。

59. Rousongrong（肉松蓉，desertliving cistanche herb，Herba Cistanches）[1]

[Original Text]

[Rousongrong（肉松蓉，desertliving cistanche herb，Herba Cistanches），] sweet in taste and slightly warm [in property], [is mainly used] to treat five [kinds of] overstrain and five [kinds of] damages, to tonify the middle（the internal organs）, to resolve cold-heat pain in the penis, to nourish the five Zang-organs, to strengthen the penis, to replenish essence and Qi [2], to increase fertility and to treat female abdominal mass. Long-term taking [of it will] relax the body. [It] grows in mountains and valleys.

[Textual Research]

[In the book entitled] *Wu Pu Ben Cao*（《吴普本草》，*Wu Pu's Studies of Materia Medica*）, [it] says [that] Roucongrong（肉苁蓉，desertliving cistanche herb，Herba Cistanches）is also called Rousongrong（肉松蓉）. [According to] Agriculture God（神农）and Yellow Emperor（黄帝）, [it is] salty [in taste]; [according to] Leigong（雷公）, [it is] sour [in taste] and slightly warm [in property]. [In the book entitled] *Tai Ping Yu Lan*（《太平御览》，*Imperial Studies in Taiping Times*）, [it] says [that it is] slightly warm [in property]. [According to] Li's（李氏）, [it can be] collected in February and August and dried in the shade.

主治五种劳伤和七种损伤,能补益人体内脏,能消解阴茎中的寒热性疾病和疼痛,能滋养五脏,能增强阴液,能补益精气,能增强生育能力,能治疗女子症瘕。长期服用能使人身体轻盈。该物生长在山谷之中。

[In the book entitled] *Ming Yi Bie Lu* (《名医别录》, *Special Record of Great Doctors*), [it] says [that Rousongrong (肉松蓉, desertliving cistanche herb, Herba Cistanches)], growing in Hexi (河西) and Yanmen (雁门) in Daijun (代郡), [can be] collected on May 5 and dried in the shade.

Notes

1. Rousongrong 肉松蓉 is another name of Roucongrong (肉苁蓉, desertliving cistanche herb, Herba Cistanches). It is a herbal medicinal，sweet and salty in taste，warm in property，entering the kidney meridian and the large intestine meridian，effective in tonifying the kidney and strengthening Yang，moistening the intestines and promoting defecation. Clinically it is used to treat impotence，sexual apathy，seminal emission，spermatorrhea，infertility，pain of the waist and spine，intestinal dryness and constipation.

2. Essence and Qi refer to kidney essence and kidney Qi.

60. 防风

【原文】

味甘,温,无毒。

主大风,头眩痛,恶风,风邪,目盲无所见,风行周身,骨节疼痹(《御览》作痛),烦满。久服轻身。一名铜芸(《御览》作芒)。生川泽。

【考据】

1.《吴普》曰:防风一名回云,一名回草,一名百枝,一名蕳根,一名百韭,一名百种,神农黄帝岐伯桐君雷公扁鹊甘无毒,李氏小寒,或生邯郸上蔡,正月生叶,细圆,青黑黄白,五月花黄,六月实黑,三月十月采根,日干,琅邪者良(《御览》)。

2.《名医》曰:一名茴草,一名百枝,一名屏风,一名蕳根,一名百蜚,生沙苑,及邯郸,琅邪,上蔡,二月十月采根,暴干。

3. 案《范子计然》云:防风出三辅,白者善。

【今译】

味甘,性温,无毒。

60. Fangfeng（防风，saposhnikovia，Radix Saposhnikoviae）[1]

[Original Text]

[Fangfeng（防 风，saposhnikovia，Radix Saposhnikoviae），] sweet in taste，warm and non-toxic [in property]，[is mainly used] to treat [disease caused by] severe [pathogenic] wind，headache with vertigo，aversion to wind，[damage due to] wind-evil，poor vision，invasion of wind in the whole body，pain and impediment of bones and joints，vexation and depression. Long-term taking [of it will] relax the body. [It is also] called Tongyun（铜芸），growing in valleys and swamps.

227

[Textual Research]

[In the book entitled] *Wu Pu Ben Cao*（《吴普本草》，*Wu Pu's Studies of Materia Medica*），[it] says [that] Fangfeng（防 风，saposhnikovia，Radix Saposhnikoviae）[is also] called Huiyun（回云，Huicao（回草），Baiji（百枝），Jiangen（茼根），Baijiu（百韭）and Baizhong（百种）. [According to] Agriculture God（神农），Yellow Emperor（黄帝），Qibo（岐伯），Tongjun（桐均），Leigong（雷公）and Bianque（扁鹊），[it is] sweet [in taste] and non-toxic [in property]；[according to] Li's（李氏），[it is] slightly cold [in property]. [According to the book entitled] *Tai Ping Yu Lan*（《太平御览》，*Imperial Studies in Taiping Times*），[it] grows in Handan

主治因严重的风邪伤人所致之症,能治疗目眩头痛,麻风之病,风邪所伤,因视力丧失而无法观看,风邪窜行全身,骨节疼痛阻痹,烦躁和郁闷。长期服用能使人身体轻盈。又称为铜芸。该物生长在山川和平泽之中。

（邯郸）and Shangcai（上蔡）.［In］January,［its］leaves begin to sprout, thin and round［in style］, green, black, yellow and white［in color］;［in］May,［it begins］to blossom［in］yellow［color］;［in］June,［it begins］to bear fruit［in］black［color］.［Its］root［can be］collected in March and October and dried in the sun.

［In the book entitled］*Ming Yi Bie Lu*（《名医别录》, *Special Record of Great Doctors*）,［it］says［that Fangfeng（防风, saposhnikovia, Radix Saposhnikoviae）is also］called Huicao（茴草）, Baiji（百枝）, Pingfeng（屏风）, Jiangen（蕳根）and Baifei（百蜚）, growing in Shayuan（沙苑）, Handan（邯郸）, Langxie（琅邪）and Shangcai（上蔡）.［Its］root［can be］collected in February and October and dried in the sun.

［In the book entitled］*Fan Zi Ji Ran*（《范子计然》, *Studies About Fan Li's Teacher*）,［it］says［that］Fangfeng（防风, saposhnikovia, Radix Saposhnikoviae）grows in three places and the white one is more effective.

Notes

1. Fangfeng（防风, saposhnikovia, Radix Saposhnikoviae）is a herbal medicinal, pungent and sweet in taste, slightly warm in property, entering the bladder meridian, the lung meridian and the spleen meridian, effective in expelling wind, drying dampness and relieving pain. Clinically it is used to treat wind-cold attack, headache with blurred vision, wind-cold and dampness impediment, aching pain of bones and joints, and tetanus.

61. 蒲黄

【原文】

味甘,平。

主心、腹、膀胱寒热,利小便,止血,消瘀血。久服,轻身益气力,延年神仙。生池泽。

【考据】

1.《名医》曰:生河东,四月采。

2. 案《玉篇》云:蒚,谓今蒲头,有台,台上有重台,中出黄,即蒲黄;陶宏景云:此即蒲厘花上黄粉也,仙经亦用此,考《尔雅》符离,其上蒚,符离与蒲厘声相近,疑即此。

【今译】

味甘,性平。

61. Puhuang（蒲黄，longbract cattail pollen，narrowleaf cattail pollen，oriental cattail pollen，Pollen Typhae）[1]

〔Original Text〕

〔Puhuang（蒲黄，longbract cattail pollen，narrowleaf cattail pollen，oriental cattail pollen，Pollen Typhae），〕sweet in taste 〔and〕mild 〔in property〕，〔is mainly used〕to treat cold-heat in the heart， abdomen and bladder， to promote urination， to cease bleeding and to resolve blood stasis. Long-term taking 〔of it will〕relax the body， replenish Qi and energy， prolong life 〔as that of〕immortals. 〔It〕grows in lakes and swamps.

〔Textual Research〕

〔In the book entitled〕*Ming Yi Bie Lu*（《名医别录》，*Special Record of Great Doctors*），〔it〕says 〔that Puhuang（蒲黄，longbract cattail pollen， narrowleaf cattail pollen， oriental cattail pollen， Pollen Typhae）〕grows in Hedong（河东）〔and can be〕collected in April.

Notes

1. Puhuang（蒲黄，longbract cattail pollen， narrowleaf cattail pollen， oriental cattail pollen， Pollen Typhae） is a herbal medicinal，sweet in taste and mild in property，entering the liver

　　主治心、腹、膀胱中的寒热性疾病,能使小便通畅,能止血,能消除瘀血。长期服用,能使人身体轻盈,能补益气力,能延年益寿,像神仙一样。该物生长在池泽中。

meridian and the heart meridian, effective in activating the blood, expelling blood stasis and ceasing bleeding. Clinically it is used to treat stagnation and obstruction caused by blood stasis, sharp pain of the heart and abdomen, blood stasis and abdominal pain after delivery of baby, flooding and spotting (metrostaxis and metrorrhagia), amenorrhea, dysmenorrhea, traumatic injury, sores, ulcers and abscesses.

62. 香蒲

【原文】

味甘,平。

主五脏,心下邪气,口中烂臭,坚齿明目聪耳。久服轻身耐老(《御览》作能老)。一名睢(《御览》云睢蒲)。生池泽。

【考据】

1.《吴普》曰:睢,一名睢石,一名香蒲,神农雷公甘,生南海,池泽中(《御览》)。

2.《名医》曰:一名醮,生南海。

3. 案《说文》云:菩,草也;玉篇云:菩,香草也,又音蒲;本草图经云:香蒲,蒲黄苗也,春初生嫩叶,未出水时,红白色茸茸然,《周礼》以为菹。

【今译】

味甘,性平。

62. Xiangpu（香蒲，longbract cattail herb，narrowleaf cattail herb，latifoliate cattail herb，david cattail herb，little cattail herb，oriental cattail herb，Herba Typhae）[1]

[Original Text]

[Xiangpu（香蒲，longbract cattail herb，narrowleaf cattail herb，latifoliate cattail herb，david cattail herb，little cattail herb，oriental cattail herb，Herba Typhae），] sweet in taste [and] mild [in property]，[is mainly used] to treat [diseases of] the five Zang-organs，[to resolve retention of] evil-Qi below the heart and oral ulceration with fetid breath，to strengthen the teeth，and to improve vision and hearing. Long-term taking [of it will] relax the body and prevent aging. [It is also] called Hui（睢）and grows in lakes and swamps.

[Textual Research]

[In the book entitled] *Wu Pu Ben Cao*（《吴普本草》，*Wu Pu's Studies of Materia Medica*），[it] says [that Xiangpu（香蒲，longbract cattail herb，narrowleaf cattail herb，latifoliate cattail herb，david cattail herb，little cattail herb，oriental cattail herb，Herba Typhae）is also] called Huishi（睢石）and Xiangpu（香蒲）. [According to] Agriculture God（神农）and Leigong（雷公），[it is] sweet [in taste] and grows in the lakes and pools in Nanhai（南海，

　　主治五脏之症,消除心下邪气,消解口中因溃烂而散发的臭气,能使牙齿坚固,眼睛明亮,听力增强。长期服用能使人身体轻盈,不易衰老。该物生长在池泽中。

Southern Sea).

[In the book entitled] *Ming Yi Bie Lu* (《名医别录》, *Special Record of Great Doctors*), [it] says [that is also] called Jiao (醮), growing in Nanhai (南海, Southern Sea).

[In] case [analysis in the book entitled] *Shuo Wen* (《说文》, *On Culture*), [it] says [that] Xiangpu (香蒲, longbract cattail herb, narrowleaf cattail herb, latifoliate cattail herb, david cattail herb, little cattail herb, oriental cattail herb, Herba Typhae) is the seedling of Puhuang (蒲黄). [In] spring, [it] begins to sprout. Before growing out of water, [it is] white.

Notes

1. Xiangpu (香蒲, longbract cattail herb, narrowleaf cattail herb, latifoliate cattail herb, david cattail herb, little cattail herb, oriental cattail herb, Herba Typhae) is a herbal medicinal, sweet in taste and mild in property, effective in promoting urination and reducing fire. Clinically it is used to treat difficulty in urination and breast carbuncle.

63. 续断

【原文】

味苦,微温。

主伤寒,补不足,金疮痈伤,折跌,续筋骨,妇人乳难(《御览》作乳痈云崩中,漏血,《大观本》,作黑字)。久服益气力。一名龙豆,一名属折。生山谷。

【考据】

1.《名医》曰:一名接骨,一名南草,一名槐,生常山,七月八月采,阴干。

2. 案《广雅》云:褱,续断也;《范子计然》云:续断,出三辅:桐君药录云:续断生蔓延,叶细,茎如荏大,根本黄白有汁,七月八月采根。

【今译】

味苦,性微温。

主治伤寒,能补充精气不足,能治疗因金属损伤而导致的痈疮,因

63. Xuduan（续断，root of Himalayan teasel，Radix Dipsaci）[1]

[Original Text]

[Xuduan（续断，root of Himalayan teasel，Radix Dipsaci），] bitter in taste and slightly warm in property], [is mainly used] to treat cold damage，to improve insufficiency，[to treat] carbuncle and injury [due to] metal attack and traumatic injury，to invigorate sinews and bones，[and to treat] dystocia. Long-term taking [of it will] replenish Qi and energy. [It is also] called Longdou（龙豆）and Shuzhe（属折），growing in mountains and valleys.

[Textual Research]

[In the book entitled] *Ming Yi Bie Lu*（《名医别录》，*Special Record of Great Doctors*），[it] says [that Xuduan（续断，root of Himalayan teasel，Radix Dipsaci) is also] called Jiegu（接骨），Nancao（南草）and Kui（槐），growing in Changshan（常山）. [It can be] collected in July and August and dried in the shade.

[In the book entitled] *Guang Ya*（《广雅》，*The First Chinese Encyclopedic Dictionary*），[it] says [that the so-called] Huai（褱）is actually Xuduan（续断，root of Himalayan teasel，Radix Dipsaci）. [In the book entitled] *Fan Zi Ji Ran*（《范子计然》，*Studies About Fan Li's Teacher*），[it] says [that] Xuduan（续断，root of Himalayan teasel，Radix Dipsaci）grows in three places[2].

外部感染所致疮痛及跌打损伤，能使跌打损伤中的筋骨续接，能消解女性分娩困难。长期服用能补益气力。又称为龙豆，又称为属折。该物生长在山谷之中。

[According to] the records about medicine [made by] Tongjun (桐均), Xuduan (续断, root of Himalayan teasel, Radix Dipsaci) grows prosperously with thin leaves and large stalks. The root is yellow and white with juice [and can be] collected in July and August.

Notes

1. Xuduan (续断, root of Himalayan teasel, Radix Dipsaci) is a herbal medicinal, bitter and pungent in taste, warm in property, entering the liver meridian and the kidney meridian, effective in tonifying the liver and kidney, cultivating injured bones and regulating vessels. Clinically it is used to treat insufficiency of the liver and kidney, pain of the waist and knees, pain of bones due to wind-dampness, traumatic injury, fracture, flooding and spotting (metrostaxis and metrorrhagia), bleeding during pregnancy and threatened abortion.

2. Three places refer to the places governed by three important officials, Jing Zhaoyi (京兆尹), Zuo Fengyi (左冯翊) and You Fufeng (右扶风), during the Han Dynasty (202 BC - 220 AC).

64. 漏芦

【原文】

味苦咸,寒。

主皮肤热,恶疮,疽痔,湿痹,下乳汁。久服轻身益气,耳目聪明,不老延年。一名野兰。生山谷。

【考据】

1.《名医》曰:生乔山,八月采根,阴干。

2. 案《广雅》云:飞廉,漏芦也;陶宠景云:俗中取根,名鹿骊。

【今译】

味苦咸,性寒。

主治身体发热,恶性痈疮,疽痛,痔疮及湿邪所致痹证,能使乳汁

64. Loulu（漏芦，uniflower swisscentaury root，Radix Rhapontici）[1]

[Original Text]

[Loulu（漏芦，uniflower swisscentaury root，Radix Rhapontici），] bitter and salty in taste and cold [in property]，[is mainly used] to treat skin heat[2]，severe sores，ulcers and dampness impediment [as well as] to promote lactation. Long-term taking [of it will] relax the body，replenish Qi，improve vision and hearing，prevent aging and prolong life. [It is also] called Yelan（野兰），growing in mountains and valleys.

[Textual Research]

[In the book entitled] *Ming Yi Bie Lu*（《名医别录》，*Special Record of Great Doctors*），[it] says [that Loulu（漏芦，uniflower swisscentaury root，Radix Rhapontici）] grows in Qiaoshan（乔山），[its] root [can be] collected in August and dried in the shade.

[In the book entitled] *Guang Ya*（《广雅》，*The First Chinese Encyclopedic Dictionary*），[it] says [that the so-called] Feilian（飞廉）refers to Loulu（漏芦，uniflower swisscentaury root，Radix Rhapontici）. Tao Hongjing（陶宏景）said，"Usually [its] root is collected [as medicinal] and called Luli（鹿骊）."

自然通畅。长期服用能使人身体轻盈，能补益精气，能使听力增强，

视力清明，能长寿不老，能延年益寿。又称为野兰。该物生长在山谷

之中。

Notes

1. Loulu （漏芦, uniflower swisscentaury root, Radix Rhapontici) is a herbal medicinal, bitter and salty in taste, cold in property, entering the stomach meridian and the large intestine meridian, effective in clearing heat, removing toxin, resolving swelling, dispelling pus and promoting lactation. Clinically it is used to treat breast carbuncle, furuncle, galactostasis, arthritis due to wind-dampness and bloody dysentery due to heat-toxin.

2. Skin heat refers to fever.

65. 营实

【原文】

味酸,温。

主痈疽恶疮,结肉,跌筋,败疮,热气,阴蚀不瘳,利关节。一名墙薇,一名墙麻,一名牛棘。生川谷。

【考据】

1.《吴普》曰:蔷薇,一名牛勒,一名牛膝,一名蔷薇,一名山枣(《御览》)。

2.《名医》曰:一名牛勒,一名蔷蘼,一名山棘,生零陵及蜀郡,八月九月采,阴干。

3. 案陶宏景云:即是墙薇子。

【今译】

味酸,性温。

65. Yingshi（营实，Japanese rose fruit，Fructus Rosae Multiflorae）[1]

［Original Text］

［Yingshi （营 实，Japanese rose fruit，Fructus Rosae Multiflorae），］sour in taste and warm ［in property］，［is mainly used］to treat carbuncle，furuncle，severe sore，lump，protrusion of sinews，severe sores ［difficult to heal］，heat-Qi and genital ulceration difficult to heal ［as well as］unobstruct joints. ［It is also］called Qiangwei （墙 薇），Qiangma （墙 麻）and Niuci （牛 棘），growing in mountain valleys and river valleys.

［Textual Research］

［In the book entitled］ *Wu Pu Ben Cao* （《吴普本草》，*Wu Pu's Studies of Materia Medica*），［it］says ［that Yingshi （营实，Japanese rose fruit，Fructus Rosae Multiflorae) is also］called Qiangwei （蔷 薇），Niule （牛 勒），）and Shanzao （山 枣）［according to the book entitled］ *Tai Ping Yu Lan* （《太平御览》，*Imperial Studies in Taiping Times*）.

［In the book entitled］ *Ming Yi Bie Lu* （《名医别录》，*Special Record of Great Doctors*），［it］says ［that Yingshi （营实，Japanese rose fruit，Fructus Rosae Multiflorae) is also］called Niule （牛 勒），Qiangmi （蔷 蘼）and Shanci （山 棘），growing in Lingling （零 陵）and Shujun （蜀郡）. ［It can be］collected in August and September，and

主治痈疽，恶性痈疮，肌肉突起，筋脉怒张，久治不愈疮痈，热邪所致病患，阴部溃疡且久治不愈，能使关节通畅。又称为墙薇，又称为墙麻，又称为牛棘。该物生长在山川河谷之中。

dried in the shade.

Notes

1. Yingshi（营 实，Japanese rose fruit，Fructus Rosae Multiflorae）is a herbal medicinal，sour in taste，cool and non-toxic in property，entering the lung meridian，the spleen meridian，the liver meridian and the bladder meridian，effective in clearing heat and removing toxin，expelling wind and activating the blood，promoting urination and resolving swelling. Clinically it is used to treat sore，carbuncle，wind-dampness impediment，inhibition of joints，irregular menstruation，edema，dysuria，beriberi and dysmenorrhea.

Agriculture
God's Canon of
Materia Medica

66. 天名精

【原文】

味甘,寒。

主瘀血,血瘕欲死,下血,止血,利小便。久服轻身耐老。一名麦句姜,一名虾蟆蓝,一名豕首。生川泽。

【考据】

1.《名医》曰:一名天门精,一名玉门精,一名彘颅,一名蟾蜍兰,一名觐。生平原,五月采。

2. 案《说文》云:薽,豕首也;《尔雅》云:茢薽豕首;郭璞云:今江东呼豨首,可以焰蚕蛹;陶宏景云:此即今人呼为豨莶;《唐本》云:鹿活草是也,别录一名天蔓菁,南文呼为地松;掌禹锡云:陈藏器别立地菘条,后人不当仍其谬。

【今译】

味甘,性寒。

66. Tianmingjing（天名精，root and leaf of common carpesium，Radix et Folium Carpesii Abrotanoidis）[1]

[Original Text]

[Tianmingjing（天名精，root and leaf of common carpesium, Radix et Folium Carpesii Abrotanoidis），] sweet in taste and cold [in property], [is mainly used] to treat blood stasis, severe lump [due to] blood stasis and bloody stool [as well as] cease bleeding and promote urination. Long-term taking [of it will] relax the body and prolong life. [It is also] called Maijujiang（麦句姜）, Xiamolan（虾蟆蓝）and Shishou（豕首）, growing in lakes and swamps.

[Textual Research]

[In the book entitled] *Ming Yi Bie Lu*（《名医别录》，*Special Record of Great Doctors*）, [it] says [that Tianmingjing（天名精，root and leaf of common carpesium, Radix et Folium Carpesii Abrotanoidis) is also] called Tianmenjing（天门精）, Yumenjing（玉门精）, Zhilu（彘颅）, Chanchulan（蟾蜍兰）and Jin（觐）, growing in Pingyuan（平原）. [It can be] collected in May.

Notes

1. Tianmingjing（天名精，root and leaf of common carpesium, Radix et Folium Carpesii Abrotanoidis）is a herbal medicinal, pungent and sweet in taste, cold and slightly toxic in property,

主治瘀血所致的下部严重出血，能阻止出血，能使小便通畅。长期服用能使人身体轻盈，不易衰老。又称为麦句姜，又称为虾蟆蓝，又称为豕首。该物生长在山川和平泽之中。

entering the liver meridian and the lung meridian, effective in clearing heat, removing toxin, expelling phlegm and ceasing bleeding. Clinically it is used to treat swelling and pain of the throat, acute iteric hepatitis, hematemesis, hematoptysis, epistaxis and hematuria.

67．决明子

【原文】

味咸,平。

主青盲,目淫,肤赤,白膜,眼赤痛,泪出。久服益精光(太平《御览》引作理目珠精,理,即治字),轻身。生川泽。

【考据】

1.《吴普》曰:决明子,一名草决明,一名羊明(《御览》)。

2.《名医》曰:生龙门,石决明生豫章,十月采,阴干百日。

3.案《广雅》云:羊蹢蹢,英光也,又决明,羊明也;《尔雅》云:蹢蹢,英光;郭璞云:英,明也,叶黄锐,赤华,实如山茱萸;陶宏景云:形似马蹄决明。

【今译】

味咸,性平。

67. Juemingzi（决明子，seed of sickle senna，Semen Cassiae）[1]

[Original Text]

[Juemingzi（决明子，seed of sickle senna，Semen Cassiae），] salty in taste and mild [in property]，[is mainly used] to treat optic atrophy，disorder of the eyes with red or white retina，redness and pain of the eyes with spontaneous tearing. Long-term taking [of it will] replenish essence and relax the body. [It] grows in mountains and lakes.

[Textual Research]

[In the book entitled] *Wu Pu Ben Cao*（《吴普本草》，*Wu Pu's Studies of Materia Medica*），[it] says [that] Juemingzi（决明子，seed of sickle senna，Semen Cassiae）[is also] called Caojueming（草决明）and Yangming（羊明）[according to the book entitled] *Tai Ping Yu Lan*（《太平御览》，*Imperial Studies in Taiping Times*）.

[In the book entitled] *Ming Yi Bie Lu*（《名医别录》，*Special Record of Great Doctors*），[it] says [that Juemingzi（决明子，seed of sickle senna，Semen Cassiae）] grows in Longmen（龙门）and Yuzhang（豫章）. [It can be] collected in October and dried in the shade in one hundred days.

Notes

1. Juemingzi（决明子，seed of sickle senna，Semen Cassiae）is a

主治青盲症，眼睛遭受赤膜和白膜的侵淫，眼睛红肿疼痛，泪流不止。长期服用能补益精气，能提高视力，能使人身体轻盈。该物生长在山川和平泽之中。

herbal medicinal，also called Mati Jueming（马蹄决明），Jialǜdou（假绿豆）and Jiahuasheng（假花生），bitter in taste and cool in property，entering the liver meridian and the kidney meridian，effective in clearing the liver and improving vision，moistening the intestines and promoting defecation. Clinically it is used to treat redness，swelling and pain of the eyes，hepatitis，intestinal dryness and constipation.

68. 丹参

【原文】

味苦,微寒。

主心腹邪气,肠鸣幽幽如走水,寒热积聚,破症除瘕,止烦满,益气。一名却蝉草。生川谷。

【考据】

1.《吴普》曰:丹参,一名赤参,一名木羊乳,一名却蝉草,神农桐君黄帝雷公扁鹊苦无毒,李氏大寒,岐伯咸,生桐柏,或生太山山陵阴,茎华小方如荏,毛,根赤,四月华紫,五月采根阴干,治心腹痛(《御览》)。

2.《名医》曰:一名赤参,一名木羊乳,生桐柏山及太山,五月采根,暴干。

3. 案《广雅》云:却蝉,丹参也。

【今译】

味苦,性微寒。

68. Danshen（丹参，root of unileaf sage，Radix Salviae Simplicifoliae）[1]

[Original Text]

[Danshen （丹参，root of unileaf sage，Radix Salviae Simplicifoliae），] bitter in taste and slightly cold [in property]，[is mainly used] to treat [disease caused by] evil-Qi in the heart and abdomen，[to resolve] borborygmus [sounding] like running water，[to expel] accumulation of cold-heat，to eliminate abdominal mass，to cease vexation and to replenish Qi. [It is also] called Chancao （蝉草），growing in mountain valleys and river valleys.

[Textual Research]

[In the book entitled] *Wu Pu Ben Cao* （《吴普本草》，*Wu Pu's Studies of Materia Medica*），[it] says [that] Danshen （丹参，root of unileaf sage，Radix Salviae Simplicifoliae）[is also] called Chishen （赤参），Muyangru （木羊乳）and Chancao （蝉草）. [According to] Agriculture God （神农），Tongjun （桐均），Yellow Emperor （黄帝），Leigong （雷公）and Bianque （扁鹊），[it is] bitter [in taste] and non-toxic [in property]；[according to] Li's （李氏），[it is] severe cold [in property]；[according to] Qibo （岐伯），[it is] salty [in property]. [It] grows in Tongbai （桐柏），or the shady side of Taishan （太山）. [Its] stalks and flowers look like common perilla and [its] leaves and roots are red. [In] April，[its] flowers are

主治心腹部邪气所致之症，治疗肠鸣幽幽如流水，寒热性疾病，腹部积聚，能破解癥瘕，能消解烦躁，能解除郁闷，能补益精气。又称为却蝉草。该物生长在山川河谷之中。

神农本草经

purple. ［In］ May，the roots ［can be］ collected and dried in the shade to treat pain of the heart and abdomen. ［According to the book entitled］ *Tai Ping Yu Lan* （《太平御览》，*Imperial Studies in Taiping Times*）.

［In the book entitled］ *Ming Yi Bie Lu* （《名医别录》，*Special Record of Great Doctors*），［it］ says ［that Danshen （丹参，root of unileaf sage，Radix Salviae Simplicifoliae） is also］ called Chishen （赤参） and Muyangru （木羊乳），growing in Tongbaishan （桐柏山） and Taishan （太山）. ［Its］ root ［can be］ collected in May and dried in the sun.

Notes

1. Danshen （丹参，root of unileaf sage，Radix Salviae Simplicifoliae） is a herbal medicinal，bitter in taste and slightly cold in property，entering the heart meridian and the liver meridian，effective in activating the blood and eliminating stasis，tranquilizing the heart and pacifying the spirit. Clinically it is used to treat irregular menstruation，amenorrhea，dysmenorrhea，blood stasis and abdominal pain after delivery of baby，coronary disease，angina，insufficiency of the blood in the heart and brain，abdominal mass，wind-dampness impediment and pain.

69. 茜根

【原文】

味苦,寒。

主寒湿,风痹,黄疸,补中。生川谷。

【考据】

1.《名医》曰:可以染绛,一名地血,一名茹藘,一名茅蒐,一名茜,生乔山,二月三月,采根,暴干。

2. 案《说文》云:茜,茅搜也,搜,茅搜,茹藘,人血所生,可以染绛,从草从鬼;《广雅》云:地血,茹藘,茜也;《尔雅》云:茹藘茅鬼;郭璞云:今茜也,可以染绛;《毛诗》云:茹藘在阪;《传》云:茹藘,茅搜也;陆玑云:一名地血,齐人谓之茜,徐州人谓之牛蔓,徐广注《史记》云:茜一名红蓝,其花染绘,赤黄也,按《名医》别出红蓝条,非。

69. Qiangen（茜根，root of Indian madder，Radix Rubiae）[1]

［Original Text］

［Qiangen（茜根，root of Indian madder，Radix Rubiae），］bitter in taste and cold［in property］，［is mainly used］to eliminate cold-dampness，［to resolve］wind impediment，［to treat］jaundice and to tonify the middle（the internal organs）.［It］grows in mountain valleys and river valleys.

［Textual Research］

［In the book entitled］*Ming Yi Bie Lu*（《名医别录》，*Special Record of Great Doctors*），［it］says［that Qiangen（茜根，root of Indian madder，Radix Rubiae）］can be dyed crimson，also called Dixue（地血），Rulǜ（茹虑），Maosou（茅蒐）and Qian（茜），growing in Qiaoshan（乔山）.［Its］root［can be］collected in February and March and dried in the sun.

Note

1. Qiangen（茜根，root of Indian madder，Radix Rubiae），also called Qiancao（茜草），Rulǘ（茹藘），Huoxuedan（活血丹），Xuejianchou（血见愁）and Huoxuecao（活血草），is a herbal medicinal，bitter in taste and cold in property，entering the liver meridian，effective in cooling the blood，ceasing bleeding，

【今译】

味苦,性寒。

主治寒湿证,治疗风湿痹证,黄疸,能补益人体内脏。该物生长在山川河谷之中。

eliminating blood stasis, stopping cough and resolving phlegm. Clinically it is used to treat hematoptysis, hematemesis, hematuria, hematochezia, flooding and spotting (metrostaxis and metrorrhagia), amenorrhea, wind-dampness impediment and pain, jaundice and bronchitis.

神农本草经

70. 飞廉

【原文】

味苦,平。

主骨节热,胫重酸疼。久服,令人身轻。一名飞轻(巳上四字,原本黑字)。生川泽。

【考据】

1.《名医》曰:一名伏兔,一名飞雉,一名木禾,生河内,正月采根,七月八月采花,阴干。

2. 案《广雅》云:伏猪,木禾也,飞廉,漏芦也;陶宠景云:今既别有漏芦,则非,此别名耳。

【今译】

味苦,性平。

主治骨节发热,小腿沉重酸疼。长期服用,能使人身体轻盈。又称为飞轻。该物生长在山川和平泽之中。

70. Feilian（飞廉，curly bristlethistle herb，Herba Cardui Crispi）[1]

[Original Text]

[Feilian（飞廉，curly bristlethistle herb，Herba Cardui Crispi），] bitter in taste and mild [in property], [is mainly used] to resolve heat in the bones and joints，and to treat heaviness and pain of the shank. Long-term taking [of it will] relax the body. [It is also] called Feiqing（飞轻）and grows in laks and swamps.

[Textual Research]

[In the book entitled] *Ming Yi Bie Lu*（《名医别录》，*Special Record of Great Doctors*），[it] says [that Feilian（飞廉，curly bristlethistle herb，Herba Cardui Crispi）is also] called Futu（伏兔），Feizhi（飞雉）and Muhuo（木禾），growing in Henei（河内）. [Its] root [can be] collected in July and August，and dried in the shade.

Notes

1. Feilian（飞廉，curly bristlethistle herb，Herba Cardui Crispi）is a herbal medicinal，bitter in taste and mild in property，effective in cooling the blood and expelling wind，clearing heat and eliminating dampness. Clinically it is used to treat hematemesis，nosebleed，hematuria，flooding and spotting（metrostaxis and metrorrhagia），vertigo due to invasion of wind into the head，acute or chronic infectious hepatitis，infection of urethra，chyluria and dampness-heat impediment.

267

71. 五味子

【原文】

味酸,温。

主益气,咳逆上气,劳伤羸瘦,补不足,强阴,益男子精(《御览》引云,一名会及,《大观本》,作黑字)。生山谷。

【考据】

1.《吴普》曰:五味子,一名元及(《御览》)。

2.《名医》曰:一名会及,一名元及,生齐山及代郡,八月,采实,阴干。

3. 案《说文》云:菋,荎猪也,荎,荎猪草也,猪,荎猪也;《广雅》云:会及,五味也;《尔雅》云:菋,荎藸;郭璞云:五味也,蔓生子,丛在茎头;《抱朴子·仙药》云:五味者五行之精,其子有五味,移门子服五味子十六年,色如玉女,入水不沾,入火不灼也。

71. Wuweizi（五味子，schisandra，Fructus Schisandrae）[1]

[Original Text]

［Wuweizi（五味子，schisandra，Fructus Schisandrae），］sour in taste and warm ［in property］，［is mainly used］to replenish Qi，to treat cough with dyspnea and upward counterflow of Qi，［to resolve］overexertion with emaciation，to improve insufficiency，to strengthen Yin and to replenish male semen. ［It］grows in mountain valleys and river valleys.

[Textual Research]

［In the book entitled］*Wu Pu Ben Cao*（《吴普本草》，*Wu Pu's Studies of Materia Medica*），［it］says［that］Wuweizi（五味子，schisandra，Fructus Schisandrae）［is also］called Yuanji（元及）［according to the book entitled］*Tai Ping Yu Lan*（《太平御览》，*Imperial Studies in Taiping Times*）.

［In the book entitled］*Ming Yi Bie Lu*（《名医别录》，*Special Record of Great Doctors*），［it］says［that Wuweizi（五味子，schisandra，Fructus Schisandrae）is also］called Huiji（会及）and Yuanji（元及），growing in Qishan（齐山）and Daijun（代郡）. ［In］August，［its］fruit［can be］collected and dried in the shade.

［In the book entitled］*Bao Pu Zi*（《抱朴子》，*Primitive and Natural View*），［it］says［that］Wuweizi（五味子，schisandra，

【今译】

味酸,性温。

能补益精气,能治疗咳嗽,呼吸困难,劳伤及身体瘦弱,能补充精气不足,能增强阴液,能补益男子之精。该物生长在山谷之中。

Fructus Schisandrae), [literally five tastes], refers to the essence of the five elements. The seeds of Wuweizi (五味子, schisandra, Fructus Schisandrae) bear five tastes. Taking it for sixteen years [will enable one to become as] beautiful as a jade girl[2], impossible to be soaked [when] jumping into water and scorched [when] falling into fire.

Notes

1. Wuweizi (五味子, schisandra, Fructus Schisandrae) is a herbal medicinal, sour in taste and warm in property, entering the lung meridian and the kidney meridian, effective in astringing the lung and nourishing the kidney, producing fluid and ceasing sweating, warming Yang and stopping diarrhea, tranquilizing the heart and pacifying the spirit. Clinically it is used to treat chronic cough with dyspnea due to deficiency, oral dryness due to insufficiency of fluid, spontaneous sweating, night sweating, seminal emission, spermatorrhea, chronic diarrhea, chronic dysentery, amnesia and insomnia.

2. The so-called jade girl refers to an immortal girl.

72. 旋华

【原文】

味甘,温。

主益气,去面皯(《御览》作黚)黑,色媚好(《御览》作令人色悦泽),其根,味辛,主腹中寒热邪气,利小便。久服不饥轻身。一名筋根华,一名金沸(《御览》引云一名美草,《大观本》,作黑字)。生平泽。

【考据】

1.《名医》曰:生豫州,五月采,阴干。

2. 案陶宏景云:东人呼为山姜,南人呼为美草;本草衍义云:世又谓之鼓子花。

【今译】

味甘,性温。

能补益精气,能祛除面部黑斑,能使人面色妩媚。

72. Xuanhua（旋华，flower of hedge glorybind，Flos Calystegiae Sepium）[1]

[Original Text]

[Xuanhua（旋华，flower of hedge glorybind，Flos Calystegiae Sepium），] sweet in taste [and] warm [in property], [is mainly used] to replenish Qi, to remove facial black spots, to luster facial expression. Its root is pungent in taste [and effective in resolving] cold and heat evil-Qi in the abdomen and promoting urination. Long-term taking [of it will make people have] no [sense of] hunger and relax the body. [It is also] called Jingenhua（筋根华）and Jinfo（金沸），growing in plains and swamps.

[Textual Research]

[In the book entitled] *Ming Yi Bie Lu*（《名医别录》，*Special Record of Great Doctors*），[it] says [that Xuanhua（旋华，flower of hedge glorybind，Flos Calystegiae Sepium）] grows in Yuzhou（豫州），[and can be] collected in May and dried in the shade.

Tao Hongjing（陶宏景）said，"People in the east call it Shanjiang（山姜）[while] people in the south call it Meicao（美草）. [In the book entitled] *Ben Cao Yan Yi*（本草衍义，*Explanation and Analysis of Materia Medica*），[it] says [that] people also call it Guzihua（鼓子花）.

其根味辛，能主治腹中寒热邪气，能使小便通畅。长期服用，能减少饥饿之感，能使身体轻盈。又称为筋根华，又称为金沸。该物生长在平川水泽之中。

Notes

1. Xuanhua（旋华，flower of hedge glorybind，Flos Calystegiae Sepium），another name of Xuanhua（旋花），is a herbal medicinal，sweet and pungent in taste，warm and non-toxic in property，effective in tonifying deficiency due to overexertion and replenishing essential Qi. Clinically it is used to treat facial black spots，cold-heat disease in the internal organs and traumatic injury，and promote urination.

275

73. 兰草

【原文】

味辛,平。

主利水道,杀蛊毒,辟不祥。久服,益气轻身,不老,通神明。一名水香。生池泽。

【考据】

1.《名医》曰:生大吴,四月五月采。

2. 案《说文》云:兰,香草也;《广雅》云:蕳,兰也,易,其臭如兰,郑云兰,香草也,《夏小正》,五月蓄兰;《毛诗》云:方秉蕳兮,《传》云蕳,兰也;陆玑云:蕳即兰,香草也,其茎叶似药草泽兰;《范子计然》云:大兰出汉中三辅,兰出河东,宏农,白者善,元杨齐贤注李白诗,引本草云:兰草,泽兰,二物同名,兰草一名水香,云,都梁是也,水经,零陵郡,都梁县西,小山上,有淳水,其中悉生兰草,绿叶紫茎,泽兰,如薄荷,微香,荆湘岭南人家多种之,与兰大抵相类,颜师古以兰草为泽兰,非也。

73. Lancao（兰草，fortune eupatorium herb，Herba Eupatorii）[1]

[Original Text]

[Lancao（兰草，fortune eupatorium herb，Herba Eupatorii），] pungent in taste and mild [in property], [is mainly used] to unobstruct waterway [in the body] [2], to eliminate worm toxin and to avoid [invasion of] unauspicious [pathogenic factors]. Long-term taking [of it will] replenish Qi, relax the body, prevent aging and cultivate spirit and mentality. [It] grows in lakes and swamps.

[Textual Research]

[In the book entitled] *Ming Yi Bie Lu*（《名医别录》，*Special Record of Great Doctors*），[it] says [that Lancao（兰草，fortune eupatorium herb，Herba Eupatorii）] grows in Dawu（大吴）[and can be] collected in April and May.

[In] case [analysis in the book entitled] *Shuo Wen*（《说文》，*On Culture*），[it] says [that Lancao（兰草，fortune eupatorium herb，Herba Eupatorii) is also called] Xiangcao（香草）. Luji（陆玑）said，"Its stalks and leaves look like those of Zelan（泽兰，hirsute shiny bugleweed herb，Herba Lycopi）." [In the book entitled] *Fan Zi Ji Ran*（《范子计然》，*Studies About Fan Li's Teacher*）[it] says [that]，"The large one grows in the three places in Hanzhong（汉中），the [small] one grows in Hedong（河东）and Hongnong（宏农）. [The

【今译】

味辛,性平。

能通利水道,能杀除虫毒,能消除不祥之气。长期服用,能补益精气,能使人身体轻盈,长寿不老,能使神志清晰,精神旺盛。又称为水香。该物生长在池泽中。

most] effective one [is] white [in color]." Yan Shigu (颜师古) said, "In ancient times [people] thought [that] Lancao (兰草, fortune eupatorium herb, Herba Eupatorii) was Zelan (泽兰, hirsute shiny bugleweed herb, Herba Lycopi). [Actually it is] not [true]."

Notes

1. Lancao (兰草, fortune eupatorium herb, Herba Eupatorii) is a herbal medicinal, pungent in taste and mild in property, entering the spleen meridian and the stomach meridian, effective in invigorating the spleen, resolving dampness and dispelling summer-heat. Clinically it is used to treat lump in the stomach due to dampness obstructing the middle energizer, nausea and vomiting, diarrhea, oral stickiness, summer-heat dampness, headache due to cold-heat, lassitude of the body, chest oppression and anorexia.

2. Waterway [in the body] refers to urethra.

74. 蛇床子

【原文】

味苦,平。

主妇人阴中肿痛,男子阴痿,湿痒,除痹气,利关节,癫痫恶疮。久服轻身。一名蛇米。生川谷及田野。

【考据】

1.《吴普》曰:蛇床一名蛇珠(《御览》)。

2.《名医》曰:一名蛇粟,一名虺床,一名思盐,一名绳毒,一名枣棘,一名墙蘼,生临淄,五月采实,阴干。

3. 案《广雅》云:蛇粟,马床,蛇床也,《尔雅》云:盱虺床,《淮南子》氾论训云:乱人者若蛇床之与蘼芜。

【今译】

味苦,性平。

74. Shechuangzi（蛇床子，fruit of common cnidium，Fructus Cnidii）[1]

[Original Text]

[Shechuangzi（蛇床子，fruit of common cnidium，Fructus Cnidii），] bitter in taste and mild [in property]，[is mainly used] to treat uterine swelling and pain and impotence，to resolve itching [due to] dampness，to eliminate impediment，to disinhibit joints and to treat epilepsy and severe sores. Long-term taking [of it will] relax the body. [It is also] called Shemi（蛇米）and grows in mountain valleys，river valleys and fields.

[Textual Research]

[In the book entitled] *Wu Pu Ben Cao*（《吴普本草》，*Wu Pu's Studies of Materia Medica*）[it] says [that] Shechuangzi（蛇床子，fruit of common cnidium，Fructus Cnidii）[is also] called Shezhu（蛇珠）[according to the book entitled] *Tai Ping Yu Lan*（《太平御览》，*Imperial Studies in Taiping Times*）.

[In the book entitled] *Ming Yi Bie Lu*（《名医别录》，*Special Record of Great Doctors*），[it] says [that Shechuangzi（蛇床子，fruit of common cnidium，Fructus Cnidii）is also called] Sheli（蛇粟），Huichuang（虺床），Siyan（思盐），Shengdu（绳毒），Zaoji（枣棘）and Qiangmi（墙蘼），growing in Linzi（临淄）. [Its] fruit [can be] collected in May and dried in the shade.

　　主治女性阴部肿痛,男子阳痿,因潮湿而导致的皮肤瘙痒,能祛除痹气,能使关节通畅,能治疗癫痫及恶性痈疮。长期服用能使人身体轻盈。又称为蛇米。该物生长在山川河谷之中及田野里。

Notes

1. Shechuangzi（蛇床子，fruit of common cnidium，Fructus Cnidii）is a herbal medicinal，pungent and bitter in taste，warm in property，entering the kidney meridian and the spleen meridian，effective in warming the kidney and assisting Yang，drying dampness and killing worms. Clinically it is used to treat impotence，sexual apathy in woman，infertility due to uterine coldness and watery leucorrhea.

75. 地肤子

【原文】

味苦,寒。

主膀胱热,利小便,补中益精气。久服,耳目聪明,轻身耐老。一名地葵(《御览》引云,一名地华,一名地脉,《大观本》无一名地华四字,脉作麦,皆黑字)。生平泽及田野。

【考据】

1. 古医曰:一名地麦,生荆州,八月十月采实,阴干。

2. 案《广雅》云:地葵,地肤也;《列仙传》云:文宾服地肤;郑樵云:地肤曰落帚,亦曰地扫;《尔雅》云:荓,马帚,即此也,今人亦用为帚。

【今译】

味苦,性寒。

75. Difuzi（地肤子，belvedere fruit，Fructus Kochiae）[1]

[Original Text]

[Difuzi（地肤子，belvedere fruit，Fructus Kochiae），] bitter in taste and cold [in property]，[is mainly used] to resolve heat in the bladder，disinhibit urination，to tonify the middle（the internal organs）and to replenish essential Qi. Long-term taking [of it will] improve hearing and vision，relax the body and prevent aging. [It is also] called Dikui（地葵）and grows in plains，swamps and fields.

[Textual Research]

[According to] medicine in ancient times，[Difuzi（地肤子，belvedere fruit，Fructus Kochiae）is also] called Dimai（地麦），growing in Jingzhou（荆州）. [Its] fruit [can be] collected in August and October and dried in the shade.

[In the book entitled] *Guang Ya*（《广雅》，*The First Chinese Encyclopedic Dictionary*），[it] says [that the so-called] Dikui（地葵）actually refers to Difuzi（地肤子，belvedere fruit，Fructus Kochiae）.

Notes

1. Difuzi（地肤子，belvedere fruit，Fructus Kochiae）is a herbal medicinal，sweet and bitter in taste，cold in property，entering the kidney meridian and the bladder meridian，effective in clearing heat

　　主治膀胱郁热症，能使小便通畅，能充实人体内脏，能补益精气。长期服用，能使人听力增强，视力清明，身体轻盈，不易衰老。又称为地葵。该物生长在平川水泽之中及田野里。

and promoting urination, eliminating dampness and ceasing itching. Clinically it is used to treat stranguira due to dampness-hat, dysuria, leucorrhea, urticaria and eczema.

76. 景天

【原文】

味苦,平。

主大热,火疮,身热烦,邪恶气。华主女人漏下赤白,轻身明目。一名戒火,一名慎火(《御览》引云,一名水母,《大观本》,作黑字,水作火)。生川谷。

【考据】

1.《名医》曰:一名火母,一名救火,一名据火,生太山,四月四日,七月七日采,阴干。

2. 案陶宏景云:今人皆盆养之于屋上,云以辟火。

【今译】

味苦,性平。

主治身体高热,能治疗火烧所致疮疡,身体发热烦躁以及邪恶

76. Jingtian（景天，common stonecrop herb，Herba Hylotelephii Erythrosticti）[1]

［Original Text］

［Jingtian（景天，common stonecrop herb，Herba Hylotelephii Erythrosticti），］bitter in taste and mild［in property］，［is mainly used］to resolve severe heat，sores and ulcers［due to］fire，fever，vexation and severe evil-Qi.［Its］flowers［can］treat metrostaxis and reddish white leucorrhea.［It can］relax the body and improve vision.［It is also］called Jiehuo（戒火）and Shenhuo（慎火），growing in mountain valleys and river valleys.

［Textual Research］

［In the book entitled］*Ming Yi Bie Lu*（《名医别录》，*Special Record of Great Doctors*），［it］says［that Jingtian（景天，common stonecrop herb，Herba Hylotelephii Erythrosticti）is also］called Huomu（火母），Jiuhuo（救火）and Juhuo（据火），growing in Taishan（太山）.［It can be］collected on April 4 and July 7，and dried in the shade.

Tao Hongjing（陶宏景）said，"People now all grow［Jingtian（景天，common stonecrop herb，Herba Hylotelephii Erythrosticti）］in the plates and put the plates on the top of houses in order to prevent fire."

之气。

　　其华主治女人阴道淋漓不断，赤白带下，能使人身体轻盈，眼睛明亮。又称为戒火，又称为慎火。该物生长在山川河谷之中。

Notes

1. Jingtian（景天，common stonecrop herb，Herba Hylotelephii Erythrosticti）is a herbal medicinal，bitter in taste and cold in property，entering the liver meridian，effective in clearing heat，resolving toxin and ceasing bleeding. Clinically it is used to treat vexation with fever，fright with mania，redness and pain of the eyes，hematemesis，hematoptysis，nosebleed，measles and dermatitis.

77. 茵陈

【原文】

味苦,平。

主风湿寒热,邪气,热结黄疸。久服轻身,益气耐老(《御览》作能老)。生邱陵阪岸上。

【考据】

1.《吴普》曰:因尘,神农岐伯雷公苦无毒,黄帝辛无毒,生田中,叶如蓝,十一月采(《御览》)。

2.《名医》曰:白兔食之仙,生太山,五月及立秋采,阴干。

3. 案《广雅》云:因尘,马先也;陶宏景云:仙经云,白蒿,白兔食之仙,而今茵陈乃云此,恐非耳;陈藏器云:茵陈,经冬不死,因旧苗而生,故名茵陈,后加蒿字也,据此,知旧作茵陈篙,非;又按《广雅》云:马先,疑即马新蒿,亦白蒿之类。

77. Yinchen（茵陈，capillaries，Herba Artemisiae Scopariae）[1]

[Original Text]

[（茵陈，capillaries，Herba Artemisiae Scopariae），] bitter in taste and mild [in property], [is mainly used] to treat [diseases caused by pathogenic] wind，dampness，cold，heat and evil-Qi [as well as] jaundice [caused by] heat bind. Long-term taking [of it will] relax the body，replenish Qi and prevent aging. [It] grows in hills and rugged areas.

[Textual Research]

[In the book entitled] *Wu Pu Ben Cao*（《吴普本草》，*Wu Pu's Studies of Materia Medica*），[it] says [that according to] Agriculture God（神农），Qibo（岐伯）and Leigong（雷公），Yinchen（茵陈，capillaries，Herba Artemisiae Scopariae）is bitter [in taste] and non-toxic [in property]；[according to] Yellow Emperor（黄帝），[it is] pungent [in taste] and non-toxic [in property]. [It] grows in the fields with green leaves. [It can be] collected in November [according to the book entitled] *Tai Ping Yu Lan*（《太平御览》，*Imperial Studies in Taiping Times*）.

[In the book entitled] *Ming Yi Bie Lu*（《名医别录》，*Special Record of Great Doctors*），[it] says [that Yinchen（茵陈，capillaries，Herba Artemisiae Scopariae）] grows in Taishan（太山）[and can

【今译】

味苦,性平。

主治风湿寒热邪气所致之症,热结,黄疸。长期服用,能使人身体轻盈,能补益精气,不易衰老。该物生长在丘陵和崎岖的岸上。

be] collected in May and autumn, and dried in the shade.

Chen Cangqi (陈藏器) said, "Yinchen (茵陈, capillaries, Herba Artemisiae Scopariae) never dies in winter and grows again [in spring] on the basis of the old seedling. That is why it is called Yinchen (茵陈, literally based on the old seedling)."

Notes

1. Yinchen (茵陈, capillaries, Herba Artemisiae Scopariae) is a herbal medicinal, bitter and pungent in taste and slightly cold in property, entering the liver meridian, the gallbladder meridian and the spleen meridian, effective in clearing heat, resolving dampness, and eliminating jaundice. Clinically it is used to treat jaundice due to heat-dampness and hepatitis at the urgent period and eliminate pathogenic wind, dampness, cold and heat.

78. 杜若

【原文】

味辛,微温。

主胸胁下逆气,温中,风入脑户,头肿痛,多涕泪出。

久服,益精(艺文类聚引作益气),明目轻身。一名杜衡(艺文类聚引作蘅,非)。生川泽。

【考据】

1.《名医》曰:一名杜连,一名白连,一名白芩,一名若芝,生武陵及冤句,二月八月采根,暴干。

2. 案《说文》云:若,杜若,香草;《广雅》云:楚蘅,杜蘅也;《西山经》云:天帝之上有草焉,其状如葵,其臭如蘼芜,名曰杜衡;《尔雅》云:杜,土卤;郭璞云:杜蘅也,似葵而香;《楚词》云:采芳州兮杜若;《范子计然》云:杜若生南郡汉中又云秦蘅,出于陇西天水;沈括补笔谈云:杜若,即今之高良姜,后人不识,又别出高良姜条,按经云一名杜蘅,是《名医》别出杜蘅条,非也,衡正字,俗加草。

78. Duruo（杜若，Japan pollia，Pollia Japonica）[1]

[Original Text]

［Duruo（杜若，Japan pollia, Pollia Japonica），］pungent in taste and slightly warm ［in property］，［is mainly used］ to regulate counterflow of Qi below the chest and rid-side，to warm the middle （the internal organs），and to treat invasion of wind into the brains，swelling and pain of the head，frequent discharge of snivel and tearing. Long-term taking ［of it will］ replenish essence，improve vision and relax the body. ［It is also］ called Duheng（杜衡），growing in mountains and lakes.

[Textual Research]

［In the book entitled］ *Ming Yi Bie Lu* （《名医别录》，*Special Record of Great Doctors*），［it］ says ［that Duruo（杜若，Japan pollia, Pollia Japonica）is also］ called Dulian（杜连），Bailian（白连），Bailing（白苓）and Ruozhi（若芝），growing in Wuling（武陵）and Yuanju（冤句）. ［Its］ root ［can be］ collected in February and August，and dried in the sun.

［In the book entitled］ *Fan Zi Ji Ran* （《范子计然》，*Studies About Fan Li's Teacher*），［it］ says ［that］ Duruo（杜若，Japan pollia, Pollia Japonica）grows in Nanjun（南郡）and Hanzhong（汉中），also called Qinheng（秦蘅），produced in Longxi（陇西）and Tianshui（天水）.

【今译】

味辛,性微温。

主治胸胁下逆气上行,能温煦人体脏器,能治疗因风邪入脑而致的头部肿痛,能消解鼻涕长流及泪流不止。

长期服用,能补益精气,能使眼睛明亮,身体轻盈。又称为杜衡。该物生长在山川和平泽之中。

Notes

1. Duruo (杜若, Japan pollia, Pollia Japonica) is a herbal medicinal, pungent in taste, slightly warm and non-toxic in property, effective in replenishing essence, resolving counterflow of Qi below the chest and rib-side, warming the middle (internal organs), dispersing cold and improving vision. Clinically it is used to treat swelling and pain of the head, frequent discharge of snivel and tearing, vertigo, common cold, panting and cough, headache, wind-cold and dampness impediment.

79. 沙参

【原文】

味苦,微寒。

主血积惊气,除寒热,补中,益肺气。久服利人。一名知母。生川谷。

【考据】

1.《吴普》曰:白沙参,一名苦心,一名识美,一名虎须,一名白参,一名志取,一名文虎,神农黄帝扁鹊无毒,岐伯咸,李氏大寒,生河内川谷,或般阳渎山,三月生如葵,叶青,实白如芥,根大白如芜菁,三月采(《御览》)。

2.《名医》曰:一名苦心,一名志取,一名虎须,一名白参,一名识美,一名文希,生河内及冤句,般阳续山,二月八月采根,暴干。

3. 案《广雅》云:苦心,沙参也,其蒿,青蘘也;《范子计然》云:白沙参,出洛阳,白者善。

79. Shashen（沙参，root of coastal glehnia，Radix Glehniae）[1]

[Original Text]

[Shashen（沙参，root of coastal glehnia，Radix Glehniae），] bitter in taste and slightly cold [in property]，[is mainly used] to resolve blood stasis with fright and convulsion，to eliminate cold-heat，to tonify the middle（the internal organs）and to replenish lung-Qi. Long-term taking [of it will be] beneficial to people's [health]. [It is also] called Zhimu（知母），growing in mountain valleys and river valleys.

[Textual Research]

[In the book entitled] *Wu Pu Ben Cao*（《吴普本草》，*Wu Pu's Studies of Materia Medica*），[it] says [that] the white Shashen（沙参，root of coastal glehnia，Radix Glehniae）[is also] called Kuxin（苦心），Shimei（识美），Huxu（虎须），Baishen（白参），Zhiqu（志取）and Wenhu（文虎）. [According to] Agriculture God（神农），Yellow Emperor（黄帝）and Bianque（扁鹊），[it is] non-toxic [in property]；[according to] Qibo（岐伯），[it is] salty [in taste]；[according to] Li's（李氏），[it is] severe cold [in property]. [According to the book entitled] *Tai Ping Yu Lan*（《太平御览》，*Imperial Studies in Taiping Times*），[it] grows in hills and valleys in Henei（河内）or Dushan（渎山）in Banyang（般阳）. [It begins] to

301

【今译】

味苦,性微寒。

主治瘀血惊恐,能治疗寒热病,能充实人体内脏,能补益肺气。长期服用有利于人体健康。又称为知母。该物生长在山川河谷之中。

blossom in March with green leaves. [Its] fruits are white like mustard. [Its] root is as large as turnip [and can be] collected in March.

[In the book entitled] *Ming Yi Bie Lu* (《名医别录》, *Special Record of Great Doctors*), [it] says [that Shashen (沙参, root of coastal glehnia, Radix Glehniae) is also] called Kuxin (苦心), Zhiqu (志取), Huxu (虎须), Baishen (白参), Shimei (识美) and Wenxi (文希), growing in Henei (河内), Yuanju (冤句) and Xushan (续山) in Banyang (般阳). [Its] root [can be] collected in February and August, and dried in the sun.

[In the book entitled] *Fan Zi Ji Ran* (《范子计然》, *Studies About Fan Li's Teacher*), [it] says [that] the white Shashen (沙参, root of coastal glehnia, Radix Glehniae) is produced in Luoyang (洛阳). The white [one is] better [in treating disease].

Notes

1. Shashen (沙参, root of coastal glehnia, Radix Glehniae) is a herbal medicinal, sweet and bitter in taste, slightly cold in property, entering the lung meridian and the stomach meridian, effective in nourishing Yang and clearing the lung, nourishing the stomach and producing fluid. Clinically it is used to treat fever due to Yin deficiency, cough due to heat in the lung, damage of fluid due to heat disease and thirst.

神农本草经

80. 白兔藿

【原文】

味苦,平。

主蛇虺,蜂虿,猘狗,菜肉蛊毒注。一名白葛。生山谷。

【考据】

1.《吴普》曰:白兔藿,一名白葛谷(《御览》)。

2.《名医》曰:生交州。

3. 案陶宏景云:都不闻有识之者,都富似葛耳;《唐本》注云:此草荆襄山谷大有,俗谓之白葛。

【今译】

味苦,性平。

主治因蛇、蜥蜴、蜜蜂、蝎子、疯狗咬伤所致之症,以及蔬菜、肉类、虫毒和怪异之邪所致之病。又称为白葛。该物生长在山谷之中。

80. Taituhuo（白兔藿，white oak，Oak Albo）[1]

［Original Text］

［Taituhuo（白兔藿，white oak，Oak Albo），］bitter in taste and mild ［in property］，［is mainly used］to treat ［injury caused by］bite of snake，lizard，bee，scorpion and insane dog ［as well as diseases caused by］vegetables，meat，worm toxin and tuberculosis. ［It is also］called Baige（白葛），growing in mountains and valleys.

［Textual Research］

［In the book entitled］*Wu Pu Ben Cao*（《吴普本草》，*Wu Pu's Studies of Materia Medica*），［it］says ［that］Taituhuo（白兔藿，white oak，Oak Albo）is also called Baigegu（白葛谷）［according to the book entitled］*Tai Ping Yu Lan*（《太平御览》，*Imperial Studies in Taiping Times*）.

［In the book entitled］*Ming Yi Bie Lu*（《名医别录》，*Special Record of Great Doctors*），［it］says ［that Taituhuo（白兔藿，white oak，Oak Albo）］grows in Jiaozhou（交州）.

Notes

1. Taituhuo（白兔藿，white oak，Oak Albo）is a herbal medicinal，bitter in taste，mild and non-toxic in proptery，effective in resolving toxin and eliminating blood stasis. Clinically it is used to treat diseases caused by various toxins and injury caused by bite of various animals and insects.

81. 徐长卿

【原文】

味辛,温。

主鬼物,百精,蛊毒,疫疾,邪恶气,温疟。久服,强悍轻身。一名鬼督邮。生山谷。

【考据】

1.《吴普》曰:徐长卿,一名石下长卿,神农雷公辛,或生陇西,三月采(《御览》)。

2.《名医》曰:生太山及陇西,三月采。

3. 案《广雅》云:徐长卿,鬼督邮也;陶宏景云:鬼督邮之名甚多,今俗用徐长卿者,其根正如细辛,小短扁扁尔,气亦相似。

【今译】

味辛,性温。

81. Xuchangqing（徐长卿，root of paniculate swallowwort，Radix Cynanchi Paniculati）[1]

[Original Text]

[Xuchangqing（徐长卿，root of paniculate swallowwort，Radix Cynanchi Paniculati），] pungent in taste and warm [in property]，[is mainly used] to resolve ghost-like evils，various unclear pathogenic factors，worm toxin，pestilence and severe evil-Qi [as well as treat] warm disease [caused by retention of summer-heat in the internal organs]. Long-term taking [of it will] strengthen the body and relax the body. [It is also] called Guiduyou（鬼督邮），growing in mountains and valleys.

[Textual Research]

[In the book entitled] *Wu Pu Ben Cao*（《吴普本草》，*Wu Pu's Studies of Materia Medica*），[it] says [that] Xuchangqing（徐长卿，root of paniculate swallowwort，Radix Cynanchi Paniculati）is also called Shixia Changqing（石下长卿）. [According to] Agriculture God（神农）and Leigong（雷公），[it is] pungent [in taste]，or growing in Longxi（陇西）. [It can be] collected in March [according to the book entitled] *Tai Ping Yu Lan*（《太平御览》，*Imperial Studies in Taiping Times*）.

[In the book entitled] *Ming Yi Bie Lu*（《名医别录》，*Special Record of Great Doctors*），[it] says [that Xuchangqing（徐长卿，root

　　主治各种鬼怪邪气所致之病，虫毒，传染病，温疟。长期服用，能使人强壮勇悍，身体轻盈。又称为鬼督邮。该物生长在山谷之中。

of paniculate swallowwort, Radix Cynanchi Paniculati)] grows in Taishan（太山）and Longxi（陇西）[and can be] collected in March.

Notes

1. Xuchangqing（徐长卿, root of paniculate swallowwort, Radix Cynanchi Paniculati）is a herbal medicinal, pungent in taste and warm in property, effective in expelling wind and ceasing pain, activating the blood and eliminating blood stasis. Clinically it is used to treat pain of joints due to wind-dampness, stomachache, intestinal inflammation, dysentery, edema, abdominal edema, traumatic injury, bite of snake and insects, eczema and urticaria.

82. 石龙刍

【原文】

味苦,微寒。

主心腹邪气,小便不利,淋闭,风湿,鬼注,恶毒。久服,补虚羸,轻身,耳目聪明,延年。一名龙须,一名草续断,一名龙珠。生山谷。

【考据】

1.《吴普》曰:龙刍,一名龙多,一名龙须,一名续断,一名龙本,一名草毒,一名龙华,一名悬莞,神农李氏小寒,雷公黄帝苦无毒,扁鹊辛无毒,生梁州,七月七日采(《御览》此条,误附续断)。

2.《名医》曰:一名龙华,一名悬莞,一名草毒,生梁州湿地,五月七月,采茎,暴干。

3. 案《广雅》云:龙木,龙须也;《中山经》云:贾超之山,其中多龙修;郭璞云:龙须也,似莞而细,生山石穴中,茎列垂,可以为席;别录云:一名方宾;郑樵云:《尔雅》所为蘼鼠莞也。

82. Shilongchu（石龙刍，common rush herb，Herba Junci）[1]

[Original Text]

[Shilongchu（石龙刍，common rush herb，Herba Junci），] bitter in taste and slightly cold [in property]，[is mainly used] to treat [disease caused by] evil-Qi in the heart and abdomen，dysuria，stranguria，wind-dampness [disease]，tuberculosis and infectious disease. Long-term taking [of it will] tonify deficiency and emaciation，relax the body，improve hearing and vision，and prolong life. [It is also] called Longxu（龙须），Caoxuduan（草续断）and Longzhu（龙珠），growing in mountains and valleys.

[Textual Research]

[In the book entitled] *Wu Pu Ben Cao*（《吴普本草》，*Wu Pu's Studies of Materia Medica*），[it] says [that] Shilongchu（石龙刍，common rush herb，Herba Junci）[is also] called Longduo（龙多），Longxu（龙须），Xuduan（续断），Longben（龙本），Ducao（草毒），Longhua（龙华）and Xuanguan（悬莞）. [According to] Agriculture God（神农）and Li's（李氏），[it is] slightly cold [in property]；[according to] Leigong（雷公）and Yellow Emperor（黄帝），[it is] bitter [in taste] and non-toxic [in property]；[according to] Bianque（扁鹊），[it is] pungent [in taste] and non-toxic [in property]. [It] grows in Liangzhou（梁州）and [can be] collected

【今译】

味苦,性微寒。

主治心腹中的邪气,小便不利,癃闭,风湿病,鬼怪恶邪所致之症,恶性传染病。长期服用,能补益虚弱消瘦,能使身体轻盈,听力增强,视力清明,能延年益寿。又称为龙须,又称为草续断,又称为龙珠。该物生长在山谷之中。

神农本草经

on July 7〔according to the book entitled〕*Tai Ping Yu Lan*（《太平御览》, *Imperial Studies in Taiping Times*）.

〔In the book entitled〕*Ming Yi Bie Lu*（《名医别录》, *Special Record of Great Doctors*）,〔it〕says〔that Shilongchu（石龙刍, common rush herb, Herba Junci）is also〕called Longhua（龙华）, Xuanguan（悬莞）and Caodu（草毒）, growing in the wet land in Liangzhou（梁州）.〔Its〕stalks〔can be〕collected in May and July and dried in the sun.

83. 薇衔

【原文】

味苦,平。

主风湿痹,历节痛,惊痫,吐舌,悸气,贼风,鼠瘘,痈肿。一名糜衔。生川泽。

【考据】

1.《吴普》曰:薇蘅,一名糜蘅,一名无颠,一名承膏,一名丑,一名无心(《御览》)。

2.《名医》曰:一名承膏,一名承肌,一名无心,一名无颠,生汉中及冤句邯郸,七月采茎。叶,阴干。

【今译】

味苦,性平。

83. Weixian（薇衔，wintergreen，Pyrola Rotundifolia）[1]

［Weixian 薇衔，wintergreen，Pyrola Rotundifolia），］bitter in taste and mild ［in property］，［is mainly used］ to treat wind-dampness impediment，arthralgia，frightened epilepsy，protrusion of tongue，palpitation，［disease caused by］ thief-wind，scrofula，carbuncle and swelling. ［It is also］ called Mixian（糜衔），growing in valleys and swamps.

［**Textual Research**］

［In the book entitled］ *Wu Pu Ben Cao*（《吴普本草》，*Wu Pu's Studies of Materia Medica*），［it］ says ［that］ Weixian（薇蓿，wintergreen，Pyrola Rotundifolia）［is also］ called Mixian（糜蓿），Wudian（无颠），Chenggao（承膏），Chou（丑）and Wuxin（无心）［according to the book entitled］ *Tai Ping Yu Lan*（《太平御览》，*Imperial Studies in Taiping Times*）.

［In the book entitled］ *Ming Yi Bie Lu*（《名医别录》，*Special Record of Great Doctors*），［it］ says ［that Weixian 薇衔，wintergreen，Pyrola Rotundifolia) is also］ called Chenggao（承膏），Chengji（承肌），Wuxin（无心）and Wudian（无颠），growing in Hanzhong（汉中）and Yuanju（冤句）in Handan（邯郸）. ［Its］ stalks and leaves ［can be］ collected in July and dried in the shade.

315

主治风湿痹证，关节疼痛，惊恐心悸，癫痫，吐舌，心悸心慌，贼风，瘰疬症，痈肿。又称为糜衔。该物生长在山川和平泽之中。

Notes

1. Weixian（薇衔，wintergreen，Pyrola Rotundifolia）is a herbal medicinal, bitter in taste, mild and non-toxic in property, entering the liver meridian and the kidney meridian, effective in improving deficiency, replenishing the kidney, expelling wind and eliminating dampness, activating the blood and regulating the meridians. Clinically it is used to treat wind-dampness impediment and pain, arthralgia, frightened epilepsy, scrofula, stranguria, hematuria, hematemesis, nosebleed, profuse menstruation, leucorrhea and bleeding due to injury.

Agriculture
God's Canon of
Materia Medica

84. 云实

【原文】

味辛,温。

主泄利(旧作痢,《御览》作泄利),肠澼,杀虫,蛊毒,去邪毒,结气,止痛,除热。花,主见鬼精物,多食令人狂走。久服,轻身通神明。生川谷。

【考据】

1.《吴普》曰:云实,一名员实,一名天豆,神农辛小温,黄帝咸,雷公苦,叶如麻,两两相值,高四五尺,大茎空中,六月花,八月九月实,十月采(《御览》)。

2.《名医》曰:一名员实,一名云英,一名天豆,生河间,十月采,暴干。案《广雅》云:天豆,云实也。

【今译】

味辛,性温。

主治泄泻和痢疾,能杀除虫子,能治疗虫毒所致之病,能祛除邪毒,

84. Yunshi（云实，mysorethorn seed，Semen Caesalpiniae Sepiariae）[1]

[Original Text]

[Yunshi（云实，mysorethorn seed，Semen Caesalpiniae Sepiariae），] pungent in taste and warm [in property]，[is mainly used] to treat diarrhea and bloody stool，to kill worms to remove worm toxin，to expel evil-toxin and Qi stagnation，and to resolve heat．[Its] flowers can treat strange vision with ghost-like phenomena. Excessive taking [of it will] make people run wildly. Long-term taking [of it will] relax the body and invigorate spirit and mentality．[It] grows in mountain valleys and river valleys.

[Textual Research]

[In the book entitled] *Wu Pu Ben Cao*（《吴普本草》，*Wu Pu's Studies of Materia Medica*），[it] says [that] Yunshi（云实，mysorethorn seed，Semen Caesalpiniae Sepiariae）[is also] called Yuanshi（员实）and Tiandou（天豆）．[According to] Agriculture God（神农），[it is] pungent [in taste] and slightly warm [in property]；[according to] Yellow Emperor（黄帝），[it is] salty [in taste]；[according to] Leigong（雷公），[it is] bitter [in taste]．[Its] leaves look like hemp，about 4 to 5 *Chi*（尺）each．[Its] large stalks are hollow and begin to blossom in June and bear fruits in August and September [which can be] collected in October

能消解气结，能消除疼痛，能治疗热邪所致之病。

　　其花能主治鬼怪邪气所致之症，用量过大则使人狂奔乱跑。长期服用，能使人身体轻盈，神志清晰，精神旺盛。该物生长在山川河谷之中。

[according to the book entitled] *Tai Ping Yu Lan* (《太平御览》, *Imperial Studies in Taiping Times*).

[In the book entitled] *Ming Yi Bie Lu* (《名医别录》, *Special Record of Great Doctors*), [it] says [that Yunshi (云实，mysorethorn seed，Semen Caesalpiniae Sepiariae) is also] called Yuanshi (员实), Yunying (云英) and Tiandou (天豆), growing in Hejian (河间). [It can be] collected in October and dried in the sun.

Notes

1. Yunshi （云实，mysorethorn seed，Semen Caesalpiniae Sepiariae) is a herbal medicinal，pungent in taste，warm and non-toxic in property，effective in killing worms，removing toxin，eliminating dampness，ceasing cough and resolving phlegm. Clinically it is used to treat dysentery，malaria，chronic tracheitis and infantile malnutrition.

85. 王不留行

【原文】

味苦,平。

主金疮,止血,逐痛,出刺,除风痹,内寒。久服,轻身耐老(《御览》作能老),增寿。生山谷。

【考据】

1.《吴普》曰:王不留行,一名王不流行,神农苦平,岐伯雷公甘,三月八月采(《御览》)。

2. 案郑樵云:王不留行,曰禁宫花,曰剪金花,叶似花,实作房。

【今译】

味苦,性平。

85. Wangbu Liuxing（王不留行，cowherb seed，Semen Vaccariae）[1]

[Original Text]

［Wangbu Liuxing（王不留行，cowherb seed，Semen Vaccariae），］bitter in taste and mild［in property］，［is mainly used］to treat sores［caused by］metal［injury］，to cease pain，to withdraw needle，to eliminate wind impediment and to treat internal cold［syndrome/pattern］. Long-term taking［of it will］relax the body，prevent aging and prolong life.［It］grows in mountains and valleys.

[Textual Research]

［In the book entitled］*Wu Pu Ben Cao*（《吴普本草》，*Wu Pu's Studies of Materia Medica*），［it］says［that］Wangbu Liuxing（王不留行，cowherb seed，Semen Vaccariae）［is also］called Wangbu Liuxing（王不流行）.［According to］Agriculture God（神农），［it is］bitter［in taste］and mild［in property］；［according to］Qibo（岐伯）and Leigong（雷公），［it is］sweet［in taste］.［It can be］collected in March and August［according to the book entitled］*Tai Ping Yu Lan*（《太平御览》，*Imperial Studies in Taiping Times*）.

Zheng Jiao said，"Wangbu Liuxing（王不留行，cowherb seed，Semen Vaccariae）［is also］called Jingonghua（禁宫花）and Jianjinhua（剪金花）.［Its］leaves look like flowers and［its］fruits

主治金属创伤，能阻止出血，能解除疼痛，能拔出刺入人体之刺，能消除风痹证，能治疗内寒症。长期服用，能使人身体轻盈，不易衰老，能增加寿命。该物生长在山谷之中。

appear like houses.

Notes

1. Wangbu Liuxing （王 不 留 行, cowherb seed, Semen Vaccariae) is a herbal medicinal, bitter in taste and mild in property, entering the liver meridian and the stomach meridian, effective in promoting blood circulation and unobstructing the meridians, promoting lactation and resolving swelling. Clinically it is used to treat amenorrhea, dysmenorrhea, acute mastitis and orchitis.

86. 升麻

【原文】

味甘,辛(《大观本》作甘平)。

主解百毒,杀百老物殃鬼,辟温疾,障,邪毒蛊。久服不夭(《大观本》作主解百毒,杀百精老物殃鬼,辟瘟疫瘴气邪气虫毒,此用《御览》文)。一名周升麻(《大观本》,作周麻)。生山谷(旧作黑字,据《吴普》有云,神农甘,则本经当有此,今增入)。

【考据】

1.《吴普》曰:升麻,神农甘(《御览》)。

2.《名医》曰:生益州,二月八月采根,日干。

3. 案《广雅》云:周麻,升麻也(此据《御览》)。

【今译】

味甘,性辛。

86. Shengma（升麻，cimicifuga，Rhizoma Cimicifuga）[1]

［Original Text］

［Shengma（升麻，cimicifuga，Rhizoma Cimicifuga），］sweet and pungent in taste，［is mainly used］to remove various toxin，to kill various ghost-like evils ［that cause various diseases］，to prevent warm disease and stagnation，［and to eliminate］evil worm toxin. Long-term taking ［of it will］prolong life. ［It］grows in mountains and valleys.

［Textual Research］

［In the book entitled］*Wu Pu Ben Cao*（《吴普本草》，*Wu Pu's Studies of Materia Medica*），［it］says ［that］Shengma（升麻，cimicifuga，Rhizoma Cimicifuga），［according to］Agriculture God（神农），is sweet ［in taste，which is also mentioned in the book entitled］*Tai Ping Yu Lan*（《太平御览》，*Imperial Studies in Taiping Times*）.

［In the book entitled］*Ming Yi Bie Lu*（《名医别录》，*Special Record of Great Doctors*），［it］says ［that Shengma（升麻，cimicifuga，Rhizoma Cimicifuga）］grows in Yizhou（益州）. ［Its］root ［can be］collected in February and August，and dried in the sun.

［In the book entitled］*Guang Ya*（《广雅》，*The First Chinese*

能消解各种毒气，能杀除各种沉痼鬼怪邪气，能祛除暑热所致之疾患，能消除郁阻之气，能剔除邪气和虫毒。长期服用不会早逝。又称为周升麻。该物生长在山谷之中。

Encyclopedic Dictionary），［it］says［that the so-called］Zhouma（周麻）refers to Shengma（升麻，cimicifuga，Rhizoma Cimicifuga）［according to the book entitled］*Tai Ping Yu Lan*（《太平御览》，*Imperial Studies in Taiping Times*）.

Notes

1. Shengma（升麻，cimicifuga，Rhizoma Cimicifuga）is a herbal medicinal, pungent and sweet in taste, slightly cold in property, entering the lung meridian, the spleen meridian, the large intestine meridian and the stomach meridian, effective in clearing heat and removing toxin, raising Yang and protruding subsidence. Clinically it is used to treat plague, headache due to cold-heat, sore-throat, oral ulcer, macula, descent of middle Qi, chronic diarrhea and dysentery, prolapse of rectum, leucorrhea, prolapse of uterus, carbuncle, swelling, sore and poisoning.

87．青蘘

【原文】

味甘,寒。

主五脏邪气,风寒湿痹,益气,补脑髓,坚筋骨。久服耳目聪明,不饥不老,增寿,巨胜苗也。生川谷(旧在米谷部,非)。

【考据】

1.《吴普》曰:青蘘,一名梦神,神农苦,雷公甘(《御览》)。

2.《名医》曰:生中原。

3. 案《抱朴子·仙药》云:孝经援神契曰,巨胜延年,又云巨胜,一名胡麻,饵服之不老,耐风湿,补衰老也。

【今译】

味甘,性寒。

主治五脏中的邪气,风寒湿邪所致之痹证,能滋补精气,能补

87. Qingxiang（青蘘，flower of Qingxiang，Flos Qingxiang）[1]

[Original Text]

[Qingxiang（青蘘，flower of Qingxiang，Flos Qingxiang），] sweet in taste and cold [in property]，[is mainly used] to treat [diseases caused by invasion of] evil-Qi into the five Zang-organs and wind-cold and dampness impediment，to replenish Qi，to tonify the brains and to strengthen the sinews and bones. Long-term taking [of it will] improve hearing and vision，[make people feel] no hunger，prevent aging and prolong life. [It is also] called Jushengmiao（巨胜苗），growing in mountain valleys.

[Textual Research]

[in the book entitled] *Wu Pu Ben Cao*（《吴普本草》，*Wu Pu's Studies of Materia Medica*），[it] says [that] Qingxiang（青蘘，flower of Qingxiang，Flos Qingxiang）[is also] called Mengshen（梦神）. [According to] Agriculture God（神农），[it is] bitter [in taste]；[according to] Leigong（雷公），[it is] sweet [in taste which is also mentioned in the book entitled] *Tai Ping Yu Lan*（《太平御览》，*Imperial Studies in Taiping Times*）.

[In the book entitled] *Ming Yi Bie Lu*（《名医别录》，*Special Record of Great Doctors*），[it] says [that Qingxiang（青蘘，flower of Qingxiang，Flos Qingxiang）] grows in Zhongyuan（中原）.

益脑髓，能使筋骨强壮。长期服用能使人听力增强，视力清明，能减少饥饿之感，能增加寿命，长生不老。该物生长在山川河谷之中。

［In the book entitled］ *Bao Pu Zi* (《抱朴子》, *Primitive and Natural View*) about magic medicinals (仙药)，［it］ says［that Qingxiang (青蘘，flower of Qingxiang，Flos Qingxiang) is also］ called Huma (胡麻). Taking it can prevent aging，tolerate wind-dampness and improve senility.

Notes

1. Qingxiang (青蘘，flower of Qingxiang，Flos Qingxiang) is a grain medicinal，sweet in taste，cold and non-toxic in property，effective in replenishing Qi，resolving pathogenic factors，expelling wind，lustering the facial expression and moistening hair and skin. Clinically it is used to treat disease caused by summer-heat，impediment caused by wind-cold，and blood stagnation during flooding and spotting (metrostaxis and metrorrhagia).

88. 姑活

【原文】

味甘,温。

主大风邪气,湿痹寒痛。久服轻身益寿耐老。一名冬葵子(旧在《唐本草》中无毒,今增)。

【考据】

1.《名医》曰:生河东。

2. 案水经注解县,引《神农本草》云:地有固活,女疏,铜芸,紫苑之族也;陶宏景云:方药亦无用此者,乃有固活丸,即是野葛,一名,此又名冬葵子,非葵菜之冬葵子,疗体乖异。

【今译】

味甘,性温。

主治大风邪气所致之症,湿邪所致之痹证及寒痛。长期服用能使人身体轻盈,增加寿命,不易衰老。又称为冬葵子。

88. Guohuo（姑活，Guohuo seed，Semen Guhuo）[1]

[Original Text]

[Guohuo（姑活，Guohuo seed，Semen Guhuo），] sweet in taste [and] warm [in property]，[is mainly used] to treat dampness impediment and cold pain [caused by] severe wind and evil-Qi. [It is also] called Dongkuizi（冬葵子）.

[Textual Research]

[In the book entitled] *Ming Yi Bie Lu*（《名医别录》，*Special Record of Great Doctors*），[it] says [that Guohuo（姑活，Guohuo seed，Semen Guhuo）] grows in Hedong（河东）

Tao Hongjing（陶宏景）said，"The formulae without this herb still contain the pill for invigorating life，i. e. Yege（野葛），also called Dongkuizi（冬葵子），[which is] not Dongkuizi（冬葵子）in Kuicai（葵菜，malva vegetable，Malva Verticillata），the therapeutic effect of which is unique."

Notes

1. Guohuo（姑活，Guohuo seed，Semen Guhuo）was used in ancient times. Now it is difficult to make sure what herb it is. In ancient times，it was also called Yege（野葛）and Dongkuizi（冬葵子）. But now Yege（野葛，kudzu，Pueraria Lobata）and Dongkuizi（冬葵子，seed of cluster mallow，Semen Malvae）are two quite different herbal medicinals.

89. 别羁

【原文】

味苦,微温。

主风寒湿痹,身重,四肢疼酸,寒邪,历节痛。生川谷(旧在《唐本草》中无毒,今增)。

【考据】

1.《名医》曰:一名别枝,一名别骑,一名鳖羁,生蓝田,二月八月采;案陶宏景云:方家时有用处,今俗亦绝耳。

【今译】

味苦,性微温。

主治风寒湿邪所致之痹证,身体沉重,四肢疼酸寒冷,关节疼痛。该物生长在山川河谷之中。

89.　Bieji（别羁，Bieji medicinal，Materia Medica Bieji）[1]

[Original Text]

[Bieji（别羁，Bieji medicinal，Materia Medica Bieji），] bitter in taste and slightly warm [in property]，[is mainly used] to treat wind-cold and dampness impediment，heaviness of the body，ache and coldness of the four limbs，[disease caused by] cold evil and pain of joints. [It] grows in mountain valleys and river valleys.

[Textual Research]

[In the book entitled] *Ming Yi Bie Lu*（《名医别录》，*Special Record of Great Doctors*），[it] says [that Bieji（别羁，Bieji medicinal，Materia Medica Bieji）is also] called Biezhi（别枝），Bieqi（别骑）and Bieji（鳖羁），growing in Lantian（蓝田）. [It can be] collected in February and August. Tao Hongjing（陶宏景）said，"Doctors use it at times. Now it is also called Jue'er（绝耳）."

Notes

1. Bieji（别羁，Bieji medicinal，Materia Medica Bieji）was a commonly used herbal medicinal in ancient China. But now it is very difficult to make clear what it is. We can only find information about its taste，property，action and application as well as its growth，collection and processing in books written in ancient times.

90. 屈草

【原文】

味苦。

主胸胁下痛,邪气,腹间寒热阴痹。久服,轻身益气,耐老(《御览》作补益能老)。生川泽(旧在《唐本草》中无毒,今增)。

【考据】

1.《名医》曰:生汉中,五月采。

2. 案陶宏景云:方药不复用,俗无识者。

【今译】

味苦,性微寒。

主治胸胁下疼痛,邪气所致之症,腹间寒热性疾病以及阴痹证。长期服用,能使人身体轻盈,能补益精气,不易衰老。该物生长在山川和河谷之中。

90. Qucao (屈草，Qucao medicinal，
Materia Medica Qucao) [1]

[Original Text]

[Qucao（屈草，Qucao medicinal，Materia Medica Qucao），] bitter in taste，[is mainly used] to relieve pain below the chest and rib-side，[to expel] evil-Qi，to resolve cold-heat in the abdomen and to treat Yin impediment. Long-taking [of it will] relax the body，replenish Qi and prevent aging.[It] grows in valleys and swamps.

[Textual Research]

[In the book entitled] *Ming Yi Bie Lu*（《名医别录》，*Special Record of Great Doctors*），[it] says [that Qucao（屈草，Qucao medicinal，Materia Medica Qucao)] grows in Hanzhong（汉中）and [can be] collected in May.

Notes

1. The problem of Qucao（屈草，Qucao medicinal，Materia Medica Qucao）is the same as Bieji（别羁，Bieji medicinal，Materia Medica Bieji）. It was a very important herbal medicinal in ancient China. But now it is very difficult to know which herb it refers to.

91. 淮木

【原文】

味苦,平。

主久咳上气,肠中虚羸,女子阴蚀,漏下赤白沃。一名百岁城中木。生山谷(旧在《唐本草》中无毒,今增)。

【考据】

1.《吴普》曰:淮木,神农雷公无毒,生晋平阳河东平泽,治久咳上气,伤中羸虚,补中益气(《御览》)。

2.《名医》曰:一名炭木,生太山,采无时。

3. 案李当之云:是樟树上寄生树,大衔枝在肌肉,今人皆以胡桃皮当之,非也;桐君云:生上洛,是木皮状如厚朴,色似桂白,其理一纵一横,今市人皆削乃以厚朴,而无正纵横理,不知此复是何物,莫测真假,何者为是也。

4. 上草,上品七十三种,旧七十二种,考六芝当为一,升麻当白字,米谷部误入青蘘,《唐本草》六种,姑活,屈草,淮木,皆当入此。

91. Huaimu（淮木，Huaimu medicinal，Materia Medica Huaimu）[1]

[Original Text]

[Huaimu（淮木，Huaimu medicinal，Materia Medica Huaimu），] bitter in taste and mild [in property], [is mainly used] to treat chronic cough with upward counterflow of Qi[2], deficiency and weakness of the intestines, vulvar ulceration and vaginal discharge of red and white liquid. [It is also] called wood in an old city, growing in mountains and valleys.

[Textual Research]

[In the book entitled] *Wu Pu Ben Cao* (《吴普本草》, *Wu Pu's Studies of Materia Medica*), [it] says [that] Huaimu（淮木，Huaimu medicinal，Materia Medica Huaimu），[according to] Agriculture God（神农）and Leigong（雷公），[is] non-toxic [in property], growing in rivers and lakes in Jinping（晋平）. [It can be used] to treat chronic cough with upward counterflow of Qi and damage of the middle（the internal organs）[due to] weakness and deficiency [as well as] tonify the middle（the internal organs）and replenish Qi [according to the book entitled] *Tai Ping Yu Lan* (《太平御览》, *Imperial Studies in Taiping Times*).

[In the book entitled] *Ming Yi Bie Lu* (《名医别录》, *Special Record of Great Doctors*), [it] says [that Huaimu（淮木，Huaimu

【今译】

味苦,性平。

主治长期咳嗽,呼吸困难,肠中损伤,虚弱消瘦,女子阴部溃疡,阴道淋漓不断,赤白带下。又称为百岁城中木。该物生长在山谷之中。

medicinal，Materia Medica Huaimu) is also] called Tanmu (炭木)，growing in Taishan (太山) and [can be] collected at any time.

Notes

1. The problem of Huaimu (淮木，Huaimu medicinal，Materia Medica Huaimu) is the same as Qucao (屈草，Qucao medicinal，Materia Medica Qucao) and Bieji (别羁，Bieji medicinal，Materia Medica Bieji). Although it was a very important herbal medicinal in ancient China，now it is very difficult to know which herb it refers to.

2. Counterflow of Qi means difficulty in breath.

92. 牡桂

【原文】

味辛,温。

主上气咳逆,结气喉痹,吐吸,利关节,补中益气。久服通神,轻身不老。生山谷。

【考据】

1.《名医》曰:生南海。

2. 案《说文》云:桂,江南木,百药之长,梫桂也;南山经云:招摇之山多桂;郭璞云:桂,叶似枇杷,长二尺余,广数寸,味辛,白花,丛生山峰,冬夏常青,间无杂木;《尔雅》云:梫,木桂;郭璞云:今人呼桂皮厚者,为木桂,及单名桂者,是也,一名肉桂,一名桂枝,一名桂心。

【今译】

味辛,性温。

92. Mugui（牡桂，Cinnamon bark，Cortex Cinnamomum Cassia）[1]

[Original Text]

[Mugui（牡桂，Cinnamon bark，Cortex Cinnamomum Cassia），] pungent in taste and warm [in property], [is mainly used] to treat cough with dyspnea [due to] counterflow of Qi, stagnation of Qi, throat impediment and breath with the mouth [due to severe impediment of the throat], to disinhibit the joints, to tonify the middle (the internal organs) and to replenish Qi. Long-term taking [of it will] invigorate the spirit and mind, relax the body and prevent aging. [It] grows in mountains and valleys.

[Textual Research]

[In the book entitled] *Ming Yi Bie Lu* (《名医别录》, *Special Record of Great Doctors*), [it] says [that Mugui（牡桂，Cinnamon bark，Cortex Cinnamomum Cassia）] grows in Nanhai （南海, Southern Sea）. [In] case [analysis in the book entitled] *Shuo Wen* (《说文》, *On Culture*), [it] says [that] Mugui（牡桂，Cinnamon bark，Cortex Cinnamomum Cassia）[is a sort of] wood in Jiangnan （江南）, the most important one among all the medicinals. Guo Pu （郭璞）said, "The leaves of Mugui（牡桂，Cinnamon bark，Cortex Cinnamomum Cassia）look like loquat, about 2 Chi（尺）in length, with pungent taste and white flowers, growing in the peaks of

主治咳嗽气逆于上，气结，喉痹之症，因呼吸困难而用口呼气，能使关节通畅，能充实人体内脏，能补益精气。长期服用能使神气通畅，身体轻盈，长寿不老。该物生长在山谷之中。

mountains, appearing green in winter and summer without any weedtree around. "

Notes

1. Mugui (牡桂,Cinnamon bark, Cortex Cinnamomum Cassia) is a herbal medicinal, pungent and sweet in taste, severe heat in property, entering the kidney meridian, the spleen meridian and the liver meridian, effective in tonifying kidney-Yang, warming the spleen and stomach, eliminating accumulation of cold, unobstructing the vessels and ceasing pain. Clinically it is used to treat impotence, frequent urination, cold pain in the waist and spine, hypotension, insufficiency of spleen-Yang, cold pain in the chest and abdomen, poor appetite and loose stool.

347

93. 菌桂

【原文】

味辛,温。

主百病,养精神,和颜色,为诸药先聘通使。久服轻身不老,面生光华,媚好常如童子。生山谷。

【考据】

1.《名医》曰:生交址桂林岩崖间,无骨,正圆如竹,立秋采。

2. 案《楚词》云:杂申椒与菌桂兮;王逸云:菜桂皆香木;《列仙传》云:范蠡好服桂。

【今译】

味辛,性温。

主治各种疾病,能滋养精神,能使面部色泽调和,可引导各种药物发挥作用。长期服用能使人身体轻盈,能长寿不老,能使面部光彩,能使形象美好如儿童。该物生长在山谷之中。

93. Jungui（菌桂，sweet osmanthus，Guepinia spathularia）[1]

[Original Text]

[Jungui（菌桂，sweet osmanthus，Guepinia spathularia），] pungent in taste and warm [in property], [is mainly used] to treat various diseases, to nourish essence and spirit, to luster facial expression and to guide all medicinals. Long-term taking [of it will] relax the body, prevent aging, luster the face and make [those who take it] as beautiful as children. [It] grows in mountains and valleys.

[Textual Research]

[In the book entitled] *Ming Yi Bie Lu*（《名医别录》，*Special Record of Great Doctors*），[it] says [that Jungui（菌桂，sweet osmanthus，Guepinia spathularia）] grows in the cliffs in Jiaozhi（交址）and Guilin（桂林）without any sticks [in it]. [It is] as round as bamboo and [can be] collected in autumn.

Notes

1. Jungui（菌桂，sweet osmanthus，Guepinia spathularia）is herbal medicinal, pungent in taste, warm and non-toxic in property, effective in nourishing essence and spirit, harmonizing the viscera, regulating vessels and meridians. Clinically it is used to treat various diseases and disorders.

94. 松脂

【原文】

味苦,温。

主疽,恶疮,头疡,白秃,疥搔,风气,安五脏,除热。久服,轻身不老,延年。一名松膏,一名松肪。生山谷。

【考据】

1.《名医》曰:生太山,六月采。

2. 案《说文》云:松木也,或作案;《范子计然》云:松脂出陇西,松胶者善。

【今译】

味苦,性温。

主治痈疽,恶性痈疮,头部溃疡,白秃,能消解风气所致之疥疮瘙

94. Songzhi（松脂，pine oleoresin，Colophonium）^[1]

〔Original Text〕

〔Songzhi（松脂，colophony，Colophonium），〕bitter in taste and warm〔in property〕,〔is mainly used〕to treat gangrene, severe sore, head ulcer, white head tinea and scabies and itching,〔to expel〕wind-Qi[2],〔to harmonize〕the five Zang-organs and to eliminate heat. Long-term taking〔of it will〕relax the body, prevent aging and prolong life.〔It is also〕called Songgao（松膏）and Songfang（松肪）, growing in mountains and valleys.

〔Textual Research〕

〔In the book entitled〕*Ming Yi Bie Lu*（《名医别录》,*Special Record of Great Doctors*）,〔it〕says〔that Songzhi（松脂，colophony, Colophonium）〕grows in Taishan（太山）and〔can be〕collected in June.

〔In the book entitled〕*Fan Zi Ji Ran*（《范子计然》,*Studies About Fan Li's Teacher*）,〔it〕says〔that〕Songzhi（松脂，colophony, Colophonium）is produced in Longxi（陇西）and larch gum is better〔than it〕.

Notes

1. Songzhi（松脂，colophony，Colophonium）is the medicinal of rosin, now known as Songxiang（松香）, bitter and sweet in taste,

痒,能安静五脏,能消除热邪所致之病。长期服用,能使人身体轻盈,长寿不老,延年益寿。又称为松膏,又称为松肪。该物生长在山谷之中。

warm in property, entering the spleen meridian and the liver meridian, effective in drying dampness and killing worms, promoting muscles and relieving pain. Clinically it is used to treat carbuncle, ulcer, furuncle, boil, scabies, itching, bleeding and scald.

    2. Wind-Qi refers to pathogenic wind.

神农本草经

95. 槐实

【原文】

味苦,寒。

主五内邪气热,止涎唾,补绝伤,五痔,火疮,妇人乳瘕,子脏急痛。生平泽。

【考据】

1.《名医》曰:生河南。

2. 案《说文》云:槐木也;《尔雅》云:櫰,槐大叶而黑。郭璞云:槐树叶大色黑者,名为櫰,又守宫槐叶,昼聂宵炕;郭璞云:槐叶昼日聂合,而夜炕布者,名为守宫槐。

【今译】

味苦,性寒。

95. Huaishi（槐实，fruit of pagodatree，Fructus Sophorae）[1]

[Original Text]

[Huaishi（槐实，fruit of pagodatree，Fructus Sophorae），] bitter in taste and cold [in property]，[is mainly used] to remove evil-Qi heat in the five Zang-organs，to cease saliva and spittle，to treat severe injury，five [kinds of] hemorrhoids，scalded sore，breast lump in woman and urgent uterine pain. [It] grows in plains and swamps.

[Textual Research]

[In the book entitled] *Ming Yi Bie Lu*（《名医别录》，*Special Record of Great Doctors*），[it] says [that Huaishi（槐实，fruit of pagodatree，Fructus Sophorae）] grows in Henan（河南）.

[In] case [analysis in the book entitled] *Shuo Wen*（《说文》，*On Culture*），[it] says [that Huaishi（槐实，fruit of pagodatree，Fructus Sophorae) is also] called Huaimu（槐木）.

Notes

1. Huaishi（槐实，fruit of pagodatree，Fructus Sophorae）is a herbal medicinal，also known as Huaijiao（槐角），bitter in taste and cold in property，entering the liver meridian and the large intestine meridian，effective in clearing heat，enriching the liver，cooling the

　　主治五脏内邪热之气,能停止涎唾,能治疗极度损伤,五种痔疮,因火烧所致疮疡,妇女腹部瘕聚,子宫拘急疼痛。该物生长在平川水泽之中。

blood and ceasing bleeding. Clinically it is used to treat enterorrhagia due to intestinal wind，bleeding due to hemorrhoids，flooding and spotting（metrostaxis and metrorrhagia），vexation，vertigo and hypertension.

96. 枸杞

【原文】

味苦,寒。

主五内邪气,热中,消渴,周痹。久服,坚筋骨,轻身不老(《御览》作耐老)。一名杞根,一名地骨,一名枸忌,一名地辅。生平泽。

【考据】

1.《吴普》曰:枸杞,一名枸已,一名羊乳。(《御览》)

2.《名医》曰:一名羊乳,一名却暑,一名仙人杖,一名西王母杖,生常山,及诸邱陵阪岸,冬采根,春夏采叶,秋采茎实,阴干。

3. 案《说文》云:继,枸杞也。杞,枸杞也;《广雅》云:地筋,枸杞也;《尔雅》云:杞,枸;郭璞云:今枸杞也;《毛诗》云:集子苞杞;《传》云:杞,枸也;陆玑云:苦杞秋熟,正赤,服之轻身益气;《列仙传》云:陆通食橐卢木实;《抱朴子·仙药》云:象柴,一名托卢,是也。或名仙人杖,或云西王母杖,或名天门精,或名却老,或名地骨,或名枸杞也。

96. Gouqi（枸杞, fruit of barbary wolfberry, Fructus Lycii）[1]

[Original Text]

[Gouqi（枸杞, fruit of barbary wolfberry, Fructus Lycii）,] bitter in taste and cold [in property], [is mainly used] to expel evil-Qi in the five Zang-organs, middle heat[2], wasting-thirst and generalized impediment. Long-term taking [of it will] strengthen the sinews and bones, relax the body and prevent aging. [It is also] called Qigen（杞根）, Digu（地骨）, Gouji（枸忌）and Dipu（地辅）, growing in plains and swamps.

[Textual Research]

[In the book entitled] *Wu Pu Ben Cao*（《吴普本草》, *Wu Pu's Studies of Materia Medica*）, [it] says [that] Gouqi（枸杞, fruit of barbary wolfberry, Fructus Lycii）[is also] called Gouji（枸已）and Yangru（羊乳）[according to the book entitled] *Tai Ping Yu Lan* (《太平御览》, *Imperial Studies in Taiping Times*).

[In the book entitled] *Ming Yi Bie Lu*（《名医别录》, *Special Record of Great Doctors*）, [it] says [that Gouqi（枸杞, fruit of barbary wolfberry, Fructus Lycii) is also] called Yangru（羊乳）, Queshu（却暑）, Xianrenzhang（仙人杖）and Xiwang Muzhang（西王母杖）, growing in Changshan（常山）, hills and scarps. [Its] root [can be] collected in winter, [its] leaves [can be] collected in

【今译】

味苦,性寒。

主治五脏邪气,能消除内脏中的热邪,能治疗消渴及全身流窜形疼痛。长期服用,能使筋骨强壮,人身体轻盈,长寿不老。又称为杞根,又称为地骨,又称为枸忌,又称为地辅。该物生长在平川水泽之中。

spring and summer, and [its] stalks and fruits [can be] collected in autumn, [which can be] dried in the shade.

[In] case [analysis in the book entitled] *Shuo Wen* (《说文》, *On Culture*), [it] says [that the so-called] Ji (继) refers to Gouqi (枸杞, fruit of barbary wolfberry, Fructus Lycii), [and the so-called] Qi (杞) also refers to Gouqi (枸杞, fruit of barbary wolfberry, Fructus Lycii). [In the book entitled] *Guang Ya* (《广雅》, *The First Chinese Encyclopedic Dictionary*), [it] says [that the so-called] Dijin (地筋) refers to Gouqi (枸杞, fruit of barbary wolfberry, Fructus Lycii).

Lu Ji (陆玑) said, "Gouqi (枸杞, fruit of barbary wolfberry, Fructus Lycii) is ripe in autumn with red color. Taking it will relax the body and replenish Qi.

Notes

1. Gouqi (枸杞, fruit of barbary wolfberry, Fructus Lycii), now known as Gouqi (枸杞子), is a herbal medicinal, sweet in taste and mild in property, entering the liver meridian and the kidney meridian, effective in tonifying the kidney and replenishing essence, nourishing the liver and improving vision. Clinically it is used to treat liver and kidney Yin deficiency, weakness of the waist and knees, seminal emission, spontaneous spermatorrhea, premature ejaculation, vertigo, hypopsia and jaundice.

2. Middle heat may refer to wasting syndrome/pattern marked by hyperphagia with frequent hunger and frequent urination, or yellowing of the eyes, or disease caused by food, overexertion, damage of the spleen and stomach as well as Yin deficiency and effulgent fire.

神农本草经

97. 柏实

【原文】

味甘,平。

主惊悸,安五脏,益气,除湿痹。久服,令人悦泽美色,耳目聪明,不饥不老,轻身延年。生山谷。

【考据】

《名医》曰:生太山,柏叶尤良,田四时各依方面采,阴干。

案《说文》云:柏,鞠也;《广雅》云:栝柏也;《尔雅》云:柏椈;郭璞云:礼《记》曰,鬯,曰以椈;《范子计然》云:柏脂出三辅,上升价七千,中三千一斗。

【今译】

味甘,性平。

主治惊恐心悸,能安静五脏,能补益精气,能祛除湿邪所致痹

97. Boshi（柏实，seed of Chinese arborvitae，Semen Platycladi）[1]

[Original Text]

[Boshi（柏实，seed of Chinese arborvitae，Semen Platycladi），] sweet in taste [and] mild [in property]，[is mainly used] to relieve fright and palpitation，to pacify the five Zang-organs，to replenish Qi and to eliminate dampness impediment. Long-term taking [of it will] luster and beautify facial expression，improve hearing and vision，[make people feel] no hunger，prevent aging，relax the body and prolong life. [It] grows in mountains and valleys.

[Textual Research]

[In the book entitled] *Ming Yi Bie Lu* （《名医别录》，*Special Record of Great Doctors*），[it] says [that Boshi （柏实，seed of Chinese arborvitae，Semen Platycladi）] grows in Taishan（太山），the leaves [of which] are better [than other parts of it]. [It can be] collected in the four seasons and dried in the shade.

Notes

1. Boshi（柏实，seed of Chinese arborvitae，Semen Platycladi） is a herbal medicinal，also known as Boziren（柏子仁），sweet in taste and mild in property，entering the heart meridian，the liver meridian and the spleen meridian，effective in nourishing the heart，

证。长期服用，能令人悦泽美色，听力增强，视力清明，能减少饥饿之感，能长寿不老，能使身体轻盈，延年益寿。该物生长在山谷之中。

invigorating wisdom, pacifying spirit and moistening dryness. Clinically it is used to treat palpitation, deficiency-vexation, insomnia, amnesia, dreaminess, intestinal dryness and constipation.

98. 伏苓

【原文】

味甘,平。

主胸胁逆气(《御览》作疝气),忧恚,惊邪,恐悸,心下结痛,寒热烦满,咳逆,口焦舌干,利小便。久服安魂养神,不饥延年。一名茯菟,(《御览》作茯神,案元本云:其有抱根者,名茯神,作黑字)生山谷。

【考据】

《吴普》曰:茯苓通神,桐君甘,雷公扁鹊甘无毒,或生茂州,大松根下,人地三丈一尺,二月七月采。(《御览》)

《名医》曰:其有抱根者名茯神,生太山大松下,二月八月采,阴干。

案《广雅》云:茯神,茯苓也;《范子计然》云:茯苓,出嵩高三辅,《列仙传》云:昌容采茯苓,饵而食之;《史记》褚先生云:传曰,下有伏灵,上有兔丝,所谓伏灵者,在兔丝之下,状似飞鸟之形,伏灵者,千岁松根也,食之不死;《淮南子》说林训云:茯苓掘,兔丝死,旧作茯,非。

98. Fuling（伏苓, poria sclerotium, Wolfiporia Cocos）[1]

〔Original Text〕

〔Fuling（伏苓, poria sclerotium, Wolfiporia Cocos），〕sweet in taste〔and〕mild〔in property〕，〔is mainly used〕to cease counterflow of Qi from the chest and rib-side，〔to relieve〕anxiety，fright and palpitation，〔to resolve〕accumulation and pain below the heart，〔to eliminate〕cold-heat，vexation and depression，〔to cease〕cough with dyspnea，〔to dispel〕parchment of the mouth and dryness of the tongue，and to promote urination. Long-term taking〔of it will〕pacify ethereal soul，nourish spirit，〔make people feel〕no hunger，and prolong life.〔It is also〕called Futu（茯菟），growing in mountains and valleys.

〔Textual Research〕

〔In the book entitled〕*Wu Pu Ben Cao*（《吴普本草》, *Wu Pu's Studies of Materia Medica*），〔it〕says〔that〕Fuling（伏苓, poria sclerotium，Wolfiporia Cocos）invigorates spirit.〔According to〕Tongjun（桐均），〔it is〕sweet〔in taste〕；〔according to〕Leigong（雷公）and Bianque（扁鹊），〔it is〕sweet〔in taste〕and non-toxic〔in property〕.〔It〕may grow in Maozhou（茂州）and〔can be〕collected in February and July〔according to the book entitled〕*Tai Ping Yu Lan*（《太平御览》, *Imperial Studies in Taiping Times*）.

【今译】

味甘,性平。

主治胸胁部气逆上行,忧愁恐怒,惊恐心悸,心下聚集疼痛,寒热疾病,烦躁郁闷,咳嗽气逆,口焦舌干,能使小便通畅。长期服用能安魂养神,能减少饥饿之感,能延年长寿。又称为茯苓。该物生长在山谷之中。

[In the book entitled] *Ming Yi Bie Lu* (《名医别录》, *Special Record of Great Doctors*), [it] says [that Fuling (伏苓, poria sclerotium, Wolfiporia Cocos) is] called Fushen (茯神) [if] it bears root. [It] grows below the high pine tree in Taishan (太山) mountain, and [can be] collected in February and August and dried in the shade. [In the book entitled] *Fan Zi Ji Ran* (《范子计然》, *Studies About Fan Li's Teacher*), [it] says [that] Fuling (伏苓, poria sclerotium, Wolfiporia Cocos) grows in three areas in Songgao (嵩高).

Notes

1. Fuling (伏苓, poria sclerotium, Wolfiporia Cocos) is a herbal medicinal, sweet and bland in taste, mild in property, entering the spleen meridian and the kidney meridian, effective in removing water and dampness, fortifying the spleen and stomach, tranquilizing the heart and pacifying the spirit. Clinically it is used to treat dysuria, edema, abdominal accumulation of water, poor appetite, diarrhea, palpitation, insomnia and dreaminess.

99. 榆皮

【原文】

味甘,平。

主大小便不通,利水道,除邪气,久服,轻身不饥。其实尤良,一名零榆。生山谷。

【考据】

《名医》曰:生颖川,三月采皮,取白,暴干,八月采实。

案《说文》云:榆,白枌,榆也;《广雅》云:柘榆,梗榆也;《尔雅》云:榆,白枌;郭璞云:枌榆先生叶,却着荚,皮色白,又莁荑.郭璞云:令云刺榆;《毛诗》云:东门之枌,《传》云枌,白榆也;又山有蓲,《传》云:枢荎也;陆玑云:其针刺如柘,其叶如榆。渝为茹,美滑如白榆之类,有十种,叶皆相似,皮及木理异矣。

【今译】

味甘,性平。

99. Yupi（榆皮，bark of Chinese elm，Cortex Ulmi Parvifoliae）[1]

［Original Text］

［Yupi（榆皮，bark of Chinese elm，Cortex Ulmi Parvifoliae），］sweet in taste［and］mild［in property］，［is mainly used］to treat dysuria，to promote urination and to eliminate evil-Qi. Long-term taking［of it will］relax the body，［make people feel］no hunger. Its fruit is more effective.［It is also］called Lingyu（零榆），growing in mountains and valleys.

［Textual Research］

［In the book entitled］*Ming Yi Bie Lu*（《名医别录》，*Special Record of Great Doctors*），［it］says［that Yupi（榆皮，bark of Chinese elm，Cortex Ulmi Parvifoliae）］grows in Yingchuan（颍川）.［Its］bark［can be］collected in March and dried in the sun.［Its］fruit［can be］collected in August.

Notes

1. Yupi（榆皮，bark of Chinese elm，Cortex Ulmi Parvifoliae），also known as Yubaipi（榆白皮），is a herbal medicinal，sweet in taste and mild in property，entering the lung meridian，the spleen meridian and the bladder meridian，effective in promoting urination，expelling stranguria and resolving swelling. Clinically it

　　主治大小便不通,能通利水道,能清除邪气。长期服用,能使人身体轻盈,能减少饥饿之感。其果实效果更好,又称为零榆。该物生长在山谷之中。

is used to treat dysuria, stranguria, leucorrhea, cough with panting and phlegm, insomnia, internal and external bleeding, dystocia, carbuncle, ulcer, scrofula and scabies.

100. 酸枣

【原文】

味酸,平。

主心腹寒热,邪结气聚,四肢酸疼,湿痹。久服安五脏,轻身延年。生川泽。

【考据】

《名医》曰:生河东,八月采实,阴干,四十日成。

案《说文》云:樲,酸枣也;《尔雅》云:樲,酸枣;郭璞云:味小实酢;孟子云:养其樲棘;赵岐云:樲棘,小棘,所谓酸枣是也。

【今译】

味酸,性平。

主治心腹部寒热病,能消解邪气停滞积聚,能治疗四肢酸疼以及湿邪所致痹证。长期服用能安静五脏,能使人身体轻盈,延年益寿。该物生长在山川和平泽之中。

100. Suanzao（酸枣，spiny jujube，Ziziphi Spinosi）[1]

[Original Text]

[Suanzao（酸枣，spiny jujube，Ziziphi Spinosi），] sour in taste and mild [in property]，[is mainly used] to treat cold-heat in the heart and abdomen，evil binding and Qi accumulation，pain of the four limbs and dampness impediment. Long-term taking [of it will] pacify the five Zang-organs，relax the body and prolong life. [It] grows in valleys and swamps.

[Textual Research]

[In the book entitled] *Ming Yi Bie Lu*（《名医别录》，*Special Record of Great Doctors*），[it] says [that Suanzao（酸枣，spiny jujube，Ziziphi Spinosi）] grows in Hedong（河东）. [It can be] collected in August and dried in the shade for forty days.

[In] case [analysis in the book entitled] *Shuo Wen*（《说文》，*On Culture*），[it] says [that the so-called] Er（樲）refers to Suanzao（酸枣，spiny jujube，Ziziphi Spinosi）.

Notes

1. Suanzao（酸枣，spiny jujube，Ziziphi Spinosi），also known as Suanzaoren（酸枣仁）and Zaoren（枣仁），is a herbal medicinal，sweet in taste and mild in property，entering the liver meridian，the heart meridian and the gallbladder meridian，effective in nourishing the heart，pacifying the spirit and restraining sweating. Clinically it is used to treat insomnia due to deficiency and vexation，palpitation and amnesia.

101. 蘖木

【原文】

味苦,寒。

主五脏,肠胃中结热,黄疸,肠痔,止泄利,女子漏下赤白,阴阳蚀疮。一名檀桓。生山谷。

【考据】

1.《名医》曰:生汉中及永昌。

2. 案《说文》云:檗,黄木也,蘖木也,《司马相如赋》有蘖;张揖云:檗木可染者;颜师古云:蘖,黄薜也。

【今译】

味苦,性寒。

101. Niemu（蘖木，root of slenderstalk mahonia，root of Chinese mahonia，Radix Mahoniae）[1]

[Original Text]

[Niemu（蘖木，root of slenderstalk mahonia，root of Chinese mahonia，Radix Mahoniae），] bitter in taste and cold [in property]，[is mainly used] to treat [diseases in] the five Zang-organs，heat binding in the intestines and stomach，jaundice，hemorrhoids，diarrhea，vaginal discharge of red and white liquid，genital ulceration and sore in man and woman. [It is also] called Tanhuan（檀桓），growing in mountains and valleys.

[Textual Research]

[In the book entitled] *Ming Yi Bie Lu*（《名医别录》，*Special Record of Great Doctors*），[it] says [that Niemu（蘖木，root of slenderstalk mahonia，root of Chinese mahonia，Radix Mahoniae）] grows in Hanzhong（汉中）and Yongchang（永昌）.

[In] case [analysis in the book entitled] *Shuo Wen*（《说文》，*On Culture*），[it] says [that the so-called] Bo（檗）and Huangmu（黄木）are other names of Niemu（蘖木，root of slenderstalk mahonia，root of Chinese mahonia，Radix Mahoniae）.

Notes

1. Niemu（蘖木，root of slenderstalk mahonia，root of Chinese

主治五脏病症，能消解肠胃中热邪聚集，能治疗黄疸，痔疮，泄泻，痢疾，女子阴道淋漓不断，赤白带下，男女阴部因虫毒损伤而生疮。又称为檀桓。该物生长在山谷之中。

mahonia, Radix Mahoniae) is a herbal medicinal, bitter in taste and cold in property, entering the kidney meridian, the bladder meridian and the large intestine meridian, effective in reducing fire and removing toxin, clearing heat and drying dampness. Clinically it is used to treat diarrhea and dysentery due to dampness-heat, jaundice, leucorrhea, stranguria, hemorrhoids, swelling and pain of the feet and knees, Yin deficiency and fire effulgence, bone steaming, fever due to overexertion and seminal emission in dream.

102. 干漆

【原文】

味辛,温,无毒。

主绝伤,补中,续筋骨,填髓脑,安五脏,五缓六急,风寒湿痹。生漆,去长虫。久服轻身耐老。生川谷。

【考据】

1.《名医》曰:生汉中,夏至后采,干之。

2. 案《说文》云:桼木汁可以髤物,象形,桼如水滴而下,以漆为漆水字;《周礼》载师云:漆林之征,郑元云:故书漆林为桼林;杜子春云:当为漆林。

【今译】

味辛,性温,无毒。

主治严重受伤,能补益人体内脏,能使跌打损伤中的筋骨续接,能

102. Ganqi（干漆，dried lacquer of true lacquertree, Resina Toxicodendri）[1]

[Original Text]

[Ganqi（干漆，dried lacquer of true lacquertree, Resina Toxicodendri），] pungent in taste, warm and non-toxic [in property], [is mainly used] to treat severe damage, tonify the middle (internal organs), to remedy [severe injury of] sinews and bones, to enrich the brains, to harmonize the five Zang-organs, to treat five [kinds of] retardations[2], six [kinds of] extreme [syndromes/patterns][3] and wind-cold dampness impediment. Raw lacquer can kill roundworms. Long-term taking [of it will] relax the body and prevent aging. [It] grows in mountain valleys and river valleys.

[Textual Research]

[In the book entitled] *Ming Yi Bie Lu*（《名医别录》，*Special Record of Great Doctors*），[it] says [that Ganqi（干漆，dried lacquer of true lacquertree, Resina Toxicodendri）] grows in Hanzhong（汉中）. [It can be] collected in Summer Solstice and dried.

Notes

1. Ganqi（干漆，dried lacquer of true lacquertree, Resina Toxicodendri) is pungent in taste, warm and non-toxic in property,

填充脑髓,能安静五脏,能治疗小儿五迟和六种极度损伤以及风寒湿邪所致之痹证。生漆能祛除蛔虫。长期服用能使人身体轻盈,不易衰老。该物生长在山川河谷之中。

entering the liver meridian and the spleen meridian, effective in breaking blood stasis, resolving accumulation and killing worms. Clinically it is used to treat amenorrhea due to blood stasis, abdominal mass, abdominal pain due to blood stasis and retention of worms.

2. Five kinds of retardations include retardations in walking, speaking, standing, fontanel closure and tooth growth.

3. Six kinds of extreme syndromes/patterns include extreme disorders of Qi, blood, sinews, bones, muscles and essence.

103. 五加皮

【原文】

味辛,温。

主心腹疝气,腹痛,益气疗躄,小儿不能行,疽疮阴蚀。一名豺漆。

【考据】

1.《名医》曰:一名豺节,生汉中及冤句,五月十月采茎,十月采根,阴干。

2. 案《大观本草》,引东华真人煮石经云:舜常登苍梧山曰,厥金玉之香草,朕那偃息正道,此乃五加也。鲁定公母,单服五加酒,以致不死。

103. Wujiapi（五加皮，root and bark of slenderstyle acanthopanax，Cortex Acanthopanacis）[1]

［Original Text］

［Wujiapi（五加皮，root and bark of slenderstyle acanthopanax，Cortex Acanthopanacis），］ pungent in taste and warm ［in property］，［is mainly used］ to treat hernia in the heart and abdomen，abdominal pain，to replenish Qi to cure limp，to treat difficulty of children in walking，carbuncle，sore and genital ulceration. ［It is also］ called Caiqi（豺漆）.

［Textual Research］

［In the book entitled］ *Ming Yi Bie Lu*（《名医别录》，*Special Record of Great Doctors*），［it］ says ［that Wujiapi（五加皮，root and bark of slenderstyle acanthopanax，Cortex Acanthopanacis）is also］ called Caijie（豺节），growing in Hanzhong（汉中）and Yuanju（冤句）. ［Its］ stalks ［can be］ collected in May and October，［its］ root ［can be］ collected in October，［both of which should be］ dried in the shade.

385

Notes

1. Wujiapi（五加皮，root and bark of slenderstyle acanthopanax，Cortex Acanthopanacis）is a herbal medicinal，pungent in taste and warm in property，entering the liver meridian and the kidney

【今译】

味辛,性温。

主治心腹部疝气,能消除腹部疼痛,能补益精气,能治疗瘸腿,小儿不能行走,疽疮及阴部溃疡。又称为豺漆。

meridian, effective in expelling wind-dampness and strengthening the sinews and bones. Clinically it is used to treat wind-cold dampness impediment, spasm of sinews and bones, pain of the waist and legs, flaccidity of lower limbs, beriberi, edema and itching of the scrotum.

104. 蔓荆实

【原文】

味苦,微寒。

主筋骨间寒热,湿痹,拘挛,明目坚齿,利九窍,去白虫。久服轻身耐老。小荆实亦等。生山谷。

【考据】

1.《名医》曰:生河间南阳冤句,或平寿都乡,高岸上,及田野中,八月九月采实,阴干。

2. 案《广雅》云:牡荆,蔓荆也;广志云:楚,荆也。牡荆,蔓荆也。据牡曼声相近,故本经于蔓荆,不载所出州土,以其见牡荆也。今或别为二条,非。

【今译】

味苦,性微寒。

主治筋骨间寒热性疾病,能治疗湿邪痹阻及肢体拘挛,能使眼睛

104. Manjingzi（蔓荆实，fruit of shrub chastetree，Fructus Viticis）[1]

［Original Text］

［Manjingzi 蔓荆实，fruit of shrub chastetree，Fructus Viticis），］bitter in taste and slightly cold ［in property］，［is mainly used］ to treat cold-heat-damp impediment in the sinews and bones，［to relieve］ spasm，to improve vision，to strengthen the teeth，to disinhibit the nine orifices and to eliminate white worms. Long-term taking ［of it will］ relax the body and prevent aging. The small fruit of it bears the same effect. ［It］ grows in mountains and valleys.

［Textual Research］

［In the book entitled］ *Ming Yi Bie Lu*（《名医别录》，*Special Record of Great Doctors*），［it］ says ［that Manjingzi 蔓荆实，fruit of shrub chastetree，Fructus Viticis）］ grows in Hejian（河间）and Yuanju（冤句）in Nanyang（南阳）or over the banks and fields in Pingshou（平寿）district. ［Its］ fruit ［can be］ collected in August and September and dried in the shade.

Notes

1. Manjingzi 蔓荆实，fruit of shrub chastetree，Fructus Viticis），known as Manjingzi（蔓荆子）now，is a herbal medicinal，bitter and pungent in taste，cool in property，entering the liver

明亮,能使牙齿坚固,能使九窍通畅,能祛除绦虫。长期服用能使人身体轻盈,不易衰老。小荆果实有同等效果。该物生长在山谷之中。

meridian and the lung meridian, effective in dispersing wind-heat, clearing and disinhibiting the head and the eyes. Clinically it is used to treat common cold due to wind-heat, migraine, redness and pain of the eyes.

105. 辛夷

【原文】

味辛,温。

主五脏,身体寒风,头脑痛,面皯。久服,下气轻身,明目,增年耐老。一名辛矧(《御览》作引),一名侯桃,一名房木。生川谷。

【考据】

1.《名医》曰:九月采实,暴干。

2. 案汉书扬雄赋云:列新雉于林薄;师古云:新雉即辛夷耳,为树甚大,其木枝叶皆芳,一名新矧;《史记·司马相如传》:杂以流夷;注《汉书音义》曰:流夷,新夷也;陶宏景云:小时气辛香,即《离骚》所呼辛夷者;陈藏起云:初发如笔,北人呼为木笔,其花最早,南人呼为迎春。按唐人名为玉蕊,又曰玉兰。

【今译】

味辛,性温。

主治五脏病症,能消解身体中寒热之气,能治疗头痛,能消除面部

105. Xinyi（辛夷，immature flower of biond magnolia，immature flower of yulan magnolia，immature flower of sprenger magnolia，Flos Magnoliae）[2]

〔Original Text〕

〔Xinyi（辛夷，immature flower of biond magnolia，immature flower of yulan magnolia，immature flower of sprenger magnolia，Flos Magnoliae），〕 pungent in taste and warm〔in property〕，〔is mainly used〕to treat〔diseases in〕the five Zang-organs, cold-wind〔disease in〕the body, headache and black facial spots. Long-term taking〔of it will〕relax the body, improve vision, prolong life and prevent aging.〔It is also〕called Xinshen（辛矧），Houtao（侯桃）and Fangmu（房木），growing in mountain valleys and river valleys.

393

〔Textual Research〕

〔In the book entitled〕*Ming Yi Bie Lu*（《名医别录》，*Special Record of Great Doctors*），〔it〕says〔that〕the fruit〔of Xinyi（辛夷，immature flower of biond magnolia，immature flower of yulan magnolia，immature flower of sprenger magnolia，Flos Magnoliae）can be〕collected in September and dried in the sun.

Shi Gu（师古）said，"〔The so-called〕Xinzhi（新雉）is another name of Xinyi（辛夷，immature flower of biond magnolia，immature flower of yulan magnolia，immature flower of sprenger magnolia，Flos Magnoliae）.〔Its〕tree is very big with fragrant stalks and

黑斑。长期服用,能使气下行,能使人身体轻盈,能使眼睛明亮,能使人延长寿命,不易衰老。又称为辛矧,又称为候桃,又称为房木。该物生长在山川河谷之中。

leaves, also called Xinshen (新矧). "Tao Hongjing (陶宏景) said, "It is pungent and fragrant when small. "

Notes

1. Xinyi (辛夷, immature flower of biond magnolia, immature flower of yulan magnolia, immature flower of sprenger magnolia, Flos Magnoliae) is herbal medicinal, pungent in taste and warm in property, entering the lung meridian and the stomach meridian, effective in dispersing wind-cold and disinhibiting nose. Clinically it is used to treat headache, nasosinusitis, stuffy nose and rhinitis.

106. 桑上寄生

【原文】

味苦,平。

主腰痛,小儿背强,痈肿,安胎,充肌肤,坚发齿,长须眉。其实,明目,轻身通神。一名寄屑,一名寓木,一名宛童。生川谷。

【考据】

1.《名医》曰:一名茑,生宏农桑树上,三月三日,采茎,阴干。

2. 案《说文》云:茑,寄生也;诗曰:茑与女萝,或作樢;《广雅》云:宛童,寄生樢也,又寄屏,寄生也;《中山经》云:龙山上多寓木;郭璞云:寄生也;《尔雅》云:寓木宛童;郭璞云:寄生树一名茑;《毛诗》云:茑与女萝;《传》云:茑,寄生山也;陆玑云:茑,一名寄生,叶似当卢,子如覆盆子,赤黑甜美。

【今译】

味苦,性平。

主治腰部疼痛,能消解小儿背部僵硬,痈肿,能安和胎儿,能充盈肌

106. Sangshang Jisheng（桑上寄生，Chinese taxillus herb，Herba Taxilli）[1]

[Original Text]

［Sangshang Jisheng（桑上寄生，Chinese taxillus herb，Herba Taxilli），］bitter in taste and mild ［in property］，［is mainly used］to treat lumbago，stiffness of infantile spine and carbuncle，to prevent abortion，to enrich muscles，to strengthen teeth and to promote eyebrow. Its fruit ［can］improve vision，relax the body and invigorate spirit. ［It is also］called Jixiao（寄屑），Yumu（寓木）and Wuantong（宛童），growing in mountain valleys and river valleys.

397

[Textual Research]

［In the book entitled］*Ming Yi Bie Lu*（《名医别录》，*Special Record of Great Doctors*），［it］says ［that Sangshang Jisheng（桑上寄生，Chinese taxillus herb，Herba Taxilli）is also］called Niao（茑），growing in mulberry. ［Its］stalks ［can be］collected on March 3 and dried in the shade.

［In］case ［analysis in the book entitled］*Shuo Wen*（《说文》，*On Culture*），［it］says ［that］Niao（茑），［i. e. Sangshang Jisheng（桑上寄生，Chinese taxillus herb，Herba Taxilli）］，is a parasite. Lu Ji（陆玑）said，"Niao（茑）is also called Jisheng（寄生）. ［Its］leaf looks like an ornament ［over the head of a horse］. ［Its］seed looks like a pot upside down. The red and black ［one is］sweet and

肤,能坚固头发和牙齿,能使须眉生长。其果实,能使眼睛明亮,能使身体轻盈,能使神气通畅。又称为寄屑,又称为寓木,又称为宛童。该物生长在山川河谷之中。

fragrant."

1. Sangshang Jisheng（桑上寄生，Chinese taxillus herb，Herba Taxilli），known as Sangjisheng（桑寄生）now，is a herbal medicinal，bitter and sweet in taste and mild in property，entering the liver meridian and the kidney meridian，effective in tonifying the liver and kidney，expelling wind-dampness，reducing blood pressure，nourishing the blood and calming fetus. Clinically it is used to treat pain of the waist and spine，flaccidity and weakness of sinews and bones，wind-cold dampness impediment，hypertension，threatened abortion and vaginal bleeding during pregnancy.

107. 杜仲

【原文】

味辛,平。

主腰脊痛,补中,益精气,坚筋骨,强志,除阴下痒湿,小便余沥。久服轻身耐老。一名思仙。生山谷。

【考据】

1.《吴普》曰:杜仲,一名木绵,一名思仲。(《御览》)

2.《名医》曰:一名思仙,一名木绵,生上虞及上党汉中,二月五月六月九月采皮。

3. 案《广雅》云:杜仲,曼榆也。《博物志》云:杜仲,皮中有丝,折之则见。

【今译】

味辛,性平。

主治腰脊部疼痛,能充实人体内脏,能补益精气,能使筋骨强壮,

107. Duzhong（杜仲，eucommia bark， Cortex Eucommiae）[1]

[Original Text]

[Duzhong （杜仲，eucommia bark，Cortex Eucommiae），] pungent in taste and mild [in property]，[is mainly used] to relieve pain in the waist and spine，to tonify the middle (internal organs)，to replenish essential Qi，to strengthen sinews and bones，to improve memory，to eliminate genital itching and dampness and to treat dribbling urination. Long-term taking [of it will] relax the body and prevent aging. [It is also] called Sixian（思仙），growing in mountains and valleys.

[Textual Research]

[In the book entitled] *Wu Pu Ben Cao*（《吴普本草》，*Wu Pu's Studies of Materia Medica*），[it] says [that] Duzhong （杜仲，eucommia bark，Cortex Eucommiae）[is also] called Mumian（木绵）and Sizhong（思仲）[according to the book entitled] *Tai Ping Yu Lan*（《太平御览》，*Imperial Studies in Taiping Times*）.

[In the book entitled] *Ming Yi Bie Lu*（《名医别录》，*Special Record of Great Doctors*），[it] says [that Duzhong（杜仲，eucommia bark，Cortex Eucommiae）is also] called Sizhong（思仲）and Mumian（木绵），growing in Shangyu（上虞），Shangdang（上党）and Hanzhong（汉中）. [Its] bark [can be] collected in February，

能增强记忆力,能消除阴部瘙痒湿腻,能治疗小便后依然淋漓不尽。长期服用能使人身体轻盈,不易衰老。又称为思仙。该物生长在山谷之中。

May，June and September.

[In the book entitled] *Guang Ya*（《广雅》，*The First Chinese Encyclopedic Dictionary*），[it] says [that] Duzhong（杜仲，eucommia bark，Cortex Eucommiae）[is also] called Manyu（曼榆）. [In the book entitled] *Bo Wu Zhi*（《博物志》，*History of All Plants*），[it] says [that] there is milk in the bark of Duzhong（杜仲，eucommia bark，Cortex Eucommiae）[which can be] seen [when] broken.

Notes

1. Duzhong（杜仲，eucommia bark，Cortex Eucommiae）is a herbal medicinal，sweet and slightly pungent in taste，warm in property，entering the liver meridian and the kidney meridian，effective in tonifying the liver and kidney，strengthening the sinews and bones，preventing abortion and reducing blood pressure. Clinically it is used to treat pain of the waist and spine，flaccidity and weakness of the sinews and bones，impotence，frequent urination，vaginal bleeding during pregnancy and threatened abortion.

108. 女贞实

【原文】

味苦,平。

主补中,安五脏,养精神,除百疾。久服肥健,轻身不老。生山谷。

【考据】

1.《名医》曰:生武陵,立冬采。

2. 案《说文》云:桢,刚木也。东山经云:太山上多桢木。郭璞云:女桢也,叶冬不凋。《毛诗》云:南山有杞。陆玑云:木杞,其树如樗(陈藏器作栗),一名狗骨,理白滑,其子为木虻子,可合药,《司马相如赋》有女贞。师古曰:女贞树,冬夏常青,未尝凋落,若有节操,故以名为焉。陈藏器云:冬青也。

【今译】

味苦,性平。

108. Nǚzhenshi（女贞实，fruit of glossy privet，Fructus Ligustri Lucidi）[1]

[Original Text]

[Nǚzhenshi（女贞实，fruit of glossy privet，Fructus Ligustri Lucidi），] bitter in taste and mild [in property], [is mainly used] to tonify the middle（internal organs），to harmonize the five Zang-organs，to nourish essence and spirit，and to eliminate all diseases. Long-term taking [of it will] cultivate health，relax the body and prevent aging. [It] grows in mountains and valleys.

[Textual Research]

[In the book entitled] *Ming Yi Bie Lu*（《名医别录》，*Special Record of Great Doctors*），[it] says [that Nǚzhenshi（女贞实，fruit of glossy privet，Fructus Ligustri Lucidi）] grows in Wuling（武陵）and [can be] collected in Winter Solstice.

[In] case [analysis in the book entitled] *Shuo Wen*（《说文》，*On Culture*），[it] says [that] Nǚzhenshi（女贞实，fruit of glossy privet，Fructus Ligustri Lucidi）usually grows in Taishan（太山）. Guo Pu（郭璞）said，"Its leaves are not withered in winter." Shi Gu（师古）said，"This tree keeps green in winter and summer，never withered."

Notes

1. Nǚzhenshi（女贞实，fruit of glossy privet，Fructus Ligustri

能补益人体内脏，能安静五脏，能滋养精神，能消除各种疾病。长期服用能使人身体康健，身体轻盈，长寿不老。该物生长在山谷之中。

Lucidi), now known as Nǔzhenzi (女贞子), is a herbal medicinal, sweet and bitter in taste, mild in property, entering the liver meridian and the kidney meridian, effective in tonifying the kidney and nourishing Yin, nourishing the liver and improving vision. Clinically it is used to treat internal heat ［disease］ due to Yin deficiency, pain and weakness of the waist and spine, vertigo, blurred vision, tinnitus, seminal emission and premature ejaculation.

109. 木兰

【原文】

味苦,寒。

主身大热在皮肤中,去面热,赤疱,酒皶,恶风,瘨疾,阴下痒湿,明耳目。一名林兰。生川谷。

【考据】

1.《名医》曰:一名杜兰,皮似桂而香,生零陵及太山,十二月采皮,阴干。

2. 案《广雅》云:木栏桂栏也。刘逵注蜀都赋云:木兰,大树也,叶似长生,冬夏荣,常以冬华,其实如小柿,甘美。南人以为梅,其皮可食。颜师古注汉书云:皮似椒而香,可作面膏药。

【今译】

味苦,性寒。

109. Mulan（木兰，lily magnolia，Magnoliae Liliflorae）[1]

[Original Text]

[Mulan（木兰，lily magnolia，Magnoliae Liliflorae），] bitter in taste and cold [in property], [is mainly used] to treat severe heat in the body，red facial spots，rosacea，severe wind[2]，epilepsy，genital itching and dampness，and to improve hearing and vision. [It is also] called Linlan（林兰），growing in mountain valleys and river valleys.

[Textual Research]

[In the book entitled] *Ming Yi Bie Lu*（《名医别录》，*Special Record of Great Doctors*），[it] says [that Mulan（木兰，lily magnolia，Magnoliae Liliflorae）is also] called Dulan（杜兰）. [Its] bark looks like cassia and is fragrant. [It] grows in Lingling（零陵）and Taishan（太山）. [Its] bark [can be] collected in December and dried in the shade.

[In] explaining Shudou Prose with Verse（蜀都赋），Liu Kui（刘逵）said，"Mulan（木兰，lily magnolia，Magnoliae Liliflorae）is a large tree. The leaves grow all the year and are prosperous in winter and summer. [It] blossoms in winter. [Its] fruits look like small persimmon，sweet and fragrant.

主治身有高热，能消除面热生红疱，能治疗酒渣鼻，麻风病，癫痫及阴下痒湿，能使听力清楚，能使视力清晰。又称为林兰。该物生长在山川河谷之中。

Notes

1. Mulan (木兰，lily magnolia，Magnoliae Liliflorae) is a herbal medicinal，pungent in taste and warm in property，entering the lung meridian，effective in dispersing wind-cold and disinhibiting the nose. Clinically it is used to treat headache due to common cold，stuffy nose and rhinitis.

2. Severe wind may refer to leprosy.

110. 蕤核

【原文】

味甘,温。

主心腹邪气,明目,目赤痛伤泪出。久服轻身益气,不饥。生川谷。

【考据】

1.《吴普》曰:蕤核,一名,神农雷公甘平无毒,生池泽,八月采,补中,强志,明目,久服不饥。(《御览》)

2.《名医》曰:生函谷,及巴西。

3. 案《说文》云:桵,白桵,棫。《尔雅》云:棫,白桵.郭璞云:桵,小木。丛生有刺,实如耳珰,紫赤可啖。一切经音义云:本草作蕤,今桵核是也。

【今译】

味甘,性温。

110. Ruihe（蕤核，hedge prinsepia mature drupe，Nux Prinsepiae）[1]

[Original Text]

[Ruihe（蕤核，hedge prinsepia mature drupe，Nux Prinsepiae），] sweet in taste and warm [in property]，[is mainly used] to expel evil-Qi in the heart and abdomen，to improve vision and to treat redness and tearing of the eyes [due to] ocular injury. Long-term taking [of it will] relax the body，replenish Qi and [make people feel] no hunger. [It] grows in mountain valleys and river valleys.

[Textual Research]

[in the book entitled] *Wu Pu Ben Cao*（《吴普本草》，*Wu Pu's Studies of Materia Medica*) Ruihe（蕤核，hedge prinsepia mature drupe，Nux Prinsepiae），[according to] Agriculture God（神农）and Leigong（雷公），[is] sweet [in property]，mild and non-toxic [in property]. [It] grows in lakes and pools，[and can be] collected in August. [It can] tonify the internal organs，strengthen memory and improve vision. Long-term taking [of it will make people feel] no hunger [according to the book entitled] *Tai Ping Yu Lan*（《太平御览》，*Imperial Studies in Taiping Times*).

[In the book entitled] *Ming Yi Bie Lu*（《名医别录》，*Special Record of Great Doctors*)，[it] says [that Ruihe（蕤核，hedge prinsepia mature drupe，Nux Prinsepiae）] grows in Hangu（函谷）

主治心腹部邪气，能使眼睛明亮，能治疗因目赤痛伤而泪流不止。长期服用能使人身体轻盈，能补益精气，能减少饥饿之感。该物生长在山川河谷之中。

and Baxi（巴西）

Notes

1. Ruihe （蕤核，hedge prinsepia mature drupe，Nux Prinsepiae），now known as Ruiren（蕤仁），is a herbal medicinal，sweet in taste and warm in property，entering the liver meridian and the heart meridian，effective in nourishing the liver and improving vision. Clinically it is used to treat redness，swelling and pain of the eyes，spontaneous tearing and insomnia.

本书为国家社科基金项目"中医名词术语英译国际标准化研究"（No.08BYY009）、国家社科基金项目"中医英语翻译理论与方法研究"（No.12BYY024）、国家中医药管理局项目"中国参与世界卫生组织ICTM方案研究"(No.YYS20090010-2)、上海市教委科研创新重点项目"中医英语翻译原则、标准与方法研究"（B-7037-12-000001）、国家外文局重点项目"中医典籍翻译的历史、现状与国际传播调研报告"、上海市教委重点课程建设项目"国学典籍英译"、上海师范大学重点科研项目"国学典籍多译本平行语料库建设"（A-7031-12-002001）的阶段性成果。

汉英对照
Classical Chinese-Modern Chinese-English

Shén Nóng Běn Cǎo Jīng

神农本草经

Agriculture God's Canon of Materia Medica

孙星衍◎考据 Textually Researched by Sun Xingyan

刘希茹◎今译 Translated in Modern Chinese by Liu Xiru

李照国◎英译 Translated in English by Li Zhaoguo

II

上海三联书店

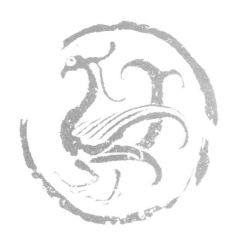

111. 橘柚

【原文】

味辛,温。

主胸中瘕热逆气,利水谷。久服,去臭下气通神,一名橘皮。生川谷。(旧在果部,非)

【考据】

1.《名医》曰:生南山,江南,十月采。

2. 案《说文》云:橘果出江南,柚条也。似橙而酢。《尔雅》云:柚条。郭璞云:似橙实酢,生江南。禹贡云:厥包橘柚。伪孔云:大曰橘,小曰柚。列子汤问篇云:吴楚之国有木焉,其名为櫾,碧树而冬生,实丹而味酸,食其皮汁,已愤厥之疾,《司马相如赋》,有橘柚。张揖曰:柚,即橙也。似橘而大,味酢皮厚。

上木,上品二十种,旧一十九种,考果部,橘柚当入此。

【今译】

味辛,性温。

111. Juyou（橘柚，tangerine pericarp, Pericarpium Citri Tangerinae）[1]

[Original Text]

[Juyou（橘柚，tangerine pericarp, Pericarpium Citri Tangerinae），] pungent in taste and warm [in property], [is mainly used] to treat accumulation of heat and counterflow of Qi in the chest and promote digestion of food. Long-term taking [of it will] remove halitosis, descend Qi and invigorate spirit. [It is also] called Jupi（橘皮），growing in mountain valleys and river valleys.

[Textual Research]

[In the book entitled] *Ming Yi Bie Lu*（《名医别录》，*Special Record of Great Doctors*），[it] says [that Juyou（橘柚，tangerine pericarp, Pericarpium Citri Tangerinae）] grows in Nanshan（南山）and Jiangnan（江南）. [It can be] collected in October.

Zhang Ji（张揖）said，"Juyou（橘柚，tangerine pericarp, Pericarpium Citri Tangerinae）actually is orange，also like tangerine [with the taste of] vinegar and thick bark."

Notes

1. Juyou（橘柚，tangerine pericarp, Pericarpium Citri Tangerinae）is a herbal medicinal, pungent and bitter in taste, warm in property, entering the spleen meridian and the lung

　　主治胸中瘕热上逆,能消化水谷。长期服用,能消除口臭,能使气下行,能使神气通畅。又称为橘皮。该物生长在山川河谷之中。

meridian, effective in regulating Qi, fortifying the spleen, drying dampness and resolving phlegm. Clinically it is used to treat abdominal distension, fullness and pain, indigestion, vomiting and panting, hiccup, chest oppression and cough with phlegm.

112. 发髲

【原文】

味苦,温。

主五癃,关格不通,利小便水道,疗小儿痫,大人痓,仍自还神化。

【考据】

1. 案《说文》云:发,根也。鬓髴也。髴鬓也。或作髲。《毛诗》云:不屑髢。《笺》云:髢鬓也。仪礼云:主妇被锡。注云:被锡,读为髲髴。古者或剔贱者刑者之发,以被妇人之紒,为饰,因名髲髴焉。李当之云:是童男发,据汉人说:发髲,当是剃刑人发,或童男发本经不忍取人发用之。故用剃余也。方家至用天灵盖,害及枯骨,卒不能治病。古人所无矣。

右人一种,旧同。

【今译】

味苦,性温。

主治五种癃闭之症及关格不通,能使小便通利,能使水外泄通畅,能治疗小儿癫痫,大人抽风,能使人恢复到神妙的美好境界。

112. Fabi（发髲，human hair，Capillus）[1]

［Original Text］

［Fabi（发髲，human hair，Capillus），］ bitter in taste and warm ［in property］，［is mainly used］ to treat five ［kinds of］ stranguria and obstruction of Guange[2]，to promote urination，to cure infantile epilepsy and convulsion in adults and to return to magic transformation.

［Textual Research］

［In］ case ［analysis in the book entitled］ *Shuo Wen*（《说文》，*On Culture*），［it］ says ［that］ Fabi（发髲，human hair，Capillus） refers to the root of hair. Li Dang（李当） said，"［Fabi（发髲，human hair，Capillus）］ refers to hair from boys."

Notes

1. Fabi（发髲，human hair，Capillus） was a special use of human hair as medicinal in ancient times. Now in the field of traditional Chinese medicine，human hair is no longer used in clinical practice.

2. Guange（关格） refers to different pathological changes，dysuria，constipation，or pathological changes revealed by pulses located in Renying（人迎） and Cunkou（寸口）.

113. 龙骨

【原文】

味甘,平。

主心腹,鬼注,精物老魅,咳逆,泄利,脓血,女子漏下,症瘕坚结,小儿热气惊痫。齿主,小儿大人惊痫瘨疾狂走,心下结气,不能喘息,诸痉,杀精物。久服,轻身通神明,延年。生山谷。

【考据】

1.《吴普》曰:龙骨生晋地,山谷阴,大水所过处,是龙死骨也,青白者善,十二月采,或无时,龙骨畏干漆,蜀椒,理石,龙齿神农李氏大寒,治惊痫,久服轻身。(《御览》《大观本》节文)

2.《名医》曰:生晋地及太山,岩水岸土穴中死龙处,采无时。

3. 案《范子计然》云:龙骨生河东。

【今译】

味甘,性平。

主治心腹部鬼怪之邪所致之症,能祛除诡异之物所致之病,能治疗

113. Longgu（龙骨，loong bone，Os Loong）[1]

[Original Text]

[Longgu（龙骨，loong bone，Os Loong），] sweet in taste and mild [in property], [is mainly used] to treat [disease in] the heart and abdomen，tuberculosis，[diseases caused by] evils，cough with dyspnea，diarrhea，blood with purulent blood，vaginal bleeding，abdominal mass with hard lump，infantile epilepsy [due to] heat.

The tooth [of loong] can treat convulsion，epilepsy and manic behavior in children and adults，accumulation of Qi below the heart，difficulty to breathe，various spasm and [disease caused by pathogenic factors like] ghost. Long-term taking [of it will] invigorate mentality and spirit，and prolong life. [It] exists in mountains and valleys.

[Textual Research]

[In the book entitled] *Wu Pu Ben Cao*（《吴普本草》，*Wu Pu's Studies of Materia Medica*），[it] says [that] Longgu（龙骨，loong bone，Os Loong）[can be] found in Jindi（晋地），shady side of mountains and the areas [where] current flood runs over. [These places are] the areas [where] loong died [in ancient times]. [Loong bones that are] blue and white are effective [in treating disease]. [These bones can be] collected in December or at any time. [According to] Agriculture God（神农）and Li's（李氏），[loong

咳嗽气逆,泄泻,痢疾,脓血,女子阴道出血淋漓不断,症瘕坚硬积聚,小儿热邪所致之病,惊恐心悸,癫痫。

其齿可主治小儿大人惊恐心悸,因癫痫症而疯狂奔跑,心下气结,不能喘息,各种痉挛,能消除妖怪之物。长期服用,能使人身体轻盈,神志清晰,精神旺盛,能延年益寿。该物生长在山谷之中。

bones and teeth are] severely cold [in property] and can treat convulsion and epilepsy. Long-term taking [of it can] relax the body [as mentioned in the book entitled] *Tai Ping Yu Lan*（《太平御览》, *Imperial Studies in Taiping Times*）.

[In the book entitled] *Ming Yi Bie Lu*（《名医别录》, *Special Record of Great Doctors*）, [it] says [that Longgu（龙骨, loong bone, Os Loong) can be] found in Jindi（晋地）, Taishan（太山）and caves in the banks of rivers [where] loong died. [It can be] collected at any time.

[In the book entitled] *Fan Zi Ji Ran*（《范子计然》, *Studies About Fan Li's Teacher*）, [it] says [that] Longgu（龙骨, loong bone, Os Loong）[can be] found in Hedong（河东）

Notes

1. Longgu（龙骨, loong bone, Os Loong）actually refers to the fossils of bones of animals died in ancient times, including elephants, rhinoceros and hipparion, sweet, astringent in taste and mild in property, enterning the heart meridian, the liver meridian and the kidney meridian, effective in harmonizing the liver and subduing Yang, ceasing fright and tranquilizing spirit. Clinically it is used to treat convulsion and epilepsy, vertigo and blurred vision, palpitation, insomnia, dreaminess, seminal emission, spontaneous spermatorrhea and premature ejaculation.

114. 麝香

【原文】

味辛,温。

主辟恶气,杀鬼精物,温疟,蛊毒,痫痉,去三虫。久服除邪,不梦寤魇寐。生川谷。

【考据】

1.《名医》曰:生中台及益州雍州山中,春风取之,生者益良。

2. 案《说文》云:麝如小麋,脐有香,黑色獐也(《御览》引多三字)。

《尔雅》云:麝父麕足。郭璞云:脚似麕有香。

【今译】

味辛,性温。

能消除邪恶之气,能杀除鬼怪之病,能治疗暑热之邪所致疟

114. Shexiang（麝香，abelmusk，Moschus）[1]

[Original Text]

[Shexiang（麝香，abelmusk，Moschus），] pungent in taste and warm [in property], [is mainly used] to avoid [invasion of] evil-Qi，expel [pathogenic factors like] ghosts，to treat warm malaria，[disease caused by] worm toxin，convulsion and epilepsy，and to kill three worms[2]. Long-term taking [of it will] eliminate evils and avoid being awakened by nightmare. [It] grows in mountain valleys and river valleys.

[Textual Research]

[In the book entitled] *Ming Yi Bie Lu*（《名医别录》，*Special Record of Great Doctors*），[it] says [that Shexiang（麝香，abelmusk，Moschus）] grows in Zhongtai（中台）and mountains in Yizhou（益州）and Yongzhou（雍州）. To collect [it] in spring is more effective for cultivating health. [In] case [analysis in the book entitled] *Shuo Wen*（《说文》，*On Culture*），[it] says [that] musk（麝）is like small elk（麋）. [If its] navel is fragrant，[it is like] black roe.

Notes

1. Shexiang（麝香，abelmusk，Moschus）is an animal medicinal，pungent in taste and warm in property，entering the heart meridian，the spleen meridian and the liver meridian，effective in opening

疾，虫毒所致之病，癫痫抽搐，能祛除三种虫子。长期服用能消除

邪气，能使人睡眠中不会有噩梦惊醒。该物生长在山川河谷

之中。

orifices, preventing filth, activating the blood and dispersing binding. Clinically it is used to treat unconsciousness caused by heat disease, phlegm stagnation due to wind stroke, convulsion and epilepsy and noxious attack.

2. Three worms include roundworm, tapeworm and pinworm.

115. 牛黄

【原文】

味苦,平。

主惊痫,寒热,热盛狂痓,除邪逐鬼。生平泽。

【考据】

1.《吴普》曰:牛黄味苦无毒。牛出入呻(《御览》作鸣吼)者有之,夜有光(《御览》作夜视有光),走(《御览》有牛字),角中,牛死入胆中,如鸡子黄。(汉后书延笃传注)

2.《名医》曰:生晋地,于牛得之,即阴干,百日,使时躁,无令见日月光。

115. Niuhuang（牛黄，cow bezoar，ox gallstone，Calculus Bovis）[1]

[Original Text]

[Niuhuang（牛黄，cow bezoar，ox gallstone，Calculus Bovis），] bitter in taste and mild [in property]，[is mainly used] to treat epilepsy，cold-heat [disease]，manic behavior and convulsion [due to] exuberant heat，and to eliminate [pathogenic factors like] evils and ghosts. [It] grows in plains and swamps.

[Textual Research]

[In the book entitled] *Wu Pu Ben Cao*（《吴普本草》，*Wu Pu's Studies of Materia Medica*），[it] says [that] Niuhuang（牛黄，cow bezoar，ox gallstone，Calculus Bovis）is bitter in taste and non-toxic. The cow [that] groans [when] coming in and going out bears [bezoar] in the ears and appears bright at night. [When] the cow is dead，[it] enters the gallbladder，looking like egg yolk.

[In the book entitled] *Ming Yi Bie Lu*（《名医别录》，*Special Record of Great Doctors*），[it] says [that Niuhuang（牛黄，cow bezoar，ox gallstone，Calculus Bovis）can be] found in Jindi（晋地）from cows. [It should be] dried in the shade for one hundred days without meeting the sun and moon.

【今译】

味苦,性平。

主治惊恐心悸,癫痫,寒热疾病,治疗因热盛而疯狂抽搐,能祛除邪恶之气、鬼怪之物。该物生于平川水泽之中。

Notes

1. Niuhuang (牛黄, cow bezoar, ox gallstone, Calculus Bovis), also called Xihuang (西黄), refers to bones in a cow's gallbladder. It is bitter and sweet in taste, cool in property, entering the heart meridian and the liver meridian, effective in clearing the heart and opening orifices, resolving phlegm and ceasing fright, clearing heat and removing toxin. Clinically it is used to treat high fever with vexation, unconsciousness, delirium, epilepsy with convulsion, mania, infantile convulsion and spasm, exuberant heat phlegm, sore-throat, oral ulcer, carbuncle, furuncle and boil.

116. 熊脂

【原文】

味甘,微寒。

主风痹,不仁,筋急,五脏腹中积聚,寒热,羸瘦,头疡,白秃,面皯疱。久服,强志不饥。轻身。生山谷。

【考据】

1.《名医》曰:生雍州,十一月取。

2. 案《说文》云:熊兽似豕,山居,冬蛰。

【今译】

味甘,性微寒。

主治风痹,麻木不仁,筋脉挛急,能消解五脏及腹中积聚,能治疗寒热疾病,身体瘦弱,头部溃疡,白秃,面部黑斑。长期服用,能增强记忆力,能减少饥饿之感,能使身体轻盈。该物生长在山谷之中。

116. Xiongzhi（熊脂，bear fat，Adeps Ursi）[1]

[Original Text]

[Xiongzhi（熊脂，bear fat, Adeps Ursi），] sweet in taste and slightly cold [in property], [is mainly used] to treat wind impediment and numbness, tension of sinews, accumulation [of pathogenic factors in] the five Zang-organs and abdomen, cold-heat [disease], emaciation, ulcer in the head and facial black spots. Long-term taking [of it will] strengthen memory，[make people feel] no hunger and relax the body. [It] grows in mountains and valleys.

[Textual Research]

[In the book entitled] *Ming Yi Bie Lu* (《名医别录》，*Special Record of Great Doctors*），[it] says [that Xiongzhi（熊脂，bear fat, Adeps Ursi)] grows in Yongzhou (雍州) and [can be] collected in December.

[In] case [analysis in the book entitled] *Shuo Wen* (《说文》，*On Culture*），[it] says [that such a] bear is like a pig. [It] stays in mountains with hibernation.

Notes

1. Xiongzhi（熊脂，bear fat, Adeps Ursi）is sweet in taste and warm in property，entering the spleen meridian，the large intestine meridian and the heart meridian，effective in tonifying deficiency，strengthening sinews and bones，and moistening muscles. Clinically it is used to treat emaciation due to deficiency and damage，wind impediment，numbness of muscles，and spasm of vessels and sinews.

117. 白胶

【原文】

味甘,平。

主伤中,劳绝,腰痛,羸瘦,补中益气,妇人血闭无子,止痛,安胎。久服轻身,延年。一名鹿角胶。

【考据】

1.《名医》曰:生云中,煮鹿角作之。

2. 案《说文》云:胶,昵也,作之以皮。考工记云:鹿胶青白,牛胶火赤。郑云:皆谓煮,用其皮,或用角。

【今译】

味甘,性平。

主治内脏损伤,劳瘵,腰痛,能治疗身体瘦弱,能充实人体内脏,能

117. Baijiao（白胶，antler glue，
Colla Cornus Cervi）[1]

［Original Text］

［Baijiao（白胶，antler glue，Colla Cornus Cervi），］ sweet in taste［and］mild［in property］，［is mainly used］to treat injury of the internal organs and lumbago，to tonify the middle（the internal organs）and to replenish Qi，to relieve amenorrhea and infertility，to stop pain and to prevent miscarriage. Long-term taking［of it will］relax the body and prolong life.［It is also］called Lujiaojiao（鹿角胶）.

［Textual Research］

［In the book entitled］*Ming Yi Bie Lu*（《名医别录》, *Special Record of Great Doctors*），［it］says［that Baijiao（白胶，antler glue，Colla Cornus Cervi）is］produced in Yunzhong（云中）by boiling antlers.

［In］case［analysis in the book entitled］*Shuo Wen*（《说文》, *On Culture*），［it］says［that］glue is produced from the skin［of beer］.［According to］the records，antler glue is blue and white［while］cow glue is red and hot. Zheng Yun（郑云）said，"All that is boiled from skin or antler."

Notes

1. Baijiao（白胶，antler glue，Colla Cornus Cervi），another

补益精气，能治疗女性因血脉闭塞所致的经闭和不孕之症，能消除疼痛，能安和胎儿。长期服用，能使人身体轻盈，能延年益寿。又称为鹿角胶。

name of Lujiaojiao（鹿角胶）, sweet and salty in taste, warm in property, entering the liver meridian and the kidney meridian, effective in tonifying kidney-Yang, producing essence and blood, and ceasing bleeding. Clinically it is used to treat emaciation due to overexertion, flaccidity of the waist and knees, impotence, spontaneous spermatorrhea, premature ejaculation, infertility due to uterine coldness and anerotism.

118. 阿胶

【原文】

味甘,平。

主心腹,内崩,劳极,洒洒如疟状,腰腹痛,四肢酸疼,女子下血,安胎。久服轻身益气,一名傅致胶。

【考据】

1.《名医》曰:生平东郡煮牛皮作之,出东阿。

2. 案二胶,本经不着所出,疑本经但作胶,《名医》增白字阿字,分为二条。

上兽,上品六种,旧同。

【今译】

味甘,性平。

主治心腹部亏损,子宫出血,劳瘵,寒战如疟疾,腰腹部疼痛,四肢酸疼,能治疗女子阴道出血,能安和胎儿。长期服用,能使人身体轻盈,能补益精气。又称为傅致胶。

118. Ejiao（阿胶，ass hide glue，Colla Corii Asini）[1]

［Original Text］

［Ejiao（阿胶，ass hide glue，Colla Corii Asini），］ sweet in taste ［and］ mild ［in property］，［is mainly used］ to treat ［disease in the］ heart and abdomen，uterine bleeding，［disease due to］ overexertion like malaria，pain of the waist and abdomen，pain of the four limbs，vaginal bleeding ［during menstruation］ and threatened abortion. Long-term taking ［of it will］ relax the body and replenish Qi. ［It is also］ called Fuzhijiao（傅致胶）.

［Textual Research］

［In the book entitled］ *Ming Yi Bie Lu*（《名医别录》，*Special Record of Great Doctors*），［it］ says ［that Ejiao（阿胶，ass hide glue，Colla Corii Asini）is］ produced in Dong'e（东阿）district in Pingdong（平东）by boiling cow skin.

Notes

1. Ejiao（阿胶，ass hide glue，Colla Corii Asini）is sweet in taste and mild in property，entering the kidney meridian，effective in tonifying the blood，ceasing bleeding，nourishing Yin and preventing threatened abortion. Clinically it is used to treat dispiritedness and jaundice due to blood deficiency，vertigo，palpitation，asthenic overstrain，hematoptysis，hematemesis，hematuria，vaginal bleeding and threatened abortion.

119. 丹雄鸡

【原文】

味甘,微温。

主女人崩中,漏下赤白沃,补虚,温中,止血,通神,杀毒,辟不祥。

头,主杀鬼,东门上者尤良。

肪,主耳聋。

肠,主遗溺。

肶胵裹黄皮,主泄利。

尿白,主消渴伤寒,寒热。

黑雌鸡,主风寒湿痹,五缓六急,安胎。

翮羽,主下血闭。

鸡子,主除热,火疮痫痓,可作虎魄,神物。

鸡白蠹,肥脂。

生平泽。

【考据】

1.《吴普》曰:丹鸡卵可作琥珀。(《御览》)

119. Danxiongji（丹雄鸡，red cock，Galli Maris Rubrum）[1]

[Original Text]

[Danxiongji（丹雄鸡，red cock，Galli Maris Rubrum），] sweet in taste and slightly warm [in property]，[is mainly used] to stop sudden internal bleeding and vaginal discharge of red and white fluid in women，to improve deficiency，to warm the middle（the internal organs），to cease bleeding，invigorate spirit，to eliminate toxin and to avoid ominous [elements].

The head [of chicken can] expel [pathogenic factors like] ghosts. [The one that stays in] the east gate is better.

The fat [of chicken can] treat deafness.

The intestines [of chicken can] treat enuresis.

The endothelium [of chicken's gizzard can] treat diarrhea.

The white droppings [of chicken can] treat wasting-thirst，cold damage and cold-heat [disease].

Black hen can treat wind-cold dampness impediment，five [kinds of] retardations[2]，six [kinds of] extreme [syndromes/patterns][3] and threatened abortion.

Stiff feathers [of chicken can] treat amenorrhea.

The egg [can] eliminate heat，treat scalded sore，epilepsy and convulsion. [It can be made into] magic product like a tiger.

White fat of chicken like moth [also can be used as medicinal].

2.《名医》曰：生朝鲜。

3. 案《说文》云：鸡知时畜也。籀文作鸡，肪，肥也。肠，大小肠也。膍鸟胵，胵鸟胃也。工菌，粪也。翮羽，茎也。羽，鸟长毛也，此作肶，省文，尿，即屎字，古文，从。亦菌假音字也。

【今译】

味甘，性微温。

主治女子体内突然出血，阴道淋漓不断和赤白带下，能补益虚弱之症，能温煦人体脏器，能阻止出血，能使神气通畅，能消杀毒气，能消除不祥之气。

鸡头，能杀除鬼怪之病，处在东门上的鸡，其头效果更好。

鸡的脂肪，能主治耳聋。

鸡肠，能主治遗尿。

鸡内金，能主治泄泻和痢疾。

鸡的白屎，能主治伤寒及寒热疾病。

黑母鸡，能主治风寒湿邪所致之痹证，小儿五迟和六种损伤，安和胎儿。

硬性鸡毛，能主治瘀血闭经。

鸡蛋，能主治热邪所致之病，能治疗因火烧所致之疮疡痈痉，可做成如虎一样的神气之物。

鸡白蠹，即鸡之肥脂，亦可入药。

该物生长在平川水泽之中。

〔This kind of chicken〕lives〔in the areas around〕plains and swamps.

〔**Textual Research**〕

〔In the book entitled〕*Wu Pu Ben Cao*（《吴普本草》，*Wu Pu's Studies of Materia Medica*），〔it〕says〔that〕Danxiongji（丹雄鸡，red cock，Galli Maris Rubrum）can be used as Hupo（琥珀，amber Succinum）〔according to the book entitled〕*Tai Ping Yu Lan*（《太平御览》，*Imperial Studies in Taiping Times*）.

〔In the book entitled〕*Ming Yi Bie Lu*（《名医别录》，*Special Record of Great Doctors*），〔it〕says〔that Danxiongji（丹雄鸡，red cock，Galli Maris Rubrum）can be〕found in Chaoxian（朝鲜）.

Notes

1. Danxiongji（丹雄鸡，red cock，Galli Maris Rubrum）refers to chicken as food，sweet in taste and warm in property，entering the spleen meridian and the stomach meridian，effective in tonifying the middle（the internal organs）and replenishing Qi. Clinically it is used to treat emaciation due to asthenic overstrain，indigestion and anorexia after illness，flooding and spotting（metrorrhagia and metrostaxis）in women and hypogalactia.

2. Please see〔2〕in 102.

3. Please see〔3〕in 102.

120. 雁肪

【原文】

味甘,平。

主风挛,拘急,偏枯,气不通利。久服,益气不饥,轻身耐老。一名
鹜肪。生池泽。

【考据】

1.《吴普》曰:雁肪神农岐伯雷公甘无毒(《御览》有鹜肪二字,当作
一名鹜肪),杀诸石药毒。(《御览》引云:采无时)

2.《名医》曰:生江南,取无时。

3. 案《说文》云:雁,鹅也。鹜,舒凫,也。《广雅》云:鸭鹜,仓鸭雁
也。凫,鹜鸭也。《尔雅》云:舒雁,鹅。郭璞云:礼《记》曰,出如舒雁。
今江东呼鸭,又舒凫,鹜。郭璞云:鸭也。方言云:雁,自关而东,谓之鸭
鹅。南楚之外,谓之鹅,或谓之仓鸭。据《说文》云:别有雁,以为鸿雁字
无鸭字,鸭,即雁之急音,此雁肪,即鹅鸭脂也。当作雁字,《名医》不晓,
别出鹜肪条,又出白鸭鹅条,反疑此为鸿雁,何其谬也。陶苏皆乱说之。

上禽,上品二种,旧同。

120. Yanfang（雁肪，fat of white fronted goose，Adeps Anseris Albifrondis）[1]

[Original Text]

［Yanfang（雁肪，fat of white fronted goose，Adeps Anseris Albifrondis），］sweet in taste［and］mild［in property］，［is mainly used］to treat wind tension，spasm，paralysis and obstruction of Qi. Long-term taking［of it will］replenish Qi，［make people feel］no hunger，relax the body and prevent aging.［It is also］called Wufang（鹜肪），growing in lakes and swamps.

[Textual Research]

447

［In the book entitled］*Wu Pu Ben Cao*（《吴普本草》，*Wu Pu's Studies of Materia Medica*），［it］says［that］Yanfang（雁肪，fat of white fronted goose，Adeps Anseris Albifrondis），［according to］Agriculture God（神农），Qibo（岐伯）and Leigong（雷公），［is］sweet［in taste］and non-toxic［in property］，and［can］remove various stone toxin.

［In the book entitled］*Ming Yi Bie Lu*（《名医别录》，*Special Record of Great Doctors*），［it］says［that Yanfang（雁肪，fat of white fronted goose，Adeps Anseris Albifrondis）is］produced in Jiangnan（江南）and can be collected at any time.

【今译】

味甘,性平。

主治因风袭所致的挛紧拘急,半身不遂,气不通利。长期服用,能补益精气,能减少饥饿之感,能使身体轻盈,不易衰老。又称为鹜肪。该物生长在池泽中。

Notes

1. Yanfang (雁肪, fat of white fronted goose, Adeps Anseris Albifrondis) is sweet in taste, mild and non-toxic in property. It can treat wind tension, spasm, paralysis, stagnation of Qi and blood, deafness, overstrain and madarosis.

121. 石蜜

【原文】

味甘,平。

主心腹邪气,诸惊痫痓,安五脏,诸不足,益气补中,止痛解毒,除众病,和百药。久服,强志轻身,不饥不老。一名石饴。生山谷。

【考据】

1.《吴普》曰:石蜜,神农雷公甘气平,生河源或河梁。(《御览》又一引云:生武都山谷)

2.《名医》曰:生武都河源及诸山石中,色白如膏者,良。

3. 案《说文》云:蠲蜂,甘饴也。一曰螟子,或作蜜。《中山经》云:平逢之山多沙石,实惟蜂蜜之庐。郭璞云:蜜,赤蜂名。西京杂记云:南越王献高帝石蜜五斛。玉篇云:蠲蠡,甘饴也。苏恭云:当去石字。

【今译】

味甘,性平。

主治心腹部邪气,能消解各种惊风、癫痫和抽搐,能安静五脏,能治

121. Shimi（石蜜，Chinese honey bee，Apis）[1]

[Original Text]

[Shimi（石蜜，Chinese honey bee，Apis），] sweet in taste [and] mild [in property], [is mainly used] to treat [disease caused by] evil-Qi in the heart and abdomen and various fright，epilepsy and convulsion，to harmonize the five Zang-organs，[to improve] insufficiency [caused by] various [diseases]，to replenish Qi，to tonify the middle (internal organs)，to stop pain，to remove toxin，to eliminate various diseases and to regulate different medicinals. Long-term taking [of it will] strengthen memory，relax the body，[make people feel] no hunger and prevent aging. [It is also] called Shiyi（石饴）and found in mountains and valleys.

[Textual Research]

[In the book entitled] *Wu Pu Ben Cao*（《吴普本草》，*Wu Pu's Studies of Materia Medica*），[it] says [that] Shimi（石蜜，Chinese honey bee，Apis），[according to] Agriculture God（神农）and Leigong（雷公），[is] sweet [in taste] and mild [in property]，to be found in rivers and bridges. [In the book entitled] *Tai Ping Yu Lan* (《太平御览》，*Imperial Studies in Taiping Times*），[it] says [that Shimi（石蜜，Chinese honey bee，Apis）can be] found in mountains and valleys in Wudu（武都）.

[In the book entitled] *Ming Yi Bie Lu*（《名医别录》，*Special*

疗各种不足之症,能补益精气,能充实人体内脏,能消除疼痛,能消解毒气,能祛除各种疾病,能调和各种药物。长期服用,能增强记忆力,能使身体轻盈,能减少饥饿之感,能长寿不老。又称为石饴。该物生长在山谷之中。

神农本草经

452

Record of Great Doctors），［it］says［that Shimi（石蜜，Chinese honey bee，Apis）can be］found in the rivers and stones in the mountains in Wudu（武都）.［If it is］as white as paste，［it is］more effective.

［In］case［analysis in the book entitled］*Shuo Wen*（《说文》，*On Culture*），［it］says［that］Shimi（石蜜，Chinese honey bee，Apis）means maltose，also called Mingzi（螟子）or Zuomi（作蜜）.

Notes

1. Shimi（石蜜，Chinese honey bee，Apis）is sweet in taste and mild in property，entering the lung meridian，the spleen meridian and the large intestine meridian，effective in moistening the lung，moistening the intestines，tonifying the middle（internal organs），removing toxin and invigorating body assistance. Clinically it is used to treat dry cough due to lung dryness，cough due to lung deficiency，constipation due to intestinal dryness and ulcer.

122. 蜂子

【原文】

味甘,平。

主风头,除蛊毒,补虚羸伤中。久服,令人光泽,好颜色,不老。

大黄蜂子,主心腹胀满痛,轻身益气。土蜂子,主痈肿。一名蜚零。生山谷。

【考据】

1.《名医》曰:生武都。

2. 案《说文》云:蜂,飞虫螫人者。古文省作蜂。《广雅》云:蠓翁,蜂也。又上蜂,蚳蜱也。《尔雅》云:土蜂。郭璞云:今江南大蜂在地中作房者为土蜂,唉其子即马蜂,今荆巴间呼为蟺,又木蜂。郭璞云:似土蜂而小,在树上作房,江东亦呼为木蜂,又食其子。礼记檀弓云:范则冠。郑云:范蜂也。方言云:蜂,燕赵之间,谓之蠓蟓,其小者,谓之蟓,或谓之蚴蜕,其大而蜜。谓之壶蜂。郭璞云:今黑蜂,穿竹木作孔,亦有蜜者,或呼笛师,按蜂名为范者声相近,若《司马相如赋》,以泛为枫。左传:沨沨即汛汛也。

122. Fengzi（蜂子，larva of Chinese honey bee，Larva Apis）[1]

［Original Text］

［Fengzi（蜂子，larva of Chinese honey bee，Larva Apis），］sweet in taste and mild［in property］，［is mainly used］to treat［invasion of pathogenic］wind into the head，to remove worm toxin，to tonify emaciation and to cure damage of the middle（the internal organs）. Long-term taking［of it will］glow the face，luster the skin and prevent aging.

Larva of yellow bee can treat distension，fullness and pain of the heart and abdomen. Larva of local bee can treat carbuncle and swelling.［It is also］called Feiling（蜚零）and［can be］found in mountains and valleys.

［Textual Research］

［In the book entitled］*Ming Yi Bie Lu*（《名医别录》，*Special Record of Great Doctors*），［it］says［that Fengzi（蜂子，larva of Chinese honey bee，Larva Apis）can be］found in Wudu（武都）

［In］case［analysis in the book entitled］*Shuo Wen*（《说文》，*On Culture*），［it］says［that Fengzi（蜂子，larva of Chinese honey bee，Larva Apis）］refers to the bee that stings people.［It was］simply called Feng（蜂）in ancient literature.［In the book entitled］*Guang Ya*（《广雅》，*The First Chinese Encyclopedic Dictionary*），

【今译】

味甘,性平。

主治因风侵袭所致头痛,能消除虫毒所致疾病,能补益虚弱消瘦,能治疗内脏损伤。长期服用,能令人面容光华,能使面部色彩美丽,能长寿不老。

大黄蜂子,主治心腹胀满疼痛,能使人身体轻盈,能补益精气。

土蜂子,主治痈肿。

又称为蜚零。该物生长在山谷之中。

［it］says ［that the so-called］Meng（蠓）actually refers to bee. Guo Pu（郭璞）said，"The large bees in Jiangnan（江南）［that］make honeycomb over land are called local bees. ［Those that］eat their larvae are called hornets." Guo Pu（郭璞）said，"［The bees that look］like local bees but are smaller ［than local bees］make honeycomb over trees. ［People in］Jiangdong（江东）call ［such bees］wood bees ［which］also eat their larvae."

Notes

1. Fengzi（蜂子，larva of Chinese honey bee，Larva Apis）is sweet in taste and mild in property，effective in expelling wind，removing toxin and killing worms. Clinically it is used to treat head-wind disease，leprosy，erysipelas，abdominal pain due to accumulation of worms and leucorrhea.

123. 蜜蜡

【原文】

味甘,微温。

主下利脓血,补中,续绝伤,金疮,益气,不饥,耐老。生山谷。

【考据】

1.《名医》曰:生武都蜜房木石间。

2. 案西京杂记云:南越王献高帝蜜蜡,二百枚。玉篇云:蜡,蜜滓。

陶宏景云:白蜡生于蜜中。故谓蜜蜡。《说文》无蜡字。张有云:腊别蜡,非,旧作蜡,今据改。

【今译】

味甘,性微温。

主治痢疾脓血,能补充人体内脏,能通过补益主治外伤所致之筋伤骨折,因金属疮伤而导致的痛疮,能补益精气,能减少饥饿感,能使人不易衰老。该物生长在山谷之中。

123. Mila（蜜蜡，beeswax，Cera Flava）[1]

[Original Text]

[Mila（蜜蜡，beeswax，Cera Flava），] sweet in taste and slightly warm [in property], [is mainly used] to relieve diarrhea with pus and blood, to tonify the middle (internal organs), to treat severe injury and trauma [caused by] metal, to replenish Qi, [to enable people to feel] no hunger and to prevent aging. [It can be] collected in mountains and valleys.

[Textual Research]

[In the book entitled] *Ming Yi Bie Lu*（《名医别录》，*Special Record of Great Doctors*），[it] says [that Mila（蜜蜡，beeswax，Cera Flava）can be] found in the honeycombs over trees and in stones in Wudu（武都）. Tao Hongjing（陶宏景）said，"White wax is produced from honey. That is why it is called beeswax."

Notes

1. Mila（蜜蜡，beeswax，Cera Flava）is sweet and bland in taste，mild in property，effective in restraining sore and ulcer，strengthening muscles，stopping pain and removing toxin. Clinically it is used to treat sore，ulcer and carbuncle that are difficult to resolve，ecthyma and scald.

124. 牡蛎

【原文】

味咸,平。

主伤寒寒热,温疟洒洒,惊恚怒气,除拘缓鼠瘘,女子带下赤白。久服,强骨节,杀邪气,延年。一名蛎蛤,生池泽。

【考据】

1.《名医》曰:一名牡蛤,生东海,采无时。

2. 案《说文》云:蚝,蚌属。似螖,微大,出海中,今民食之,读苦赖又云:蜃属,有三,皆生于海,蛤厉,千岁雀所化,秦谓之牡蛎。

【今译】

味咸,性平。

主治伤寒病,寒热疾病,暑热之邪所致的疟疾,颤栗恶寒,惊恐愤

124. Muli（牡蛎，oyster shell，Concha Ostreae）[1]

[Original Text]

[Muli（牡蛎，oyster shell，Concha Ostreae），] salty in taste and [in property], [is mainly used] to treat cold damage [with aversion to] cold and fever，warm malaria [with aversion to cold and] shivering and [disease marked by] fright，resentment and anger，to eliminate contracture，to relieve scrofula，and to resolve red and white leucorrhea. Long-term taking [of it will] strengthen joints，expel evil-Qi and prolong life. [It is also] called Lige（蛎蛤）[and can be] found in lakes and swamps.

[Textual Research]

[In the book entitled] M*ing Yi Bie Lu* (《名医别录》，*Special Record of Great Doctors*)，[it] says [that Muli（牡蛎，oyster shell，Concha Ostreae）]，also called Muge（牡蛤），[can be] found in Donghai（东海，East Sea）and collected at any time.

[In] case [analysis in the book entitled] *Shuo Wen* (《说文》，*On Culture*)，[it] says [that] Chai（虿，scorpion），pertaining to Bang（蚌，clam）and looking like Lian（蠊，similar to clam），is a little big [and can be] collected from the sea and edible.

Notes

1. Muli（牡蛎，oyster shell，Concha Ostreae）is salty in taste，

怒,能消除拘急,能使其和缓,能治疗瘰疬及女子赤白带下。长期服用,

能强壮骨节,能消杀邪气,能使人延年益寿。又称为蛎蛤,该物生长在

池泽中。

astringent and cool in property, entering the liver meridian and the kidney meridian, effective in relieving vertigo, epilepsy, convulsion, palpitation and insomnia. Clinically it is used to treat night sweating, seminal emission, spontaneous spermatorrhea, premature ejaculation, flooding and spotting (metrorrhagia and metrostaxis) in women, leucorrhea, scrofula, goiter, tumor and excessive gastric acid.

125. 龟甲

【原文】

味咸,平。

主漏下赤白,破症瘕,痎疟,五痔,阴蚀,湿痹,四肢重弱,小儿囟不合。久服,轻身不饥。一名神屋。生池泽。

【考据】

1.《名医》曰:生南海及湖水中,采无时。

2. 案《广雅》云:介,龟也。高诱注淮南云:龟壳,龟甲也。

【今译】

味咸,性平。

主治阴道出血淋漓不断,赤白带下,能破除症瘕,能治疗疟疾,五种痔,阴部溃疡,湿邪所致之痹证,四肢沉重虚弱,小儿囟门不合。长期服用,能使人身体轻盈,能减少饥饿感。又称为神屋。该物生长在池泽中。

125. Guijia (龟甲, tortoise shell and plastron, Carapax et Plastrum Testudinis) [1]

[Original Text]

[Guijia (龟甲, tortoise shell and plastron, Carapax et Plastrum Testudinis),] salty in taste and mild [in property], [is mainly used] to treat red and white flooding and spotting, in women, abdominal mass, malaria, five [kinds of] hemorrhoids, vulva ulcer, dampness impediment, heaviness and weakness of the four limbs and infantile metopism. Long-term taking [of it will] relax the body and [make people feel] no hunger. [It is also] called Shenwu (神屋) and [can be] found in lakes and swamps.

[Textual Research]

[In the book entitled] *Ming Yi Bie Lu* (《名医别录》, *Special Record of Great Doctors*), [it] says [that Guijia (龟甲, tortoise shell and plastron, Carapax et Plastrum Testudinis) can be] found in Nanhai (南海, Southern Sea) and lakes, and collected at any time.

Notes

1. Guijia (龟甲, tortoise shell and plastron, Carapax et Plastrum Testudinis) is salty and sweet in taste, mild in property, entering the liver meridian and the kidney meridian, effective in enriching Yin and subduing Yang, tonifying Yin and stopping bleeding, replenishing the kidney and fortifying bones. Clinically it is used to treat seminal emission, spontaneous spermatorrhea, premature ejaculation, wilting of bones, five kinds of retardation and five kinds of flaccidity in children.

126. 桑蜱蛸

【原文】

味咸,平。

主伤中,疝瘕,阴痿,益精生子,女子血闭,腰痛,通五淋,利小便水道。一名蚀疣,生桑枝上,采,蒸之。

【考据】

1.《吴普》曰:桑蛸条,一名(今本脱此二字),蚀疣,一名害焦,一名致,神农咸无毒。(《御览》)

2.《名医》曰:螳螂子也,二月三月采,火炙。

3. 案《说文》云:蜱,蜱蛸也,或作蜱蛸,虫蛸,螂子。《广雅》云:蟥蟭,乌涕,冒焦,螵蛸也。《尔雅》云:不过蟷蠰,其子蜱蛸。郭璞云:一名蟥焦,螳蠰卵也。范子计然云:螵蛸出三辅,上价三百,旧作螵,声相近,字之误也。玉篇云:蜱同螵。

【今译】

味咸,性平。

126. Sangpixiao（桑蜱蛸，mantis larva，
Larva Tenodera seu Statilia）[1]

[Original Text]

[Sangpixiao（桑蜱蛸，mantis larva，Larva Tenodera seu Statilia），] salty in taste and mild [in property]，[is mainly used] to relieve damage of the internal organs，abdominal mass and impotence，to replenish essence to conceive baby，to treat amenorrhea，lumbago and five [kinds of] stranguria[2]，and to disinhibit urination. [It]，also called Shiyou（蚀疣），grows in the branches of mulberry and [can be] collected and steamed [for medical purpose].

467

[Textual Research]

[In the book entitled] *Wu Pu Ben Cao*（《吴普本草》，*Wu Pu's Studies of Materia Medica*），[it] says [that] Sangpixiao（桑蜱蛸，mantis larva，Larva Tenodera seu Statilia）[is also] called Shiyou（蚀疣），Haijiao（害焦）and Zhi（致）. [According to] Agriculture God（神农），[it is] salty [in taste] and non-toxic [in property].

[In the book entitled] *Ming Yi Bie Lu*（《名医别录》，*Special Record of Great Doctors*），[it] says [that Sangpixiao（桑蜱蛸）] refers to the larva of mantis. [It can be] collected in February and March，and broiled [for medical purpose].

主治内脏损伤，疝瘕，阳痿，能补益精气，能使人生育子女，能治疗女子经闭，腰痛，能消解五种淋证，能使小便通畅，能疏通水道。又称为蚀疣，生长在桑枝之上，采集后要蒸一下。

Notes

1. Sangpixiao （桑蜱蛸，mantis larva, Larva Tenodera seu Statilia) is sweet and salty in taste, mild in property, entering the liver meridian and the kidney meridian, effective in tonifying the kidney, assisting Yang, securing essence and restraining urination. Clinically it is used to treat seminal emission due to insufficiency of kidney-Yang, spontaneous spermatorrhea, premature ejaculation, leucorrhea, frequent urination and enuresis.

2. Five kinds of stranguria include heat stranguria, stony stranguria, bony stranguria, overstrained stranguria and bloody stranguria.

127. 海蛤

【原文】

味苦,平。

主咳逆上气,喘息烦满,胸痛,寒热。一名魁蛤。

【考据】

1.《吴普》曰:海蛤,神农苦,岐伯甘,扁鹊咸,大节头有文,文如磨齿,采无时。

2.《名医》口:生南海。

3. 案《说文》云:蛤,蜃属,海蛤者,百岁燕所化,魁蛤,一名复累老服翼所化。《尔雅》云:魁陆。郭璞云:本草云,魁,状如海蛤,园而厚朴有理纵横,即今之蚶也。《周礼》鳖人供蠯郑司农云:蠯,蛤也。杜子春云:蠯蜯也。周书王会云:东越海蛤。孔晁云:蛤,文蛤。按《名医》别出海蛤条云:一名魁陆,一名活东,非。

127.　Haige（海蛤，clam shell，
Concha Meretricis seu Cyclinae）[1]

[Original Text]

[Haige（海蛤，clam shell，Concha Meretricis seu Cyclinae），] bitter in taste and mild [in property], [is mainly used] to treat cough with dyspnea and upward counterflow of Qi, panting, vexation, chest pain and cold-heat [disease]. [It is also] called Kuige（魁蛤）.

[Textual Research]

[In the book entitled] *Wu Pu Ben Cao*（《吴普本草》，*Wu Pu's Studies of Materia Medica*），[it] says [that] Haige（海蛤，clam shell，Concha Meretricis seu Cyclinae），[according to] Agriculture God （神农），[it is] bitter [in taste]；[according to Qibo（岐伯），[it is] sweet [in taste]；[according to] Bianque（扁鹊），[it is] salty [in taste]. There is texture like rubbed teeth at the tip of the large shell. [It can be] collected at any time.

[In the book entitled] *Ming Yi Bie Lu*（《名医别录》，*Special Record of Great Doctors*），[it] says [that Haige（海蛤，clam shell，Concha Meretricis seu Cyclinae）] exists in Nanhai（南海，South Sea）.

【今译】

味苦,性平。

主治咳嗽及呼吸困难,能消除喘息,烦躁,郁闷,胸痛,能治疗寒热性疾病。又称为魁蛤。

Notes

1. Haige（海蛤，clam shell，Concha Meretricis seu Cyclinae）is bitter and salty in taste，mild and non-toxic in property. Clinically it is used to treat cough with dyspnea，panting，vexation，chest pain，cold-heat disease，wind stroke，paralysis，cold damage and edema with fever.

128. 文蛤

【原文】

主恶疮,蚀(《御览》作除阴蚀),五痔(《御览》下有大孔出血,《大观本》,作黑字)。

神农本草经

【考据】

1.《名医》曰:生东海,表有文,采无时。

【今译】

主治恶性痈疮,阴部蚀疮及五种痔疮。

128. Wenge（文蛤，meretrix clam shell，Concha Meretricis）[1]

［**Original Text**］

［Wenge（文蛤，meretrix clam shell，Concha Meretricis）］ treats severe sore and five ［kinds of］ hemorrhoids.

［**Textual Research**］

［In the book entitled］ *Ming Yi Bie Lu*（《名医别录》，*Special Record of Great Doctors*），［it］ says ［that Wenge（文蛤，meretrix clam shell，Concha Meretricis）］ exists in Donghai（东海，East Sea）with texture in the superficies and ［can be］ collected at any time.

Notes

1. Wenge（文蛤，meretrix clam shell，Concha Meretricis）is salty in taste，mild and non-toxic in property. Clinically it is used to treat severe sore，five kinds of hemorrhoids，cough with dyspnea，chest impediment，lumbago and ulcerated scrofula.

129. 蠡鱼（初学记引作鳢鱼）

【原文】

味甘,寒。

主湿痹,面目浮肿,下大水。一名鲖鱼。生池泽。

【考据】

1.《名医》曰:生九江,采无时。

2. 案《说文》云:鳢,鲖也。鲖,鳢也。读若裤桄。《广雅》云:鲡,鳎鲖也。《尔雅》云:鳢。郭璞云:鲖也。《毛诗》云:鲂鳢。《传》云:鳢鲖也。据《说文》云:鳢鳢也。与鳢不同,而毛苌。郭璞以鲖释鳢,与许不合。然初学记引此亦作鳢,盖二字音同,以讹舛,不可得详。《广雅》又作鲡,亦音之讹。又广志云:豚鱼,一名鲖(《御览》),更异解也。

3. 又陆玑云:鳢即鲍鱼也。似鳢,狭厚,今京东人犹呼鳢鱼,又本草衍义曰。蠡鱼,今人谓之黑鲤鱼,道家以为头有星为厌,据此诸说,若作鲤字,《说文》所云鲖。

4. 广志以为江豚,本草衍义以为黑鲤鱼,若作鲤字,《说文》以为

129. Liyu（蠡鱼，serpent-head meat，Caro Ophiocephalus Argus Cantor）[1]

［Original Text］

［Liyu（蠡鱼，serpent-head meat，Caro Ophiocephalus Argus Cantor），］sweet in taste and cold［in property］，［is mainly used］to treat dampness impediment，to relieve dropsy of face and eyes and to eliminate severe dampness.［It can be］found in lakes and swamps.

［Textual Research］

［In the book entitled］*Ming Yi Bie Lu*（《名医别录》，*Special Record of Great Doctors*），［it］says［that Liyu（蠡鱼，serpent-head meat，Caro Ophiocephalus Argus Cantor）can be］found in Jiujiang（九江）and［can be］collected at any time.

Notes

1. Liyu（蠡鱼，serpent-head meat，Caro Ophiocephalus Argus Cantor）is sweet in taste and cold in property，entering the spleen meridian，the stomach meridian，the lung meridian and the kidney meridian，effective in tonifying the spleen and replenishing the stomach，promoting urination and resolving swelling. Clinically it is used to treat dropsy of the body and face，edema during pregnancy，dampness impediment，beriberi，lack of milk after delivery of

477

鲡。《广雅》以为鳗鲡。陆玑以为鲍鱼,说各不同,难以详究。

【今译】

味甘,性寒。

主治湿邪所致痹证,能消除面目浮肿,能清除严重水肿。又称为鲖
鱼。该物生长在池泽中。

baby, habitual abortion, tuberculosis, distension and fullness of the gastric region, bloody stool due to wind in the intestines, hemorrhoids and scabies.

130. 鲤鱼胆

【原文】

味苦,寒。

主目热赤痛青盲,明目。久服,强悍益志气。生池泽。

【考据】

1.《名医》曰:生九江,采无时。

2. 案《说文》云:鲤,鱣也。鱣,鲤也。《尔雅》云:鲤鱣.舍人云:鲤,一名鱣.郭璞注鲤云:今赤鲤鱼。注鱣云:大鱼似鲟。《毛诗》云:鱣鲔发发。《传》云:鱣,鲤也,据此知郭璞别为二,非矣。古今注云:兖州人呼赤鲤为赤骥,谓青鲤为青马,黑鲤为元驹,白鲤为白骐,黄鲤为黄雉。

上虫,鱼。上品一十种,旧同。

【今译】

味苦,性寒。

主治热邪伤眼,眼睛赤痛,能治疗青盲症,能使眼睛明亮。长期服用,能使人强壮勇悍,能使记忆力增强。该物生长在池泽中。

130. Liyudan（鲤鱼胆，carp gall，Fel Cyprinus Carpio）[1]

[Original Text]

[Liyudan（鲤鱼胆，carp gall，Fel Cyprinus Carpio），] bitter in taste and cold [in property], [is mainly used] to treat redness, pain and blue blindness of the eyes [caused by] heat, and to improve vision. Long-term taking [of it will] forcefully strengthen the body and replenish will. [It] exists in lakes and swamps.

[Textual Research]

[In the book entitled] *Ming Yi Bie Lu* （《名医别录》，*Special Record of Great Doctors*），[it] says [that Liyudan（鲤鱼胆，carp gall，Fel Cyprinus Carpio）] exists in Jiujiang（九江）and [can be] collected at any time.

Notes

1. Liyudan（鲤鱼胆，carp gall，Fel Cyprinus Carpio）is sweet in taste and mild in property, entering the spleen meridian and the kidney meridian, effective in promoting urination and resolving swelling, descending Qi and promoting lactation. Clinically it is used to treat edema, distension, jaundice, diarrhea, dysentery, cough with dyspnea and agalactia.

131. 藕实茎

【原文】

味甘,平。

主补中养神,益气力,除百疾。久服,轻身耐老,不饥延年。一名水芝丹。生池泽。

【考据】

1.《名医》曰:一名莲,生汝南,八月采。

2. 案《说文》云:藕,夫渠根。莲,夫渠之实也。茄,夫渠茎。《尔雅》云:荷,芙渠。郭璞云:别名芙蓉,江东呼荷,又其茎茄,其实莲。郭璞云:莲谓房也,又其根藕。

【今译】

味甘,性平。

131. Oushijing（藕实茎，large rhizome of hindu lotus，Rhizoma Nelumbinis）[1]

［Original Text］

［Oushijing（藕实茎，large rhizome of hindu lotus，Rhizoma Nelumbinis），］sweet in taste ［and］ mild ［in property］，［is mainly used］ to tonify the middle (internal organs)，to nourish the spirit，to replenish Qi and energy，and to eliminate all diseases. Long-term taking ［of it will］ relax the body，prevent aging，［make people feel］ no hunger and prolong life. ［It is also］ called Shuizhidan（水芝丹），growing in lakes and swamps.

［Textual Research］

［In the book entitled］ *Ming Yi Bie Lu*（《名医别录》，*Special Record of Great Doctors*），［it］ says ［that Oushijing（藕实茎，large rhizome of hindu lotus，Rhizoma Nelumbinis），also］ called Lian（莲），grows in Runan（汝南）and ［can be］ collected in August.

Guo Pu（郭璞云）said，"［Its］ another name is Furong（芙蓉）. ［It is also］ called He（荷）in Jiangdong（江东）. ［Its］ stalk ［is called］ Qie（茄）and ［its］ fruit ［is called］ Lian（莲）."

Notes

1. Oushijing（藕实茎，large rhizome of hindu lotus，Rhizoma Nelumbinis）is a herbal medicinal，sweet in taste and cold in

能充实人体内脏，能滋养神气，能补益气力，能消除百病。长期服用，能使人身体轻盈，不易衰老，能减少饥饿感，能延年益寿。又称为水芝丹。该物生长在池泽中。

property, entering the heart meridian, the spleen meridian and the kidney meridian, effective in clearing heat and producing fluid, cooling the blood and dispersing stasis. Clinically it is used to treat heat disease with vexation, hemoptysis, hematemesis, hematochezia and hematuria.

132. 大枣

【原文】

味甘,平。

主心腹邪气,安中,养脾,助十二经,平胃气,通九窍,补少气,少津液,身中不足,大惊,四肢重,和百药。久服轻身长年。

叶,覆麻黄,能令出汗。生平泽。

【考据】

1.《吴普》曰:枣主调中,益脾气,令人好颜色,美志气。(《大观本草》引吴氏本草)

2.《名医》曰:一名干枣,一名美枣,一名良枣,八月采,曝干,生河东。

3. 案《说文》云:枣,羊枣也。《尔雅》云:遵羊枣。郭璞云:实小而圆,紫黑色,今俗呼之为羊矢枣,又洗大枣。郭璞云:今河东猗氏县,出大枣子,如鸡卵。

132. Dazao（大枣，jujube，Fructus Ziziphi Jujubae）[1]

[Original Text]

[Dazao（大枣，jujube，Fructus Ziziphi Jujubae），] sweet in taste and mild [in property], [is mainly used]] to relieve evil-Qi in the heart and abdomen, to harmonize the middle (internal organs), to nourish the spleen, to assist the twelve meridians, to pacify stomach-Qi, to disinhibit the nine orifices, to improve insufficiency of Qi, fluid and [energy in] the body, to treat severe fright [disorder] and heaviness of the four limbs, and to regulate all medicinals. Long-term taking [of it will] relax the body and prolong life.

[In] inducing sweating, [the effect of its] leaves is better [than that of] Mahuang（麻黄，ephedra，Herba Ephedrae）. [It] grows in plains and swamps.

[Textual Research]

[In the book entitled] *Wu Pu Ben Cao*（《吴普本草》，*Wu Pu's Studies of Materia Medica*），[it] says [that] jujube can regulate the middle (internal organs), replenish spleen-Qi, luster facial expression and invigorate memory.

[In the book entitled] *Ming Yi Bie Lu*（《名医别录》，*Special Record of Great Doctors*），[it] says [that Dazao（大枣，jujube，Fructus Ziziphi Jujubae）is also] called Ganzao（干枣，dry jujube），

【今译】

味甘,性平。

主治心腹部邪气,能安和内脏,能滋养脾气,能充实十二经,能平和胃气,能使九窍畅通,能治疗少气,津液不足,身体虚弱,惊恐,四肢沉重,能调和各种药物。长期服用能使人身体轻盈,能增加寿命。

大枣叶能发汗,其作用超过麻黄。该物生长在平川水泽之中。

Meizao（美枣，fragrant jujube）and Liangzao（良枣，excellent jujube）. [It] grows in Hedong（河东）and [can be] collected in August and dried in the sun.

Notes

1. Dazao（大枣，jujube，Fructus Ziziphi Jujubae）is sweet in taste and warm in property，entering the spleen meridian and kidney meridian，effective in tonifying the internal organs，replenishing Qi，nourishing the blood and pacifying the spirit. Clinically it is used to treat deficiency of the spleen and kidney，poor appetite，floppy stool，lassitude，insufficiency of Qi and blood，palpitation，sensitive peliosis and hysteria.

133. 葡萄

【原文】

味甘,平。

主筋骨湿痹,益气,倍力,强志,令人肥健,耐饥忍风寒。久食轻身,不老延年,可作酒。生山谷。

【考据】

1.《名医》曰:生陇西五原敦煌。

2. 案史纪大宛列《传》云:大宛左右,以葡萄为酒,汉使取其实来,于是天子始种苜蓿,葡萄,肥饶地,或疑此本经不合有葡萄,《名医》所增,当为黑字。

3. 然《周礼》场人云:树之查蔬,珍异之物。郑元云:珍异,葡萄枇杷之属,则古中国本有此,大宛种类殊常,故汉特取来植之,旧作葡,据《史记》作蒲。

【今译】

味甘,性平。

133. Putao（葡萄，fruit of European grape， Fructus Vitis Viniferae）[1]

[Original Text]

[Putao （葡萄，fruit of European grape， Fructus Vitis Viniferae），] sweet in taste and mild [in property]，[is mainly used] to treat dampness impediment in the sinews and bones，to replenish Qi，increase energy，to strengthen memory，to cultivate health，and to tolerate hunger and wind-cold. Long-term taking [of it will] relax the body，prevent aging and prolong life. [It] can be made into wine. [It] grows in mountains and valleys.

[Textual Research]

[In the book entitled] Ming Yi Bie Lu（《名医别录》），[it]says [that it] grows in Wuyuan（五原）and Dunhuang（敦煌）in Longxi （陇西）.

[In the book entitled] *Shi Ji*（《史记》，*Records of History*），[it] says [that]，around Dawan（大宛），Putao（葡萄，fruit of European grape，Fructus Vitis Viniferae）was made into wine. The emissary from the Han Dynasty brought some of the fruits to the Han Empire and the Han Emperor began to plant clover and grape in fertile land. Perhaps what it talked about in this Canon is not grape. [In the book entitled] *Ming Yi Bie Lu*（《名医别录》，*Special Record of Great Doctors*），[it] says [that this medicinal is] called black grape.

　　主治筋骨湿邪所致痹证,能补益精气,能增强力气和记忆力,能使人身体康健,能减退饥饿感,能增强对风寒的抵抗能力。长期食用能使人身体轻盈,能长寿不老,能延年益寿。可以用其酿酒。该物生长在山谷之中。

Zheng Yuan (郑元) said, "[This is] really unique. In ancient times, grape and loquat already grew in China. [However the grape] growing in Dawan (大宛) is unique. That was why it was brought to China in the Han Dynasty."

Notes

1. Putao (葡萄, fruit of European grape, Fructus Vitis Viniferae) is sweet and sour in taste, mild in property, entering the lung meridian, the spleen meridian and the kidney meridian, effective in tonifying Qi and blood, strengthening sinews and bones, and promoting urination. Clinically it is used to treat cough due to lung deficiency, palpitation, night sweating, wind-dampness impediment and pain, stranguria, edema and dysuria.

神农本草经

494

134. 蓬蘽

【原文】

味酸,平。

主安五脏,益精气,长阴令坚,强志,倍力有子。久服轻身不老。一名覆盆。生平泽。

【考据】

1.《吴普》曰:缺盆,一名决盆(《御览》)。甄氏本草曰:覆盆子,一名马瘘,一名陆荆。(同上)

2.《名医》曰:一名陵蘽,一名阴药,生荆山及冤句。

3. 案《说文》云:蘽,木也。茥,缺盆也。《广雅》云:蒛盆陆英,莓也。《尔雅》云:茥蒛盆。郭璞云:覆盆也,实似莓而小,亦可食。《毛诗》云:葛苗苗之。陆玑云:一名巨瓜,似燕薁,亦连蔓,叶似艾,白色,其子赤可食。

4.《列仙传》云:昌容食蓬蘽根。李当之云:即是人所食莓。陶宏景云:蓬蘽是根名,覆盆是实名。

134. Penglei（蓬蔂，fruit of palmleaf raspberry， Fructus Rubi）[1]

[Original Text]

[Penglei（蓬蔂，fruit of palmleaf raspberry，Fructus Rubi），] sour in taste and mild [in property]，[is mainly used] to harmonize the five Zang-organs，to replenish essential Qi，to invigorate and harden penis，to strengthen memory，to increase energy and [to enable people to] conceive baby. Long-term taking [of it will] relax the body and prevent aging. [It is also] called Fupen（覆盆）and grows in plains and swamps.

[Textual Research]

[In the book entitled] *Ming Yi Bie Lu*（《名医别录》，*Special Record of Great Doctors*），[it] says [that Penglei（蓬蔂，fruit of palmleaf raspberry，Fructus Rubi）is also] called Linglei（陵蔂）and Yinyao（阴药），growing in Jingshan（荆山）and Yuanju （冤句）.

Lu Ji（陆玑）said，"[It is] also called Jugua（巨瓜，large melon） like Yan'ao（燕薁，Vitis Bryoniifolia），growing prosperously. [Its] leaves are white like mugwort. [Its] seed is red and edible." Tao Hongjing（陶宏景）said，"[Its] root is called Penglei（蓬蔂）and [its] fruit is called Fupen（覆盆）."

【今译】

味酸,性平。

能安和五脏,能补益精气,能增加阴液,能增强记忆力,能充实力气,能使人生养子女。长期服用能使人身体轻盈,能长寿不老。又称为覆盆。该物生长在平川水泽之中。

神农本草经

Notes

1. Penglei (蓬蘽, fruit of palmleaf raspberry, Fructus Rubi) is a herbal medicinal, bitter and sweet in taste, slightly cold in property, effective in clearing heat, removing toxin and activating the blood. Clinically it is used to treat hepatitis, swelling and pain of the throat, phlebitis, pain due to abnormal circulation of Qi and blood, urticaria, paddy-field dermatitis, carbuncle, sore, boil and traumatic injury.

135. 鸡头实

【原文】

味甘,平。

主湿痹,腰脊膝痛,补中,除暴疾,益精气,强志,令耳目聪明。久服,轻身不饥,耐老,神仙。一名雁啄实。生池泽。

【考据】

1.《名医》曰:一名芡,生雷泽,八月采。

2. 案《说文》云:芡,鸡头也。《广雅》云:莜芡,鸡头也,《周礼》,笾人加笾之实芡。郑元云:芡,鸡头也。方言云:莜芡,鸡头也,北燕谓之莜,青徐淮泗之间,谓之芡。

3. 南楚江湘之间,谓之鸡头,或谓之雁头,或谓之乌头。《淮南子》说山川云:鸡头已瘘。高诱云:水中芡,幽州谓之雁头。古今注云:叶似荷而大,叶上蹙绉如沸,实有芒刺,其中有米,可以度饥,即今莴子也。

上果,上品五种,旧六种,今以橘柚入木。

135. Jitoushi（鸡头实，seed of gordon Euryale，semen Euryale Ferox）[1]

［Original Text］

［Jitoushi（鸡头实，seed of gordon Euryale，semen Euryale Ferox），］ sweet in taste ［and］ mild ［in property］，［is mainly used］ to treat dampness impediment and pain of the waist，spine and knees，to tonify the middle（the internal organs），to eliminate severe disease，to replenish essential Qi，to strengthen memory and to improve hearing and vision. Long-term taking ［of it will］ relax the body，［make people feel］ no hunger，prevent aging like immortals. ［It is also］ called Yanzhuoshi（雁啄实），growing in lakes and swamps.

499

［Textual Research］

［In the book entitled］ *Ming Yi Bie Lu*（《名医别录》，*Special Record of Great Doctors*），［it］ says ［that Jitoushi（鸡头实，seed of gordon Euryale，semen Euryale Ferox），］ also called Qian（芡），grows in Leize（雷泽）and ［can be］ collected in August.

［According to］ explanations made in the past and present，［its］ leaves are as large as that of lotus with astringent texture. ［In its］ fruits，there are awns over the surface. Inside there are seeds ［that are］ edible.

【今译】

味甘,性平。

主治湿邪所致痹证,能治疗腰部、脊部、膝部疼痛,能充实人体内脏,能解除暴疾,能补益精气,能增强记忆力,能令人耳目聪明。长期服用,能使人身体轻盈,能减少饥饿感,能使人不易衰老,像神仙一样。又称为雁啄实。该物生长在池泽中。

Notes

1. Jitoushi (鸡头实, seed of gordon Euryale, semen Euryale Ferox) is a herbal medicinal, sweet in taste, astringent and mild in property, entering the spleen meridian and the kidney meridian, effective in replenishing the kidney and securing essence, tonifying the spleen and ceasing diarrhea. Clinically it is used to treat seminal emission, spontaneous spermatorrhea, premature ejaculation, frequent urination, enuresis, leucorrhea and chronic diarrhea.

神农本草经

136. 胡麻

【原文】

味甘,平。

主伤中虚羸,补五内(《御览》作藏),益气力,长肌肉,填髓脑。久服,轻身不老。一名巨胜。叶名青蘘。生川泽。

【考据】

1.《吴普》曰:胡麻一名方金,神农雷公甘无毒,一名狗虱,立秋采。

2.《名医》曰:一名狗虱,一名方茎,一名鸿藏,生上党。

3. 案《广雅》云:狗虱,巨胜,藤苰,胡麻也。孝经援神契云:钜胜延年。宋均云:世以钜胜为苟杞子。陶宏景云:本生大宛,故曰胡麻。按本经已有此,陶说非也,且与麻蕡并列,胡之言大或以叶大于麻,故名之。

【今译】

味甘,性平。

136. Huma（胡麻，seed of oriental sesame，Semen Sesami Nigrum）[1]

[Original Text]

[Huma （胡麻，seed of oriental sesame，Semen Sesami Nigrum），] sweet in taste and mild [in property]，[is mainly used] to treat emaciation and weakness [caused by] injury，to tonify the five internal [Zang-organs]，to replenish Qi and energy，to promote growth of muscles and to enrich the brains. Long-term taking [of it will] relax the body and prevent aging. [It is also] called Jusheng （巨胜）.[Its] leaf is called Qingguan （青蘘），growing in valleys and swamps.

[Textual Research]

[In the book entitled] *Wu Pu Ben Cao* （《吴普本草》，*Wu Pu's Studies of Materia Medica* ），[it] says [that] Huma （胡麻，seed of oriental sesame，Semen Sesami Nigrum） [is also] called Fangjin （方金）.[According to] Agriculture God（神农） and Leigong（雷公），[it is] sweet [in taste] and non-toxic [in property].[It is also] called Goushi （狗虱） and [can be] collected in the Autumn Solstice.

[In the book entitled] *Ming Yi Bie Lu* （《名医别录》，*Special Record of Great Doctors* ），[it] says [that Huma （胡麻，seed of oriental sesame，Semen Sesami Nigrum） is also] called Goushi（狗虱），Fangjing（方茎） and Hongzang（鸿藏），growing in Shangdang

　　主治内脏损伤，身体虚弱消瘦，能滋补五脏，能补益气力，能增长肌肉，能填充脑髓。长期服用，能使人身体轻盈，能长寿不老。又称为巨胜。叶名青蘘。该物生长在山川和平泽之中。

（上党）.

Tao Hongjing（陶宏景）said，"It originally grows in Dawan（大宛）. That is why it is called Huma（胡麻）."This Canon has already mentioned this herb. Hence what Tao Hongjing（陶宏景）said was not correct.

Notes

1. Huma（胡麻，seed of oriental sesame，Semen Sesami Nigrum）is a herbal medicinal，sweet in taste and mild in property，entering the liver meridian and the kidney meridian，effective in tonifying the liver and kidney，moistening the five Zang-organs. Clinically it is used to treat insufficiency of the liver and kidney，vertigo due to deficiency and wind attack，tinnitus，headache，blood stasis，wind impediment，numbness，constipation due to intestinal dryness，white hair，loss of hair after illness and lack of lactation.

137. 麻蕡

【原文】

味辛,平。

主五劳七伤,利五脏,下血,寒气,多食,令人见鬼狂走。久服,通神明,轻身。一名麻勃。麻子,味甘平,主补中益气,肥健不老神仙。生川谷。

【考据】

1.《吴普》曰:麻子中仁,神农岐伯辛,雷公扁鹊无毒,不欲牡蛎白薇,先藏地中者食杀人,麻蓝一名麻蕡,一名青欲,一名青葛,神农辛,岐伯有毒,雷公甘,畏牡蛎白薇,叶上有毒,食之杀人,麻勃,一名花,雷公辛无毒,畏牡蛎。(《御览》)

2.《名医》曰:麻勃,此麻花上勃勃者,七月七日采。良,子九月采,生太山。

3. 案《说文》元:麻与枲同,人所治在屋下,枲麻也,萉枲实也,或作黂荸,麻母也,荜,枲也,以蕡为杂香草。《尔雅》云:蕡,枲实,枲,麻孙。炎云:茡麻子也。郭璞云:别二名,又芋,麻母。郭璞云:苴,麻盛子者,

137．Mafen（麻蕡，seed of hemp fimble，Semen Cannabis）[1]

[Original Text]

［Mafen（麻蕡，seed of hemp fimble，Semen Cannabis），］pungent in taste and mild［in property］，［is mainly used］to treat five［kinds of］overstrain[2] and seven［kinds of］damage[3]，to regulate the five Zang-organs，bleeding，cold Qi，and wildly running like a ghost［due to］overeating. Long-term taking［of it will］invigorate spirit light and relax the body.［It is also］called Mabo（麻勃）.

［Its］seed，sweet in taste and mild［in property］，can tonify the middle（internal organs），replenish Qi，fortify the body and prolong life like immortals.［It］grows in mountain valleys and river valleys.

507

[Textual Research]

［In the book entitled］*Wu Pu Ben Cao*（《吴普本草》，*Wu Pu's Studies of Materia Medica*），［it］says［that］Mafen（麻蕡，seed of hemp fimble，Semen Cannabis），［according to］Agriculture God（神农）and Qibo（岐伯），［is］pungent［in taste］；［according to］Leigong（雷公）and Bianque（扁鹊），［it is］non-toxic［in property］；［according to］Qibo（岐伯），［it is］toxic［in property］；［according to］Leigong（雷公），［it is］sweet［in property］.

《周礼》,笾朝事之笾,其实麷蕡,郑云:蕡枲实也,郑司农云麻麻曰蕡.《淮南子》齐俗训云:胡人见筦,不知其可以为布。高诱云:蕡,麻实也,据此则宏景以为牡麻无实,非也,《唐本》以为麻实,是。

上米,谷,上品二种,旧三种,今以青蘘入草。

【今译】

味辛,性平。

主治五种劳伤和七种损伤,能通利五脏,能治疗下血,能清除寒气,吃多了会使人精神恍惚,如同遇到鬼一样的狂奔乱跑。长期服用,能使神志清晰,精神旺盛,人身体轻盈。又称为麻勃。

麻子,味甘,性平,能充实人体内脏,能补益精气,能使人身体康健,长寿不老,像神仙一样。该物生长在山川河谷之中。

[In the book entitled] *Ming Yi Bie Lu* (《名医别录》，*Special Record of Great Doctors*)，[it] says [that] the flower of Mafen（麻蕡，seed of hemp fimble, Semen Cannabis）[can be] collected on July 7. [It is] better to collect [its] seed in September. [It] grows in Taishan（太山）.

Notes

1. Mafen（麻蕡，seed of hemp fimble, Semen Cannabis）is pungent in taste and mild in property, entering the spleen meridian, the stomach meridian and the large intestine meridian, effective in moistening the intestines and promoting defecation, moistening dryness and killing worms. Clinically it is used to treat hypertension, diarrhea, constipation and stagnation due to accumulation of pathogenic factors.

2. Five kinds of overstrain refer to either seeing, walking, standing, sitting and sleeping for a long time, or damage of the heart, liver, spleen, lung and kidney, or damage of sinews, muscles, bones, Qi and blood.

3. Seven kinds of damage refer to either damage caused by eating, anxiety, drinking, sexual intercourse, hunger, overstrain and meridians, or damage caused by Yin cold, Yin wilting, tenesmus, seminal emission, oligospermia, vulva dampness and frequent urination, or damage of the spleen, liver, kidney, lung, heart, body and mind.

138. 冬葵子

【原文】

味甘,寒。

主五脏六腑,寒热羸瘦,五癃,利小便。久服坚骨长肌肉,轻身延年。

【考据】

1.《名医》曰:生少室山,十二月采之。

2. 案《说文》云:昇,古文终,葵菜也。《广雅》云:菚,葵也,考升与终形相近,当即《尔雅》蔏葵,《尔雅》云蔏,葵繁露。郭璞云:承露也,大茎小叶,华紫黄色。

3. 本草图经云:吴人呼为繁露,俗呼胡燕支,子可妇人涂面及作口脂,按《名医》别有落葵条,一名繁露,亦非也,陶宏景以为终冬至春作子,谓之冬葵,不经甚矣。

【今译】

味甘,性寒。

138. Dongkuizi（冬葵子，seed of cluster mallow，Semen Malvae）[1]

〔**Original Text**〕

〔Dongkuizi（冬葵子，seed of cluster mallow，Semen Malvae），〕sweet in taste and cold 〔in property〕，〔is mainly used〕to regulate the five Zang-organs and six Fu-organs，〔to improve〕weakness and emaciation 〔caused by〕cold-heat 〔disease〕，〔to treat〕five 〔kinds of〕urine retention and to promote urination. Long-term taking 〔of it will〕strengthen bones，promote muscles，relax the body and prolong life.

〔**Textual Research**〕

〔In the book entitled〕*Ming Yi Bie Lu*（《名医别录》，*Special Record of Great Doctors*），〔it〕says 〔that Dongkuizi（冬葵子，seed of cluster mallow，Semen Malvae）〕grows in Shaoshi（少室）mountain and 〔can be collected〕in December. Guo Pu（郭璞）said，"〔It〕receives dew，〔characterized by〕large stalks，small leaves and purplish yellow flowers."

Notes

1. Dongkuizi（冬葵子，seed of cluster mallow，Semen Malvae）is a herbal medicinal，sweet in taste and cold in property，entering the large intestine meridian，the small intestine meridian，the liver

主治五脏六腑的寒热性疾病,能缓解身体瘦弱,能治疗五种淋证,能使小便通畅。长期服用,能使骨骼坚强,能增长肌肉,能使人身体轻盈,能延年益寿。

meridian, the lung meridian, the stomach meridian and the bladder meridian, effective in promoting urination and relieving stranguria, moistening the intestines and promoting defecation. Clinically it is used to treat stranguria, edema, constipation, lack of lactation and sweating.

139. 苋实

【原文】

味甘,寒。

主青盲,明目除邪,利大小便,去寒热。久服,益气力,不饥,轻身。一名马苋。

【考据】

1.《名医》曰:一名莫实,生淮阳及田中,叶如蓝,十一月采。

2. 案《说文》云:苋,苋菜也。《尔雅》云蒉,赤苋。郭璞云:今苋叶之赤茎者。

3. 李当之云:苋实,当是今白苋,《唐本》注云:赤苋一名䔖,今名莫实字误。

【今译】

味甘,性寒。

主治青盲症,能使眼睛明亮,能消除邪气,能通利大小便,能祛除寒热疾病。长期服用,能补益气力,能减少饥饿感,能使身体轻盈。又称为马苋。

139. Xianshi（苋实，seed of three-coloured amaranth，Semen Amaranthi Tricoloris） [1]

［Original Text］

［Xianshi（苋实，seed of three coloured amaranth，Semen Amaranthi Tricoloris），］ sweet in taste and cold ［in property］, ［is mainly used］ to treat blue blindness，improve vision，to eliminate evils，to promote urination and defecation，and to remove cold and heat. Long-term taking ［of it will］ replenish Qi and energy，［make people feel］ no hunger and relax the body. ［It is also］ called Maxian（马苋）.

［Textual Research］

［In the book entitled］ *Ming Yi Bie Lu*（《名医别录》，*Special Record of Great Doctors*），［it］ says ［that Xianshi（苋实，seed of three coloured amaranth，Semen Amaranthi Tricoloris）is also］ called Moshi（莫实），growing in Huaiyang（淮阳）and Tianzhong（田中）. ［It can be］ collected in November.

Notes

1. Xianshi（苋实，seed of three coloured amaranth，Semen Amaranthi Tricoloris）is sweet in taste and cold in property，entering the liver meridian，the large intestine meridian and the bladder meridian，effective in clearing the liver，improve vision and promoting urination and defecation. Clinically it is used to treat glaucoma，blurred vision，hematuria，dysuria and constipation.

140. 瓜蒂

【原文】

味苦,寒。

主大水身面四肢浮肿,下水,杀蛊毒,咳逆上气。及食诸果,病在胸腹中,皆吐下之。生平泽。

【考据】

1.《名医》曰:生嵩高,七月七日采,阴干。

2. 案《说文》云:瓜,胍瓜也,象形。蒂,瓜当也。《广雅》云:水芝,瓜也。陶宏景云:甜瓜蒂也。

【今译】

味苦,性寒。

主治恶性水肿,身体、面部和四肢浮肿,能消除水湿,能杀除虫毒,能治疗咳嗽及呼吸困难。食用各种果实所引起胸腹中疾病,都可以通过呕吐和下泻予以治疗。该物生长在平川水泽之中。

140. Guadi（瓜蒂, fruit pedicel of muskmelon, Pedicellus Melo Fructus）[1]

［**Original Text**］

［Guadi（瓜蒂, fruit pedicel of muskmelon, Pedicellus Melo Fructus）,］bitter in taste and cold［in property］,［is mainly used］to relieve dropsy of the body, face and four limbs［caused by］severe edema, to discharge water, to remove worm toxin, to treat cough with dyspnea and upward flow of Qi. Disease in the chest and abdomen［caused by］eating various fruits［can be treated by］vomiting and purgative［therapies］.［It］grows in plains and swamps.

［**Textual Research**］

［In the book entitled］*Ming Yi Bie Lu*（《名医别录》, *Special Record of Great Doctors*）,［it］says［that Guadi（瓜蒂, fruit pedicel of muskmelon, Pedicellus Melo Fructus）］grows in Songgao（嵩高）,［and can be］collected on July 7 and dried in the shade.

Notes

1. Guadi（瓜蒂, fruit pedicel of muskmelon, Pedicellus Melo Fructus）is a herbal medicinal, bitter in taste, cold and toxic in property, entering the spleen meridian, the stomach meridian, the heart meridian and the lung meridian, effective in promoting vomiting and removing toxin. Clinically it is used to treat epilepsy, profuse phlegm, jaundice, chronic and acute hepatitis, and hepatocirrhosis.

141. 瓜子

【原文】

味甘,平。

主令人悦泽,好颜色,益气不饥。久服轻身耐老。一名水芝。(《御览》作土芝)生平泽。

【考据】

1.《吴普》曰:瓜子一名瓣,七月七日采,可作面脂。(《御览》)

2.《名医》曰:一名白瓜子,生嵩高,冬瓜仁也,八月采。

3. 案《说文》云:瓣,瓜中实。《广雅》云:冬瓜瓝也,其子谓之瓤。

陶宏景云:白当为甘,旧有白字。据《名医》云:一名白瓜子,则本名当无。

【今译】

味甘,性平。

141. Guazi（瓜子，muskmelon seed，Semen Melo）[1]

[Original Text]

[Guazi（瓜子，muskmelon seed，Semen Melo），] sweet in taste and mild [in property], [is mainly used] to amuse [people], to luster complexion, to replenish Qi and [to make people feel] no hunger. Long-term taking [of it will] relax the body and prevent aging. [It is also] called Shuizhi（水芝）, growing in plains and swamps.

[Textual Research]

[In the book entitled] Wu Pu Ben Cao（《吴普本草》，Wu Pu's Studies of Materia Medica）, [it] says [that] Guazi（瓜子，muskmelon seed，Semen Melo）is also called Ban（瓣）. [It can be] collected on July 7 and used as grease to luster the face [according to the book entitled] Tai Ping Yu Lan（《太平御览》，Imperial Studies in Taiping Times）.

[In the book entitled] Ming Yi Bie Lu（《名医别录》，Special Record of Great Doctors）, [it] says [that Guazi（瓜子，muskmelon seed，Semen Melo）is also] called Baiguazi（白瓜子）, growing in Songgao（嵩高）. [It is] the seed of white gourd and [can be] collected in August.

[In] case [analysis in the book entitled] Shuo Wen（《说文》，On Culture）, [it] says [that the so-called] Ban（瓣）is the seed in

能使人愉悦润泽,能使面部色彩美丽,能补益精气,能使人减少饥饿感。长期服用能使人身体轻盈,不易衰老。又称为水芝。该物生长在平川水泽之中。

the melon. [According to the book entitled] *Guang Ya* (《广雅》, *The First Chinese Encyclopedic Dictionary*), the seed of white gourd is called Rang (瓤).

Notes

1. Guazi (瓜子, muskmelon seed, Semen Melo) is sweet in taste and mild in property, effective in clearing heat, resolving phlegm, moistening dryness, expelling wind and removing worms. Clinically it is used to treat cough with profuse sputum, ascaridiasis, constipation, arteriosclerosis, hypertension, fracture, sinew injury, oxyuriasis and wind-dampness impediment.

142. 苦菜

【原文】

味苦,寒。

主五脏邪气,厌谷,胃痹。久服,安心益气,聪察少卧,轻身耐老。一名荼草,一名选。生川谷。

【考据】

1.《名医》曰:一名游冬,生益州山陵道旁,凌冬不死,三月三日采,阴干。

2. 案《说文》云:荼,苦菜也。《广雅》云:游冬,苦菜也。《尔雅》云:荼,苦菜,又槚,苦荼。郭璞云:树小如栀子,冬生叶,可煮作羹,今呼早采者为荼,晚取者为茗,一名荈,蜀人名之苦菜。陶宏景云:此即是今茗,茗一名荼又令人不眠,亦凌冬不凋而兼其止,生益州,《唐本》注驳之非矣,选与荈,音相近。

上菜,上品五种旧同。

142. Kucai（苦菜，common sowthistle herb，Herba Sonchi Oleracei）[1]

[Original Text]

[Kucai（苦菜，common sowthistle herb，Herba Sonchi Oleracei），] bitter in taste and cold [in property]，[is mainly used] to treat [disease caused by] evil-Qi in the five Zang-organs，anorexia and stomach impediment. Long-term taking [of it will] harmonize the heart，replenish Qi，improve hearing [and ability] to analyze，relax the body and prevent aging. [It is also] called Tucao（荼草）and Xuan（选），growing in mountain valleys and river valleys.

523

[Textual Research]

[In the book entitled] *Ming Yi Bie Lu*（《名医别录》，*Special Record of Great Doctors*），[it] says [that Kucai（苦菜，common sowthistle herb，Herba Sonchi Oleracei) is also] called Youdong（游冬），growing in the sides of roads around the hills in Yizhou（益州）. [It does] not die in winter and [can be] collected on March 3 and dried in the shade.

[In] case [analysis in the book entitled] *Shuo Wen*（《说文》，*On Culture*），[it] says [that the so-called] Tu（荼）is Kucai（苦菜，common sowthistle herb，Herba Sonchi Oleracei）. [In the book entitled] *Guang Ya*（《广雅》，*The First Chinese Encyclopedic*

【今译】

味苦,性寒。

主治五脏中的邪气,能缓解食欲不振,能治疗胃痹证。长期服用,能使人心安神静,能补益精气,能使人聪明而有才智,可治疗彻夜难眠,能使身体轻盈,不易衰老。又称为荼草,又称为选。该物生长在山川河谷之中。

Dictionary), [it] says [that the so-called] Youdong (游冬) is Kucai (苦菜, common sowthistle herb, Herba Sonchi Oleracei).

Notes

1. Kucai (苦菜, common sowthistle herb, Herba Sonchi Oleracei) is a herbal medicinal, pungent and bitter in taste, slightly cold in property, entering the kidney meridian, the large intestine meridian and the liver meridian, effective in clearing heat and removing toxin, dispersing stasis and eliminating pus. Clinically it is used to treat intestinal disease, pulmonary ulcer, hepatitis, enteritis, dysentery, metritis and abdominal pain after delivery of baby due to blood stasis.

中卷 中品

1. 雄黄

【原文】

味苦,平寒。

主寒热,鼠瘘,恶疮,疽,痔,死肌,杀精物恶鬼,邪气,百虫毒,胜五兵。炼食之,轻食神仙。一名黄食石。生山谷。

【考据】

1.《吴普》曰:雄黄,神农苦,山阴有丹雄黄,生山之阳,故曰雄,是丹之雄,所以名雄黄也。

2.《名医》曰:生武都敦煌山之阳,采无时。

3. 案《西山经》云:高山其下多雄黄。郭璞云:晋大兴三年,高平郡界有山崩,其中出数千斤雄黄。《抱朴子·仙药》云:雄黄当得武都山所出者,纯而无杂,其赤如鸡冠,光明晔晔乃可用耳,其但纯黄似雄黄,色无赤光者,不任以作仙药,可以合理病药耳。

【今译】

味苦,性平寒。

主治寒热病,治疗瘰疬,恶疮,痈疽,痔疮,肌肉坏死,能清除妖魔

Volume 2   The middle Grade

1. Xionghuang（雄黄，realgar；Realgar）[1]

[Original Text]

[Xionghuang（雄黄，realgar；Realgar），] bitter in taste，mild and cold [in property]，[is mainly used] to treat cold-heat [disease]，atrophy [caused by scrofula]，severe sore，carbuncle，hemorrhoids and putrescence of muscles，to expel [severe pathogenic factors like] monster and ghost，[and to eliminate] evil-Qi and all worm toxin. [It is] much better than five [kinds of important] weapons. To take refined [Xionghuang（雄黄，realgar；Realgar）will enable people] to relax the body [as dexterous as] immortals. [It is also] called Huangshishi（黄食石）and [can be] found in mountains and valleys.

527

[Textual Research]

[In the book entitled] *Wu Pu Ben Cao*（《吴普本草》，*Wu Pu's Studies of Materia Medica*），[it] says [that] Xionghuang（雄黄，realgar；Realgar），[according to] Agriculture God（神农），[is] bitter [in taste]. [In] Shanyin（山阴），there is red realgar in the sunny side. That is why [it is] called Xiong（雄）[which means great and bright in] red [color]. For this reason，[it is] named Xionghuang（雄黄，realgar；Realgar）.

[In the book entitled] *Ming Yi Bie Lu*（《名医别录》，*Special Record of Great Doctors*），[it] says [that Xionghuang（雄黄，

鬼怪邪气,能消除各种虫毒,其效果胜过五种兵器。冶炼之后服用,能使身体轻盈,像神仙一样。又称为黄食石。该物生长在山谷之中。

realgar; Realgar)] exists in the sunny side of mountains in Dunhuang（敦煌） in Wudu（武都）. [It can be] collected at any time.

[In the book entitled] *Xi Shan Jing* (《西山经》, *Canon About the West Mountain*), [it] says [that] there are many Xionghuang （雄黄, realgar; Realgar） in the areas below the mountains. Guo Pu （郭璞） said, "In the third year of Taixing（太兴） period in the Jin Dynasty（晋朝, 265 AD - 420 AD）, there was landslide in Gaoping （高平） region, thousands *Jin*（斤） of Xionghuang（雄黄, realgar; Realgar） appeared."

[In the book entitled] *Bao Pu Zi* (《抱朴子》, *Primitive and Natural View*) about magic medicinals（仙药）, [it] says [that] Xionghuang （雄黄, realgar; Realgar） exists in Wudu （武都） mountain [which is] pure without any other elements [in it], red [in color] like cockscomb and bright like the sun. [This is the best one]. [If it is] quite yellow, but not red [in color], [it is] not a panacea, just an appropriate element for medical purpose.

529

Notes

1. Xionghuang（雄黄, realgar; Realgar） is a mineral medicinal, pungent in taste, warm and toxic in property, entering the heart meridian and the liver meridian, effective in drying dampness, killing worms and removing toxin. Clinically it is used to treat carbuncle, sore, swelling, bite by viper, scabies, erysipelas, epilepsy, malaria, cough and panting.

2. 石流黄（流旧作硫，《御览》引作流，是）

【原文】

味酸，温。

主妇人阴蚀，疽痔恶血，坚筋骨，除头秃，能化金银铜铁奇物（《御览》引云：石流青、白色，主益肝气明目，石流赤，生羌道山谷）。生山谷。

【考据】

1.《吴普》曰：硫黄一名石留黄，神农黄帝雷公咸有毒，医和扁鹊苦无毒，或生易阳，或河西，或五色，黄是潘水石液也（潘，即矾，古字），烧令有紫焰者，八月九日采，治妇人血结（《御览》云：治妇人绝阴，能合金银铜铁）。

2.《名医》曰：生东海牧羊山，及太山河西山，矾石液也。

3. 案《范子计然》云：石流黄出汉中，又云刘冯饵石流黄而更少。刘逵注吴都赋云：流黄，土精也。

2. Shiliuhuang（石流黄，sulphur，Sulfur）[1]

［Original Text］

［Shiliuhuang（石流黄，sulphur，Sulfur），］sour in taste and warm［in property］，［is mainly used］to treat vulva ulcer, carbuncle，hemorrhoids and blood stasis，to strengthen sinews and bones，to eliminate sores on the head，and to transform［it into］unique gold, silver, copper and iron.［It］exists in mountains and valleys.

［Textual Research］

531

［In the book entitled］*Wu Pu Ben Cao*（《吴普本草》，*Wu Pu's Studies of Materia Medica*），［it］says［that］Shiliuhuang（石流黄，sulphur，Sulfur）［is also］called Shiliuhuang（石留黄）.［According to］Agriculture God（神农），Yellow Emperor（黄帝）and Leigong（雷公），［it is］salty［in taste］and toxic［in property］；［according to］Yihe（医和）and Bianque（扁鹊），［it is］bitter［in taste］and non-toxic［in property］.［It］may exist in Yiyang（易阳），or Hexi（河西），or Wuse（五色）. Yellow（黄）means liquid in stones.［When］burnt，［it］becomes purple.［It can be］collected on August 9 and［used］to treat amenorrhea［according to the book entitled］*Tai Ping Yu Lan*（《太平御览》，*Imperial Studies in Taiping Times*）.

［In the book entitled］*Ming Yi Bie Lu*（《名医别录》，*Special Record of Great Doctors*），［it］says［that Shiliuhuang（石流黄，

【今译】

味酸,性温。

主治妇人阴部溃疡,痈疽,痔疮,因瘀滞所致的死血证,能使筋骨强壮,能祛除头生秃疮,能使其转化为金、银、铜、铁等奇特物质。该物生长在山谷之中。

sulphur, Sulfur)] exists in Muyang (牧羊) mountain in Donghai (东海, East Sea) and Hexi (河西) mountain in Taishan (太山). [It is] the liquid in Fanshi (矾石, chalcanthite, Chalcanthitum).

[In the book entitled] *Fan Zi Ji Ran* (《范子计然》, *Studies About Fan Li's Teacher*), [it] says [that] Shiliuhuang (石流黄, sulphur, Sulfur) exists in Hanzhong (汉中). Liu Feng (刘冯) said, "Yellow Shiliuhuang (石流黄, sulphur, Sulfur) is rare." [In] explaining verse about Wudu (吴都) [written by Zuo Si (左思)], Liu Kui (刘逵) said, "Shiliuhuang (石流黄, sulphur, Sulfur) refers to essence of earth."

Notes

1. Shiliuhuang (石流黄, sulphur, Sulfur) is a mineral medicinal, sour in taste, warm and toxic in property, entering the kidney meridian and large intestine meridian, effective in killing worms, fortifying fire and replenishing Yang. Clinically it is used to treat scabies, eczema, impotence, abdominal pain due to deficiency-cold, diarrhea, dysentery and constipation.

3. 雌黄

【原文】

味辛,平。

主恶疮头秃痂疥,杀毒虫虱,身痒,邪气诸毒。炼之,久服,轻身增年不老。生山谷。

【考据】

1.《名医》曰:生武都,与雄黄同山生,其阴山有金,金精熏,则生雌黄,采无时。

【今译】

味辛,性平。

主治恶疮,头秃,痂疥,杀死毒性虫虱,消除身痒和毒邪之气。冶炼后长期服用,能使人身体轻盈,能延长寿命,能长寿不老。该物生长在山谷之中。

3. Cihuang（雌黄，orpiment ore，Orpimentum）[1]

［**Original Text**］

［Cihuang（雌黄，orpiment ore，Orpimentum），］ pungent in taste and mild ［in property］，［is mainly used］ to treat severe sore，scalp favus and scabies，to kill worms with toxin，［to relieve］ itching and ［to eliminate］ evil-Qi and various toxin. Long-term taking ［of it will］ relax the body, prolong life and prevent aging. ［It］ exists in mountains and valleys.

［**Textual Research**］

［In the book entitled］ *Ming Yi Bie Lu*（《名医别录》，*Special Record of Great Doctors*），［it］ says ［that Cihuang（雌黄，orpiment ore，Orpimentum）］ exists in the mountains in Wudu（武都）together with Xionghuang（雄黄，realgar；Realgar）．［In］ the shady side of the mountains，there is gold. ［When］ gold is fumigated，Cihuang（雌黄，orpiment ore，Orpimentum）appears. ［It can be］ collected at any time.

Notes

1. Cihuang（雌黄，orpiment ore，Orpimentum）is a mineral medicinal，pungent in taste，mild and toxic in property，entering the liver meridian，effective in drying dampness，killing worms，resolving phlegm，relieving fright and removing toxin. Clinically it is used to treat scabies，severe sore，polypus，vulva ulcer，bite by snake and worms，epilepsy and cough with dyspnea due to cold phlegm.

神农本草经

4. 水银

【原文】

味辛,寒。

主疗痵痂疡白秃,杀皮肤中虱,堕胎,除热,杀金银铜锡毒。熔化还复为丹,久服神仙不死。生平土。

【考据】

1.《名医》曰:一名汞,生符陵,出于丹砂。

2.案《说文》云:澒,丹沙所化为水银也。《广雅》云:水银谓之汞。《淮南子》地形训云:白旁,九百岁生白旁,白(上兴下石),九百岁生百金。高诱云:白旁,水银也。

【今译】

味辛,性寒。

主治疥疮溃烂,痂疡,白秃,能杀死皮肤中的虫虱,能堕胎,能

4. Shuiyin（水银，mercury，Hydrargyrum）[1]

［Original Text］

［Shuiyin（水银，mercury，Hydrargyrum），］pungent in taste and cold ［in property］，［is mainly used］ to treat scabies，ulcer and tinea tonsure，to kill worms in the skin，to induce abortion，to expel heat，and to remove toxin in gold，silver，copper and tin. ［When］ heated，［it will］ become red again. Long-term taking ［of it will］ prolong life like immortals. ［It］ exists in plain land.

［Textual Research］

［In the book entitled］ *Ming Yi Bie Lu*（《名医别录》，*Special Record of Great Doctors*），［it］ says ［that Shuiyin（水银，mercury，Hydrargyrum）is also］ called Gong（汞），existing in Fuling（符陵）and originating from Dansha（丹砂，cinnabar，Cinnabaris）.

［In］ case ［analysis in the book entitled］ *Shuo Wen*（《说文》，*On Culture*），［it］ says ［that the so-called］ Hong（澒）refers to Dansha（丹砂，cinnabar，Cinnabaris）［that has］ transformed into Shuiyin（水银，mercury，Hydrargyrum）. ［In the book entitled］ *Guang Ya*（《广雅》，*The First Chinese Encyclopedic Dictionary*），［it］ says ［that］ Shuiyin（水银，mercury，Hydrargyrum）is called Gong（汞）. ［In the book entitled］ *Huai Nan Zi*（《淮南子》，*A Philosophy Book Compiled by Liu An，King in Huainan*），［it］ says ［that it takes］ nine hundred years to form Baihong（白澒）and

消除热邪所致之病，杀能祛除金、银、铜、锡之毒。烧熔后能再变为红色，长期服用能像神仙一样不死。该物生长在平坦的土地上。

hundred ［kinds of］ metal. Gao You （高诱） said，"［The so-called］ Baihong （白澒） refers to Shuiyin （水银，mercury，Hydrargyrum）."

Notes

1. Shuiyin （水银，mercury，Hydrargyrum） is a mineral medicinal，pungent in taste，cold with severe toxin in property，entering the liver meridian and the kidney meridian，effective in removing toxin，eliminating water and promoting defecation. Clinically it is used to treat scabies，ringworm，scrofula，syphilis，skin ulcer and edema.

5. 石膏

【原文】

味辛,微寒。

主中风寒热,心下逆气惊喘,口干,舌焦,不能息,腹中坚痛,除邪鬼,产乳,金疮。生山谷。

【考据】

1.《名医》曰:一名细石,生齐山及齐卢山,鲁蒙山,采无时。

【今译】

味辛,性微寒。

主治因感受风邪所致疾病,寒热病,心下逆气上行,惊风,喘息,口干舌焦,不能安息,腹中坚硬疼痛,能消除鬼怪邪气,能促使女子分娩,能治疗因金属疮伤而导致的痈疮。该物生长在山谷之中。

5. Shigao（石膏，gypsum，Gypsum Fibrosum）[1]

[Original Text]

[Shigao（石膏，gypsum，Gypsum Fibrosum），] pungent in taste and slightly cold [in property], [is mainly used] to treat [disease caused by pathogenic] wind, cold and heat, fright and panting [due to] upward counterflow of Qi from below the heart, dryness of the mouth with scorched tongue [as well as] stiffness and pain of the abdomen, to eliminate [pathogenic factors like] evil and ghost, to promote lactation and to cure injury [caused by] metal. [It] exists in mountains and valleys.

[Textual Research]

[In the book entitled] *Ming Yi Bie Lu*（《名医别录》，*Special Record of Great Doctors*），[it] says [that Shigao（石膏，gypsum，Gypsum Fibrosum) is also] called Xishi（细石），existing in Qishan （齐山）mountain，Qilou（齐卢）mountain and Loumeng（鲁蒙） mountain. [It can be] collected at any time.

Notes

1. Shigao（石膏，gypsum，Gypsum Fibrosum）is a mineral medicinal, pungent and sweet in taste, severe cold in property, entering the lung meridian and the stomach meridian, effective in clearing heat and purging fire. Clinically it is used to treat stomach heat, headache, toothache, oral ulcer and fulminant conjunctivitis.

6. 慈石

【原文】

味辛,寒。

主周痹,风湿,肢节中痛不可持物,洗洗,酸消,除大热烦满及耳聋。一名元石。生山谷。

【考据】

1.《吴普》曰:慈石,一名磁君。

2.《名医》曰:一名处石,生太山,及慈山山阴,有铁处则生其阳,采无时。

3. 案《北山经》云:灌题之山其中,多磁石。郭璞云:可以取铁。管子地数篇云:山上有慈石者,下必有铜。吕氏春秋精通篇云:慈石召铁。《淮南子》说山训云:慈石能引铁,只作慈,旧作磁,非,《名医》别出元石条,亦非。

【今译】

味辛,性寒。

6. Cishi（慈石，magnetite ore，Magnetitum）[1]

[Original Text]

[Cishi（慈石，magnetite ore，Magnetitum），] pungent in taste and cold [in property]，[is mainly used] to treat generalized impediment，wind-dampness [syndrome/pattern]，pain of limbs [that are] difficult to hold anything and chilliness with ache，and to eliminate severe heat，vexation，fullness and deafness. [It is also] called Yuanshi（元石），existing in mountains and valleys.

[Textual Research]

[In the book entitled] *Wu Pu Ben Cao*（《吴普本草》，*Wu Pu's Studies of Materia Medica*），[it] says [that] Cishi（慈石，magnetite ore，Magnetitum) is also called Cishi（磁石）. [In the book entitled] *Ming Yi Bie Lu*（《名医别录》，*Special Record of Great Doctors*），[it] says [that Cishi（慈石，magnetite ore，Magnetitum）is also] called Chushi（处石），existing in the shady sides of Taishan（太山）mountain and Cishan（慈山）. [Where] there is iron，there is Yang. [It can be] collected at any time.

[In the book entitled] *Shan Hai Jing*（《山海经》，*Canon of Mountains and Seas*) about north mountain，[it] says [that] there are many Cishi（磁石，magnetite ore，Magnetitum) in it. Guo Pu（郭璞）said，"Iron can be obtained from it." In the chapter about lands，Guan Zi（管子）said，"The mountain with Cishi（磁石，

主治全身流窜性疼痛，风湿证，肢节因疼痛而不能持物，发冷酸痛，能消除高热、烦躁、郁闷、耳聋。又称为元石。该物生长在山谷之中。

magnetite ore，Magnetitum）must contain copper in it." ［In the book entitled］ *Lǔ Shi Chun Qiu*（《吕氏春秋》，*Lǔ's History About Spring and Autumn Period*），［it］says［that］Cishi（磁石，magnetite ore，Magnetitum）keeps iron. ［In the book entitled］ *Huai Nan Zi* （《淮南子》，*A Philosophy Book Compiled by Liu An，King in Huainan*），［it］says［that］Cishi（磁石，magnetite ore，Magnetitum） can attract iron.

Notes

1. Cishi（磁石，magnetite ore，Magnetitum）is a mineral medicinal，pungent in taste and cold in property，entering the kidney meridian，the liver meridian and the lung meridian， effective in subduing Yang，receiving Qi，relieving fright and tranquilizing spirit. Clinically it is used to treat vertigo，blurred vision， tinnitus， deafness， panting， epilepsy， convulsion， palpitation and insomnia.

7. 凝水石

【原文】

味辛,寒。

主身热,腹中积聚,邪气,皮中如火烧,烦满。水饮之。久服不饥。一名白水石。生山谷。

【考据】

1.《吴普》曰:神农辛,岐伯医和扁鹊甘无毒。李氏大寒,或生邯郸,采无时,如云母色(《御览》引云,一名寒水石)。

2.《名医》曰:一名寒水石,一名凌水石,盐之精也,生常案及凝山,又中水县邯郸。

3.《范子计然》云:水石出河东,色泽者善。

【今译】

味辛,性寒。

7. Ningshuishi（凝水石，calcitum，Gypsum Rubrum）[1]

［Original Text］

［Ningshuishi（凝水石，calcitum，Gypsum Rubrum），］ pungent in taste and cold ［in property］，［is mainly used］ to treat fever，accumulation of evil-Qi in the abdomen，severe heat in the skin like scald and vexation.［It should be］ washed with water for taking. Long-term taking ［of it will make people feel］ no hunger. ［It is also］ called Baishuishi（白水石），existing in mountains and valleys.

［Textual Research］

［In the book entitled］ *Wu Pu Ben Cao*（《吴普本草》，*Wu Pu's Studies of Materia Medica*），［it］ says ［that Ningshuishi（凝水石，calcitum，Gypsum Rubrum），according to］ Agriculture God（神农），［is］ pungent ［in taste；［according to］ Qibo（岐伯），Yihe（医和）and Bianque（扁鹊），［it is］ sweet ［in taste] and non-toxic ［in property］；［according to］ Li's（李氏），［it is］ severe cold ［in property］.［It］ may exist in Handan（邯郸）and ［can be］ collected at any time，appearing like Yunmu（云母，muscovite，Muscovitum）in color.［According to the book entitled］ *Tai Ping Yu Lan*（《太平御览》，*Imperial Studies in Taiping Times*），［it is also］ called Hanshuishi（寒水石）.

［In the book entitled］ *Ming Yi Bie Lu*（《名医别录》，*Special*

547

主治身体发热,腹中积聚邪气,皮中热如火烧,烦躁郁闷。可用水冲饮凝水石。长期服用能减少饥饿感。又称为白水石。该物生长在山谷之中。

Record of Great Doctors），［it］says［that Ningshuishi（凝水石，calcitum，Gypsum Rubrum）is also］called Hanshuishi（寒水石）and Lingshuishi（凌水石），［seeming to be］the essence of salt.［It］may exist in Chang'an（常案）and Nishan（凝山）or Handan（邯郸）in Zhongshui（中水）county.

［In the book entitled］*Fan Zi Ji Ran*（《范子计然》，*Studies About Fan Li's Teacher*），［it］says［that Ningshuishi（凝水石，calcitum，Gypsum Rubrum）is］collected from Hedong（河东）with excellent color.

Notes

1. Ningshuishi（凝水石，calcitum，Gypsum Rubrum）is a mineral medicinal，pungent and salty in taste，severe cold in property，entering the heart meridian，the stomach meridian and the kidney meridian，effective in clearing heat，purging fire，disinhibiting orifices and resolving swelling. Clinically it is used to treat high fever，vexation and thirst，swelling and pain of the throat，erysipelas，scald and gingival bleeding.

549

8. 阳起石

【原文】

味咸,微温。

主崩中漏下,破子臧中血,症瘕结气,寒热,腹痛无子,阴痿不起(《御览》引,作阴阳不合),补不足(《御览》引,有句孪二字)。一名白石。生山谷。

550

【考据】

1.《吴普》曰:阳起石,神农扁鹊酸无毒,桐君雷公岐伯咸无毒,李氏小寒,或生太山(《御览》引云,或阳起山,采无时)。

2.《名医》曰:一名石生,一名羊起石,云母根也,生齐山及琅邪,或云山阳起山,采无时。

【今译】

味咸,性微温。

8. Yangqishi（阳起石，actinolite，Actinolitum）[1]

[Original Text]

[Yangqishi（阳起石，actinolite，Actinolitum），] salty in taste and slightly warm [in property], [is mainly used] to treat flooding and spotting (metrostaxis and metrorrhagia), vaginal bleeding [due to] uterine injury, abdominal mass [due to] stagnation of Qi, cold-head [disease], infertility [due to] abdominal pain and impotence. [It is also] called Baishi（白石），existing in mountains and valleys.

[Textual Research]

[in the book entitled] *Wu Pu Ben Cao*（《吴普本草》，*Wu Pu's Studies of Materia Medica*），[it] says [that] Yangqishi（阳起石，actinolite，Actinolitum），[according to] Agriculture God（神农）and Bianque（扁鹊），[is] sour [in taste] and non-toxic [in property]；[according to] Tongjun（桐均），Leigong（雷公）and Qibo（岐伯），[it is] salty [in taste] and non-toxic [in property]；[according to] Li's（李氏），[it is] slightly cold [in property]. [It] may exist in Taishan（太山）. [According to the book entitled] *Tai Ping Yu Lan*（《太平御览》，*Imperial Studies in Taiping Times*），[it] may exist in Yangqi（阳起）mountain and [can be] collected at any time.

[In the book entitled] *Ming Yi Bie Lu*（《名医别录》，*Special Record of Great Doctors*），[it] says [that Yangqishi（阳起石，actinolite，Actinolitum）is also] called Shisheng（石生）and

551

　　主治阴道突然出血,淋漓不断,能消除子宫中的瘀血,能治疗症瘕,

气结,寒热病,腹部疼痛,不孕之症以及因阳痿而阴茎不能勃起。又称

为白石。该物生长在山谷之中。

Yangqishi（羊起石）. [It is] the root of Yunmu（云母, muscovite, Muscovitum）, existing in Qishan（齐山）and Langxie（琅邪）, or Yunshan（云山）and Yangqishan（阳起山）. [It can be] collected at any time.

Notes

1. Yangqishi（阳起石, actinolite, Actinolitum）is a mineral medicinal, salty in taste and warm in property, entering the kidney meridian, effective in warming the kidney and reinforcing Yang. Clinically it is used to treat impotence, seminal emission, premature ejaculation, infertility and uterine coldness.

9. 孔公蘗

【原文】

味辛,温。

主伤食不化,邪结气,恶疮,疽瘘痔,利九窍,下乳汁(《御览》引云,一名通石,《大观本》,作黑字)。生山谷。

【考据】

1.《吴普》曰:孔公蘗,神农辛,岐伯咸,扁鹊酸无毒,色青黄。

2.《名医》曰:一名通石,殷蘗根也,青黄色生梁山。

【今译】

味辛,性温。

主治食积不化,邪气结滞,恶性疮,疽瘘,痔疮,能使九窍畅通,能使乳汁通畅。该物生长在山谷之中。

9. Konggongnie（孔公蘖，stalactites，Stalactitum） [1]

[Original Text]

[Konggongnie（孔公蘖，stalactites，Stalactitum），] pungent in taste and warm [in property], [is mainly used] to treat indigestion, stagnation of Qi, severe sore, carbuncle, scabies and hemorrhoids, to disinhibit nine orifices and to promote lactation. [It] exists in mountains and valleys.

[Textual Research]

[In the book entitled] *Wu Pu Ben Cao*（《吴普本草》，*Wu Pu's Studies of Materia Medica*），[it] says [that] Konggongnie（孔公蘖，stalactites，Stalactitum），[according to] Agriculture God（神农），[is] pungent [in taste]；[according to] Qibo（岐伯），[it is] salty [in property]；[according to] Bianque（扁鹊），[it is] sour [in taste]，non-toxic [in property]，yellow and green in color.

[In the book entitled] *Ming Yi Bie Lu*（《名医别录》，*Special Record of Great Doctors*），[it] says [that Konggongnie（孔公蘖，stalactites，Stalactitum），also] called Tongshi（通石），[is] the root of Yinnie（殷孽）[2]. [It is] green and yellow in color，existing in Liangshan（梁山）.

Notes

1. Konggongnie（孔公蘖，stalactites，Stalactitum），also known as Shizhongru（石钟乳），is a mineral medicinal，pungent in taste and warm in property，entering the stomach meridian，the lung meridian and the kidney meridian，effective in warming the lung，assisting Yang，replenishing Qi and enriching essence. Clinically it is used to treat cough with dyspnea，agalactostasis，damage and exhaustion of the lower energizer，pain of the waist and knees，infertility，impotence，disorder of the five Zang-organs and obstruction of the orifices.

10. 殷蘖

【原文】

味辛,温。

主烂伤瘀血,泄利,寒热,鼠瘘,症瘕,结气。一名姜石。生山谷(按此当与孔公蘖为一条)。

【考据】

1.《名医》曰:钟乳根也生赵国,又梁山及南海,采无时。

【今译】

味辛,性温。

主治因外伤及烂伤所引起的瘀血,泄泻,痢疾,寒热病,鼠瘘,症瘕,气结。又称为姜石。该物生长在山谷之中。

10. Yinnie（殷孽，Yinnie medicinal， Materia Medica Yinnie）[1]

[Original Text]

[Yinnie（殷孽），Yinnie medicinal，Materia Medica Yinnie] pungent in taste and warm [in property]，[is mainly used to] treat blood stasis [due to] severe traumatic injury，diarrhea，cold-head [disease]，cold ulcerated scrofula，abdominal mass and stagnation of Qi. [It is also] called Jiangshi（姜石），existing in mountains and valleys.

[Textual Research]

[In the book entitled] *Ming Yi Bie Lu*（《名医别录》，*Special Record of Great Doctors*），[it] says [that Yinnie（殷孽，Yinnie medicinal，Materia Medica Yinnie) is] the root of Zhongru（钟乳）[2]，existing in Zhaoguo（赵国），or Liangshan（梁山）mountain and Nanhai（南海，South Sea）. [It can be] collected at any time.

557

Notes

1. Yinnie（殷孽，Yinnie medicinal，Materia Medica Yinnie) shares the same source with Konggongnie（孔公蘗，stalactites，Stalactitum）which is also known as Shizhongru（石钟乳）. That means Yinnie（殷孽，Yinnie medicinal，Materia Medica Yinnie) and Konggongnie（孔公蘗，stalactites，Stalactitum) are practically the same. The difference is that they are collected from different parts of the same source.

2. Zhongru（钟乳）is a simplified name of Shizhongru（石钟乳）.

神农本草经

11. 铁精

【原文】

平。

主明目化铜。

铁落,味辛,平,主风热,恶疮,疡疽疮痂,疥气在皮肤中。

铁,主坚肌耐痛,生平泽(旧为三条,今并)。

【考据】

1.《名医》曰:铁落一名铁液,可以染皂,生牧羊及祊城或析城,采无时。

2. 案《说文》云:铁,黑金也,或省作铁,古文作铁。

【今译】

性平。

能使眼睛明亮,能变化成铜。

铁落,味辛,性平,主治风热病,恶性痈疮,疡疽,疮痂,皮肤中的

11. Tiejing（铁精，iron powder，Ferrum Pulveratum）[1]

[Original Text]

[Tiejing（铁精，Ferrum Pulveratum；iron powder），] mild [in property]，[is mainly used] to improve vision. [It can be] transformed into copper.

Tieluo（铁落，iron filing），pungent [in taste] and mild [in property]，[is mainly used] to treat wind-heat [disease]，severe sore，ulcer，carbuncle，scab and scabies in the skin.

Tie（铁，iron）[is mainly used] to strengthen the muscles and relieve pain.

[It] exists in plains and swamps.

[Textual Research]

[In the book entitled] *Ming Yi Bie Lu*（《名医别录》，*Special Record of Great Doctors*），[it] says [that] Tieluo（铁落，iron filing），also called Tieye（铁液），can dye black. [It] exists in Muyang（牧羊），Bengcheng（祊城）or Xicheng（析城），and [can be] collected at any time.

[In] case [analysis in the book entitled] *Shuo Wen*（《说文》，*On Culture*），[it] says [that] Tie（铁，iron）is a black metal，simply called Tie（铁，iron）.

疠气。

铁，能使肌肉坚强，能耐受疼痛。

该物存在于平川水泽之中。

Notes

1. Tiejing (铁精, Ferrum Pulveratum; iron powder), including Tieluo (铁落, iron filing) and Tie (铁, iron), is pungent in taste and mild in property, entering the liver meridian, effective in harmonizing the liver, relieving fright and nourishing muscles. Clinically it is used to treat epilepsy, mania, severe sore, wind-heat disease, ulcer and retention of pathogenic factors in the skin.

12. 理石

【原文】

味辛,寒。

主身热,利胃解烦,益精明目,破积聚,去三虫。一名石立制石。生山谷。

【考据】

1.《名医》曰:一名饥石,如石膏,顺理而细,生汉中,及卢山,采无时。

【今译】

味辛,性寒。

主治身体发热,能使胃和顺,能解除烦躁,能补益精气,能使眼睛明亮,能破解积聚,能祛除三种虫子。又称为石立制石。该物存在于山谷之中。

12. Lishi（理石，fibrous gypsum，Gypsum et Anhydritum） [1]

［**Original Text**］

［Lishi （理石，fibrous gypsum，Gypsum et Anhydritum），］pungent in taste and cold ［in property］，［is mainly used］ to treat fever，to soothe the stomach，to relieve vexation，to replenish essence，to improve vision，to dispel accumulation ［of pathogenic factors］ and to eliminate three worms. ［It is also］ called Lizhishi （立制石）and exists in mountains and valleys.

［**Textual Research**］

［In the book entitled］ *Ming Yi Bie Lu* （《名医别录》，*Special Record of Great Doctors*），［it］ says ［that Lishi（理石，fibrous gypsum，Gypsum et Anhydritum）is also］ called Jishi（饥石）like Shigao（石膏，gypsum，Gypsum Fibrosum），smooth and fine，existing in Hanzhong（汉中）and Lushan（卢山）. ［It can be］ collected at any time.

Notes

1. Lishi（理石，fibrous gypsum，Gypsum et Anhydritum）is a mineral medicinal，pungent in taste，cold and non-toxic in property，entering the stomach meridian，effective in clearing heat and eliminating vexation，nourishing the stomach and replenishing Yin，resolving accumulation of pathogenic factors and breaking stagnation. Clinically it is used to treat fever，flaccidity，impediment，wasting-thirst and wind stroke.

13. 长石

【原文】

味辛,寒。

主身热,四肢寒厥,利小便,通血脉,明目,去翳眇,下三虫,杀蛊毒。久服不饥。一名方石。生山谷。

【考据】

1.《吴普》曰:长石一名方石,一名直石,生长子山谷,如马齿,润泽玉色长鲜,服之不饥(《御览》)。

2《名医》曰:一名土石,一名直石,理如马齿,方面润泽,玉色,生长子山,及太山临溜采无时。

【今译】

味辛,性寒。

13. Changshi（长石，fieldspar，Adularia）[1]

[Original Text]

[Changshi（长石，fieldspar，Adularia），] pungent in taste and cold [in property]，[is mainly used] to treat fever and coldness of limbs，to promote urination，to disinhibit vessels，to improve vision，to dispel nebula，to eliminate three worms and to expel worm toxin. Long-term taking [of it will make people feel] no hunger. [It is also] called Fangshi（方石），existing in mountains and valleys.

[Textual Research]

[In the book entitled] *Wu Pu Ben Cao*（《吴普本草》，*Wu Pu's Studies of Materia Medica*），[it] says [that] Changshi（长石，fieldspar，Adularia) is also called Fangshi（方石）and Zhishi（直石），existing in the mountains and valleys in Changzi（长子）like the teeth of a horse. [It is like] jade，smooth，moist and fresh. [When one has] taken it，[he will feel] no hunger,[according to the book entitled] *Tai Ping Yu Lan*（《太平御览》，*Imperial Studies in Taiping Times*）.

[In the book entitled] *Ming Yi Bie Lu*（《名医别录》，*Special Record of Great Doctors*），[it] says [that Changshi（长石，fieldspar，Adularia) is also] called Tushi（土石）and Zhishi（直石），looking like the teeth of a horse [as well as a] smooth and fresh jade，

　　主治身体发热,四肢厥冷,能使小便通畅,能使血脉畅通,能使眼睛

明亮,能祛除翳膜所致的偏盲,能杀除三种虫子和虫毒。长期服用能使

人减少饥饿感。又称为方石。该物存在于山谷之中。

existing in Changzi (长子) mountain and Linliu (临溜) in Taishan (太山). [It can be] collected at any time.

Notes

1. Changshi (长石, fieldspar, Adularia) is mineral medicinal, pungent and bitter in taste, cold in property, effective in clearing heat and producing fluid, descending Qi and promoting urination, improving vision and expelling nebula. Clinically it is used to treat fever, vexation, flaccidity of limbs, heat stranguria, dysuria, pterygium and blurred vision.

14. 肤青

【原文】

味辛,平。

主蛊毒,及蛇菜肉诸毒,恶疮。生川谷。

【考据】

1.《名医》曰:一名推青,一名推石,生益州。

2. 案陶宏景云:俗方及仙经,并无用此者,亦相与不复识。

上玉石,中品一十四种,旧十六种,考铁落、铁,宜与铁精为一。

【今译】

味辛,性平。

主治虫毒及蛇、菜、肉等毒素所致之病,能治疗恶性痈疮。该物生长在山川河谷之中。

神农本草经

14. Fuqing（肤青，Fuqing medicinal，Fuqing Materia Medica）[1]

[Original Text]

[Fuqing（肤青），] pungent in taste and mild [in property]，[is mainly used] to treat [disease caused by] worm toxin and other toxin from snake，vegetables and meat [as well as] severe sore. [It] exists in mountain valleys and river valleys.

[Textual Research]

[In the book entitled] *Ming Yi Bie Lu* (《名医别录》, *Special Record of Great Doctors*)，[it] says [that Fuqing（肤青）is also] called Tuiqing（推青）and Tuishi（推石），existing in Yizhou（益州）.

Tao Hongjing（陶宏景）said，"In ordinary formulae and *Xian Jing* (《仙经》, *Immortal Canon*)，there is no record of such a medicinal. [It is] not clear [what it] is." Perhaps it is one category of Tieluo（铁落，iron filing）and Tie（铁，iron）.

Notes

1. Fuqing（肤青）is still unclear now. According to some of the ancient literature，this medicinal is effective in expelling various toxin from worms，snakes and vegetables，and can be used to treat severe sores，scabies and ringworm.

15. 干姜

【原文】

味辛,温。

主胸满咳逆上气,温中止血,出汗,逐风,湿痹,肠澼,下利。生者尤良,久服去臭气,通神明。生川谷。

【考据】

1.《名医》曰:生楗为及荆州扬州,九月采。

2.案《说文》云:姜,御湿之菜也。《广雅》云:蔟廉姜也。吕氏春秋本味篇云:和之美者,阳朴之姜,高诱注,阳朴地名在蜀郡,司马相如上林赋,有茈姜云云。

【今译】

味辛,性温。

主治胸满,咳嗽,呼吸困难,能温煦人体脏器,能止血,能引起出

15. Ganjiang（干姜，dry ginger，Rhizoma Zingiberis）[1]

[Original Text]

[Ganjiang（干姜，dry ginger，Rhizoma Zingiberis），] pungent in taste and warm [in property], [is mainly used] to relieve chest fullness，cough with dyspnea and upward counterflow of Qi，to warm the middle（the internal organs），to cease bleeding，[to promote] sweating，to expel wind，to treat dampness impediment，dysentery and diarrhea. The raw one is more effective. Long-term taking [of it will] remove foul smell and invigorate spirit and mentality. [It] grows in mountain valleys and river valleys.

571

[Textual Research]

[In the book entitled] *Ming Yi Bie Lu*（《名医别录》，*Special Record of Great Doctors*），[it] says [that Ganjiang（干姜，dry ginger，Rhizoma Zingiberis）] grows in Jianwei（楗为），Jingzhou（荆州）and Yangzhou（扬州）. [It can be] collected in September.

[In] case [analysis in the book entitled] *Shuo Wen*（《说文》，*On Culture*），[it] says [that] ginger is a vegetable preventing dampness.

Notes

1. Ganjiang（干姜，dry ginger，Rhizoma Zingiberis）is a herbal

汗,能祛除风湿所致之痹证,能治疗泄泻,痢疾。生姜的疗效更好,长期服用能祛除臭气,能使神志清晰、精神旺盛。该物生长在山川河谷之中。

medicinal, pungent in taste, hot in property, entering the heart meridian, the spleen meridian, the lung meridian and the kidney meridian, effective in warming the middle (the internal organs) and expelling cold, restoring Yang and disinhibiting vessels, resolving lump and descending Qi. Clinically it is used to treat abdominal and gastric pain, vomiting due to deficiency-cold, coldness of limbs with weak pulse, cough and panting due to drinking cold water, wind-cold and dampness impediment.

16. 枲耳实

【原文】

味甘,温。

主风头,寒痛,风湿,周痹,四肢拘挛,痛,恶肉死肌。久服益气,耳目聪明,强志轻身。一名胡枲,一名地葵。生川谷。

【考据】

1.《名医》曰:一名葹,一名常思,生安陆及六安田野,实熟时采。

2. 案《说文》云:葹,卷耳也。苓,卷耳也。《广雅》云:苓,耳葹,常枲,胡枲,枲耳也。《尔雅》云:苍耳,苓耳。郭璞云:江东呼为常枲,形似鼠耳,丛生如盘。《毛诗》云:采采卷耳。《传》云:卷耳,苓耳也。陆玑云:叶青,白色,似胡荽,白华,细茎蔓生,可煮为茹,滑而少味,四月中生子,正如妇人耳珰,今或谓之耳珰草,郑康成谓是白胡荽,幽州人谓之爵耳。《淮南子》览冥训云:位贱尚枲。高诱云:枲者,枲耳,菜名也。幽冀谓之檀菜,锥下谓之胡枲。

16. Xi'ershi（枲耳实，fruit of Siberian cocklebur，Fructus Xanthii）[1]

[Original Text]

[Xi'ershi（枲耳实，fruit of Siberian cocklebur，Fructus Xanthii），] sweet in taste [and] warm [in property]，[is mainly used] to treat coldness and pain of the head [caused by attack of] wind，generalized impediment，spasm and pain of the four limbs，severely damaged muscles and putrescent muscles. Long-term taking [of it will] replenish Qi，improve hearing and vision，strengthen memory and relax the body. [It is also] called Huxi（胡枲）and Dikui（地葵），growing in mountain valleys and river valleys.

[Textual Research]

[In the book entitled] *Ming Yi Bie Lu*（《名医别录》，*Special Record of Great Doctors*），[it] says [that Xi'ershi（枲耳实，fruit of Siberian cocklebur，Fructus Xanthii) is also] called Mingshi（名菕）and Changsi（常思），growing in the fields in Anlu（安陆）and Liu'an（六安）. [It can be] collected [when its] fruit is ripe.

Lu Ji（陆玑）said，"[Its] leaves are green，[its] flowers are as white as coriander，[its] stalks are thin，and [it] sprawls all the way. [It] can be boiled for eating. [When boiled，it is] smooth and tasteless. [It begins] to bear seeds in April，like women's ear pendants. Now [it] may be called ear pendant herb."

575

【今译】

味甘,性温。

主治伤风头痛,冷痛,风湿证,全身流窜性疼痛,四肢拘挛疼痛,肌肉坏死。长期服用能补益精气,能使听力敏锐,视力清明,能增强记忆力,能使人身体轻盈。又称为胡枲,又称为地葵。该物生长在山川河谷之中。

Notes

1. Xi'ershi（枲耳实，fruit of Siberian cocklebur，Fructus Xanthii) is a herbal medicinal，sweet and bitter in taste，warm and slightly toxic in property，entering the lung meridian and the liver meridian，effective in inducing sweating and relieving pain，disinhibiting nostrils and expelling wind-dampness. Clinically it is used to treat headache due to wind-cold attack，nasosinusitis，wind-dampness impediment and pain，spasm of limbs，leprosy，scabies，ringworm and itching.

17. 葛根

【原文】

味甘,平。

主消渴,身大热,呕吐,诸痹,起阴气,解诸毒,葛谷,主下利十岁已上。一名鸡齐根。生川谷。

【考据】

1.《吴普》曰:葛根,神农甘,生太山(《御览》)。

2.《名医》曰:一名鹿藿,一名黄斤,生汶山,五月采根,暴干。

【今译】

味甘,性平。

主治消渴病,身体高热,呕吐,各种痹证,能使阴茎勃起,能消解各种毒气。

葛谷,主治十年以上的慢性痢疾,使之痊愈。又称为鸡齐根。该物生长在山川河谷之中。

17. Gegen（葛根，pueraria，Radix Puerariae）[1]

[Original Text]

[Gegen（葛根，pueraria，Radix Puerariae），] sweet in taste [and] mild [in property], [is mainly used] to treat wasting-thirst, severe fever, vomiting, nausea and various impediment, to invigorate Yin Qi[2] and to remove various toxin. The seed of Gegen（葛根，pueraria，Radix Puerariae) can effectively treat diarrhea [continuing for] over ten years. [It is also] called Jiqigen（鸡齐根），growing in mountain valleys and river valleys.

[Textual Research]

[In the book entitled] *Wu Pu Ben Cao*（《吴普本草》，*Wu Pu's Studies of Materia Medica*），[it] says [that] Gegen（葛根，pueraria，Radix Puerariae），[according to] Agriculture God（神农），[is] sweet [in taste], growing in Taishan（太山）[as mentioned in the book entitled] *Tai Ping Yu Lan*（《太平御览》，*Imperial Studies in Taiping Times*).

[In the book entitled] *Ming Yi Bie Lu*（《名医别录》，*Special Record of Great Doctors*），[it] says [that Gegen（葛根，pueraria，Radix Puerariae) is also] called Luhuo（鹿藿）and Huangjin（黄斤），growing in Wenshan（汶山）. [Its] root [can be] collected in May and dried in the sun.

579

Notes

1. Gegen（葛根，pueraria，Radix Puerariae) is a herbal medicinal, sweet and pungent in taste, mild in property, entering the spleen meridian and the stomach meridian, effective in solving hunger and reducing heat, producing fluid and ceasing thirst. Clinically it is used to treat common cold, fever, thirst, headache, stiff neck, measles that are difficult to be resolved, diarrhea and dysentery.

---

[2]　Yin Qi here refers penis.

神农本草经

18. 括楼根

【原文】

味苦,寒。

主消渴,身热,烦满,大热,补虚安中,续绝伤。一名地楼。生川谷,及山阴。

【考据】

1.《吴普》曰:括楼,一名泽巨,一名泽姑(《御览》)。

2.《名医》曰:一名果裸,一名天瓜,一名泽姑,实名黄瓜,二月八月,采根,暴干,三十日成,生宏农。

3. 案《说文》云:菩,菩蒌,果蓏也。《广雅》云:王白,菩也。(党为王菩)《尔雅》云:果裸之实,括楼。郭璞云:今齐人呼之为天瓜。《毛诗》云:果裸之实,亦施于宇。《传》云:果裸,括楼也。吕氏春秋云:王善生。高诱云:善或作瓜,舐瓝也。案吕氏春秋善字乃菩之误。

【今译】

味苦,性寒。

18. Kuolougen（括楼根，root of Mongolian snakegourd，Radix Trichosanthis）[1]

[Original Text]

[Kuolougen（括楼根，root of Mongolian snakegourd，Radix Trichosanthis），] bitter in taste and cold [in property]，[is mainly used] to treat wasting-thirst，fever，vexation and severe heat，to improve deficiency，to harmonize the middle（the internal organs）and to cure severe injury. [It is also] called Dilou（地楼），growing in mountain valleys，river valleys and the shady sides of mountains.

[Textual Research]

[In the book entitled] *Wu Pu Ben Cao*（《吴普本草》，*Wu Pu's Studies of Materia Medica*），[it] says [that] Kuolougen（括楼根，root of Mongolian snakegourd，Radix Trichosanthis）is also called Zeju（泽巨）and Zegu（泽姑）[according to the book entitled] *Tai Ping Yu Lan*（《太平御览》，*Imperial Studies in Taiping Times*）.

[In the book entitled] *Ming Yi Bie Lu*（《名医别录》，*Special Record of Great Doctors*），[it] says [that Kuolougen（括楼根，root of Mongolian snakegourd，Radix Trichosanthis）is also] called Guoluo（果裸），Tiangua（天瓜）and Zegu（泽姑）. The actual name is Huanggua（黄瓜）. [Its] root [can be] collected in February and August，and dried in the sun for thirty days. [It] grows in Hongnong（宏农）.

　　主治消渴病，身体发热，烦躁，郁闷，身体高热，能补益虚弱，能安静内脏，能通过补益主治外伤所致之筋伤骨折。又称为地楼。该物生长在山川河谷之中及山的阴面。

Notes

1. Kuolougen（括楼根，root of Mongolian snakegourd，Radix Trichosanthis）is a herbal medicinal，sweet and slightly bitter in taste，slightly cold in property，entering the lung meridian and the kidney meridian，effective in clearing heat and producing fluid，reducing fire and moistening dryness，eliminating pus and resolving swelling. Clinically it is used to treat heat disease that damages fluid and causes thirst，cough due to dryness and heat in the lung，hemoptysis，wasting-thirst，jaundice，carbuncle，acute mastitis，scabies and hemorrhoids.

19. 苦参

【原文】

味苦,寒。

主心腹结气,症瘕积聚,黄疸,溺有余沥,逐水,除痈肿,补中,明目,止泪。一名水槐,一名苦识。生山谷及田野。

【考据】

1.《名医》曰:一名地槐,一名菟槐,一名骄槐,一名白茎,一名虎麻,一名芩茎,一名禄曰,一名陵郎,生汝南,三月八月十月,采根,暴干。

【今译】

味苦,性寒。

主治心腹结气,症瘕积聚,黄疸,尿后淋漓不尽,能祛除水湿,能消除痈肿,能充实人体内脏,能使眼睛明亮,能止泪。又称为水槐,又称为苦识。该物生长在山谷之中及田野。

19. Kushen（苦参，flavescent sophora，

Radix Sophorae Flavescentis）[1]

［Original Text］

［Kushen （苦参，flavescent sophora，Radix Sophorae Flavescentis），］bitter in taste and cold ［in property］，［is mainly used］ to treat stagnation of Qi in the heart and abdomen，abdominal mass and accumulation ［of pathogenic factors］，jaundice and dribbling after urination，to expel water，to eliminate carbuncle and swelling，to tonify the middle（the internal organs），to improve vision and to stop tearing. ［It is also］ called Shuihuai（水槐）and Kushi（苦识），growing in mountains，valleys and fields.

［Textual Research］

［In the book entitled］ *Ming Yi Bie Lu*（《名医别录》，*Special Record of Great Doctors*），［it］ says ［that Kushen（苦参，flavescent sophora，Radix Sophorae Flavescentis）is also］ called Dihuai（地槐），Tuhuai（菟槐），Jiaohuai（骄槐），Baijing（白茎），Huma（虎麻），Qinjing（芩茎），Luyue（禄曰）and Lingliang（陵郎），growing in Runan（汝南）. ［Its］ root ［can be］ collected in March，August and October，and dried in the sun.

585

Notes

1. Kushen（苦参，flavescent sophora，Radix Sophorae Flavescentis）is a herbal medicinal，bitter in taste and cold in property，entering the lung meridian，the large intestine meridian and the small intestine meridian，effective in clearing heat and drying dampness，killing worms and relieving itching. Clinically it is used to treat dysentery due to dampness-heat，jaundice，infantile malnutrition，bloody hemorrhoids，dysuria，dribbling urination and red and white leucorrhea.

20. 当归

【原文】

味甘,温。

主咳逆上气,温疟,寒热洗洗在皮肤中(《大观本》,洗音癣)。妇人漏下绝子,诸恶疮疡金疮。煮饮之。一名干归。生川谷。

【考据】

1.《吴普》曰:当归,神农黄帝桐君扁鹊甘无毒,岐伯雷公辛无毒,李氏小温,或生羌胡地。

2.《名医》曰:生陇西,二月八月,采根阴干。

3. 案《广雅》云:山靳,当归也。《尔雅》云:薜,山靳。郭璞云:今似靳而粗大,又薜,白靳。郭璞云:即上山靳。《范子计然》云:当归,出陇西,无枯者善。

【今译】

味甘,性温。

20. Danggui（当归，Chinese angelica，Radix Angelicae Sinensis）[1]

［Original Text］

［Danggui（当归，Chinese angelica，Radix Angelicae Sinensis），］ sweet in taste［and］warm［in property］，［is mainly used］to treat cough with dyspnea and upward counterflow of Qi，warm malaria with cold and heat in the skin，infertility with vaginal bleeding，various severe sores， ulcers and injury［caused by］metal.［It is also］called Gangui（干归），growing in mountain valleys and river valleys.

［Textual Research］

［In the book entitled］*Wu Pu Ben Cao*（《吴普本草》，*Wu Pu's Studies of Materia Medica*），［it］says［that］Danggui（当归，Chinese angelica，Radix Angelicae Sinensis），［according to］Agriculture God（神农），Yellow Emperor（黄帝），Tongjun（桐均）and Bianque（扁鹊），［is］sweet［in taste］and non-toxic［in property］；［according to］Qibo（岐伯）and Leigong（雷公），［it is］pungent［in taste］and non-toxic［in property］；［according to］Li's（李氏），［it is］slightly warm［in property］.［It］may grow in Qianghu（羌胡）.

［In the book entitled］*Ming Yi Bie Lu*（《名医别录》，*Special Record of Great Doctors*），［it］says［that Danggui（当归，Chinese angelica，Radix Angelicae Sinensis）］grows in Longxi（陇西）.［Its］

　　主治咳嗽及呼吸困难，温疟，皮肤中寒热颤栗，能治疗妇人阴道出血淋漓不断，不孕症，能消除各种恶性疮疡及因金属创伤而导致的痈疮。煮汁饮用。又称为干归。该物生长在山川河谷之中。

root〔can be〕collected in February and August，and dried in the shade.

〔In the book entitled〕*Guang Ya*（《广雅》，*The First Chinese Encyclopedic Dictionary*），〔it〕says〔that the so-called〕Shanjin（山靳）refers to Danggui（当归，Chinese angelica，Radix Angelicae Sinensis）.〔In the book entitled〕*Fan Zi Ji Ran*（《范子计然》，*Studies About Fan Li's Teacher*），〔it〕says〔that〕Danggui（当归，Chinese angelica，Radix Angelicae Sinensis）grows in Longxi（陇西）.〔It is〕more effective〔if it is〕not withered.

Notes

1. Danggui（当归，Chinese angelica，Radix Angelicae Sinensis）is a herbal medicinal，sweet and pungent in taste，warm in property，entering the heart meridian，the spleen meridian and the liver meridian，effective in tonifying the blood，activating the blood，regulating meridians，unobstructing collaterals and moistening the intestines. Clinically it is used to treat irregular menstruation，amenorrhea，dysmenorrhea，flooding and spotting（metrostaxis and metrorrhagia），anemia，headache due to blood deficiency，vertigo，constipation，abdominal mass，wind-dampness impediment and pain，carbuncle，scabies，ulcer and traumatic injury.

21. 麻黄

【原文】

味苦,温。

主中风,头痛,伤寒,温疟,发表出汗,去邪热气,止咳逆上气,除寒热,破症坚积聚。一名龙沙。

【考据】

1.《吴普》曰:麻黄一名卑相,一名卑坚,神农雷公苦无毒,扁鹊酸无毒,李氏平,或生河东,四月,立秋采(《御览》)。

2.《名医》曰:一名卑相,一名卑盐,生晋地及河东,立秋采茎,阴干令青。

3. 案《广雅》云:龙沙,麻黄也。麻黄茎,狗骨也。《范子计然》云:麻黄出汉中三辅。

【今译】

味苦,性温。

21. Mahuang（麻黄，ephedra，Herba Ephedrae）[1]

[Original Text]

[Mahuang（麻黄，ephedra，Herba Ephedrae），] bitter in taste and warm [in property], [is mainly used] to treat wind stroke, headache, cold damage and malaria, to relieve superficies, to induce sweating, to eliminate evil-heat Qi, to stop cough with dyspnea with upward counterflow of Qi, to eliminate cold-heat and to resolve abdominal lump and accumulation [of pathogenic factors]. [It is also] called Longsha（龙沙）.

[Textual Research]

[In the book entitled] *Wu Pu Ben Cao*（《吴普本草》，*Wu Pu's Studies of Materia Medica*）, [it] says [that] Mahuang（麻黄，ephedra，Herba Ephedrae）[is also] called Beixiang（卑相）and Beijian（卑坚）. [According to] Agriculture God（神农）and Leigong（雷公），[it is] bitter [in taste] and non-toxic [in property]; [according to] Bianque（扁鹊），[it is] sour [in taste] and non-toxic [in property]; [according to] Li's（李氏），[it is] mild [in property]. [It] may grow in Hedong（河东）and [can be] collected in April and the Autumn Solstice [according to the book entitled] *Tai Ping Yu Lan*（《太平御览》，*Imperial Studies in Taiping Times*）.

[In the book entitled] *Ming Yi Bie Lu*（《名医别录》，*Special*

　　主治中风,伤寒,头痛,温疟,发表出汗,能祛除邪热所致之症,能消除咳嗽及呼吸困难,能治疗寒热病,能消散坚硬痞块和体内积聚。又称为龙沙。

Record of Great Doctors），［it］says［that Mahuang（麻黄，ephedra，Herba Ephedrae）is also］called Beixiang（卑相）and Beiyan（卑盐），growing in Jindi（晋地）and Hedong（河东）.［Its］stalks［can be］collected in the Autumn Solstice and dried in the shade.

［In the book entitled］*Guang Ya*（《广雅》，*The First Chinese Encyclopedic Dictionary*），［it］says［that the so-called］Longsha（龙沙）refers to Mahuang（麻黄，ephedra，Herba Ephedrae）and the stalk of Mahuang（麻黄，ephedra，Herba Ephedrae）is called Gougu（狗骨）.［In the book entitled］*Fan Zi Ji Ran*（《范子计然》，*Studies About Fan Li's Teacher*），［it］says［that］Mahuang（麻黄，ephedra，Herba Ephedrae）grows in the three places in Hanzhong（汉中）.

Notes

1. Mahuang（麻黄，ephedra，Herba Ephedrae）is a herbal medicinal，bitter and pungent in taste，warm in property，entering the lung meridian and the bladder meridian，effective in inducing sweating，relieving asthma and promoting urination. Clinically it is used to treat common cold due to wind-cold，fever with sweating，measles，urticaria，bronchitis，asthma，pneumonia and edema at the early period of nephritis.

22. 通草 (《御览》作蓪草)

【原文】

味辛,平。

主去恶虫,除脾胃寒热,通利九窍,血脉关节,令人不忘。一名附支。生山谷。

【考据】

1.《吴普》曰:蓪草,一名丁翁,一名附支,神农黄帝辛,雷公苦,生石城山谷,叶菁蔓延,止汗,自正月采(《御览》)。

2.《名医》曰:一名丁翁,生石城及山阳,正月采枝,阴干。

3. 案《广雅》云:附支,蓪草也。《中山经》云:升山其草多寇脱。郭璞云:寇脱草,生南方,高丈许,似荷叶,而茎中有瓤,正白,零陵人植而日灌之,以为树也。《尔雅》云:离南活莧.郭璞注同,又倚商,活脱。郭璞云:即离南也。《范子计然》云:蓪草,出三辅。

22. Tongcao（通草，ricepaperplant stempith，Medulla Tetrapanacis）[1]

[Original Text]

[Tongcao （通草，ricepaperplant stempith，Medulla Tetrapanacis），] pungent in taste and mild [in property]，[is mainly used] to expel evil worms，to eliminate cold-heat in the spleen and stomach，to disinhibit the nine orifices，blood vessels and joints，and to prevent amnesia. [It is also] called Fuzhi（附支），growing in mountains and valleys.

[Textual Research]

[In the book entitled] *Wu Pu Ben Cao* （《吴普本草》，*Wu Pu's Studies of Materia Medica* ），[it] says [that] Tongcao （通草，ricepaperplant stempith，Medulla Tetrapanacis）[is also] called Dingweng（丁翁）and Fuzhi（附支）. [According to] Agriculture God（神农）and Yellow Emperor（黄帝），[it is] pungent [in taste]；[according to] Leigong（雷公），[it is] bitter [in taste]. [It] grows in the mountains and valleys in Shicheng（石城）. [Its] leaf is green，sprawls all the way and [can be used] to stop sweating. [It can be] collected in January [according to the book entitled] *Tai Ping Yu Lan* （《太平御览》，*Imperial Studies in Taiping Times* ）.

[In the book entitled] *Ming Yi Bie Lu* （《名医别录》，*Special Record of Great Doctors* ），[it] says [that Tongcao （通草，

【今译】

味辛,性平。

能祛除肠道中的寄生虫,能消除脾胃中的寒热,能通畅九窍,血脉和关节,能消除健忘之症。又称为附支。该物生长在山谷之中。

ricepaperplant stempith，Medulla Tetrapanacis）is also］called Dingweng（丁翁），growing in Shicheng（石城）and Shanyang（山阳）.［Its］branches［can be］collected in January and dried in the shade.

［In the book entitled］*Guang Ya*（《广雅》，*The First Chinese Encyclopedic Dictionary*），［it］says［that the so-called］Fuzhi（附支）refers to Tongcao （通 草，ricepaperplant stempith，Medulla Tetrapanacis）.［In the book entitled］*Fan Zi Ji Ran*（《范子计然》，*Studies About Fan Li's Teacher*），［it］says［that］Tongcao（通草，ricepaperplant stempith，Medulla Tetrapanacis）grows in three places.

Notes

1. Tongcao （通 草，ricepaperplant stempith，Medulla Tetrapanacis）is a herbal medicinal，sweet and bland in taste，and cold in property，entering the lung meridian，the stomach meridian and the bladder meridian，effective in clearing heat，promoting urination and lactation. Clinically it is used to treat dysuria，edema，infection of urethra and agalactostasis.

23. 芍药

【原文】

味苦,平。

主邪气腹痛,除血痹,破坚积寒热,疝瘕,止痛,利小便,益气(艺文类聚引云:一名白术,《大观本》,作黑字)。生川谷及丘陵。

【考据】

1.《吴普》曰:芍药,神农苦,桐君甘,无毒,岐伯咸。李氏小寒,雷公酸,一名甘积,一名解仓,一名诞,一名余容,一名白术,三月三日采。(《御览》)

2.《名医》曰:一名白术,一名余容,一名犁食,一名解食,一名铤,生中岳,二月八月,采根,暴干。

3. 案《广雅》云:挛夷,芍药也。白术、牡丹也。北山经云:绣山其草多芍药。郭璞云:芍药一名辛夷,亦香草属。《毛诗》云:赠之以芍药。《传》云:芍药,香草。《范子计然》云:芍药出三辅。崔豹古今注云:芍药有三种,有草芍药,有木芍药,木有花,大而色深,俗呼为牡丹,非也。又云:一名可离。

23. Shaoyao（芍药，peony，Radix Paeoniae）[1]

[Original Text]

[Shaoyao（芍药，peony，Radix Paeoniae），] bitter in taste and mild [in property]，[is mainly used] to expel evil-Qi，to relieve abdominal pain，to eliminate blood impediment，to dispel hard accumulation of cold and heat，to cease pain，to promote urination and to replenish Qi. [It] grows in mountain valleys，river valleys and hills.

[Textual Research]

[In the book entitled] *Wu Pu Ben Cao*（《吴普本草》，*Wu Pu's Studies of Materia Medica*），[it] says [that] Shaoyao（芍药，peony，Radix Paeoniae），[according to] Agriculture God（神农），[is] bitter [in taste]；[according to] Tongjun（桐均），[it is] sweet [in taste] and non-toxic [in property]；[according to] Qibo（岐伯），[it is] salty [in taste]；[according to] Li's（李氏），[it is] slightly cold [in property]；[according to] Leigong（雷公），[it is] sour [in taste]. [It is also] called Ganji（甘积），Jiecang（解仓），Dan（诞），Yurong（余容）and Baizhu（白术），[and can be] collected on March 3 [according to the book entitled] *Tai Ping Yu Lan*（《太平御览》，*Imperial Studies in Taiping Times*）.

[In the book entitled] *Ming Yi Bie Lu*（《名医别录》，*Special Record of Great Doctors*），[it] says [that Shaoyao（芍药，peony，Radix Paeoniae）is also] called Baizhu（白术），Yurong（余容），Lishi（犁食），

【今译】

味苦,性平。

主治邪气所致之症,腹部疼痛,能消除因血虚所致之痹证,能破除坚硬积聚和寒热病,能治疗疝瘕,能解除疼痛,能使小便通畅,能补益精气。该物生长在山川河谷之中及丘陵。

Jieshi（解食）and Ting（铤）, growing in Zhongyue（中岳）. ［Its］root ［can be］collected in February and August, and dried in the sun.

［In the book entitled］ *Guang Ya* （《广雅》, *The First Chinese Encyclopedic Dictionary*）, ［it］says ［that the so-called］Luanyi（挛夷）refers to Shaoyao（芍药, peony, Radix Paeoniae）and ［the so-called］Baizhu（白术）refers to Mudan（牡丹, moutan, Cortex Moutan Radicis）. ［In the book entitled］ *Shan Hai Jing* （《山海经》, *Canon of Mountains and Seas*）about］North Mountain, ［it］says ［that］most of the herbs in Xiushan（绣山）are Shaoyao（芍药, peony, Radix Paeoniae）. Guo Pu（郭璞）said, "Shaoyao（芍药, peony, Radix Paeoniae）［is also］called Xinyi（辛夷）, a kind of fragrant herb." ［In the book entitled］ *Fan Zi Ji Ran* （《范子计然》, *Studies About Fan Li's Teacher*）, ［it］says ［that］Shaoyao（芍药, peony, Radix Paeoniae）grows in three places. ［In］explaining the ancient and present, Cui Bao（崔豹）said, "There are three kind of Shaoyao（芍药, peony, Radix Paeoniae）, grass, wood, and wood with flowers. ［It is］large and deep in color. People call it Mudan（牡丹, moutan, Cortex Moutan Radicis）. ［Actually it is］not true."

Notes

1. Shaoyao （芍药, peony, Radix Paeoniae） is a herbal medicinal, bitter and sour in taste, slightly cold in property, entering the liver meridian and the spleen meridian, effective in nourishing the blood and subduing Yin, soothing the liver and stopping pain. Clinically it is used to treat headache, vertigo, pain in the chest, rib-side, gastric region and abdomen, diarrhea, dysentery, irregular menstruation, dysmenorrhea, flooding and spotting（metrostaxis and metrorrhagia）, leucorrhea, spasm of muscles, hands and feet, spontaneous sweating and night sweating.

24. 蠡实

【原文】

味甘,平。

主皮肤寒热,胃中热气,寒湿痹,坚筋骨,令人嗜食。久服轻身。花叶,去白虫。一名剧草,一名三坚,一名豕首。生川谷。

【考据】

1.《吴普》曰:蠡实,一名剧草,一名三坚,一名剧荔华(《御览》),一名泽蓝,一名豕首,神农黄帝甘辛无毒,生宛句,五月采。(同上)

2.《名医》曰:一名荔实,生河东,五月采,实阴干。

3. 案《说文》云:荔,草也,似蒲而小,根可作刷。《广雅》云:马薤,荔也。月令云:仲冬之月,荔挺出。郑云:荔挺,马薤也。高诱注《淮南子》云:荔马,荔草也。通俗文云:一名马兰。颜之推云:此物河北平泽率生之,江东颇多种于阶庭,但呼为旱蒲,故不识马薤。

【今译】

味甘,性平。

24. Lishi（蠡实，seed of swordlike iris，Semen Iridis Ensatae）[1]

[Original Text]

[Lishi（蠡实，seed of swordlike iris，Semen Iridis Ensatae），] sweet in taste [and] mild [in property]，[is mainly used] to treat cold and heat in the skin and heat-Qi in the stomach，to strengthen the sinews and bones，and to increase appetite. Long-term taking [of it will] relax the body.

[Its] flowers and leaves can expel tapeworm. [It is also] called Jucao（剧草），Sanjian（三坚）and Shishou（豕首），growing in mountain valleys and river valleys.

[Textual Research]

[In the book entitled] *Wu Pu Ben Cao*（《吴普本草》，*Wu Pu's Studies of Materia Medica*），[it] says [that] Lishi（蠡实，seed of swordlike iris，Semen Iridis Ensatae）[is also] called Jucao（剧草），Sanjian（三坚）and Julihua（剧荔华）. [In the book entitled] *Tai Ping Yu Lan*（《太平御览》，*Imperial Studies in Taiping Times*），[it] says [that it is also] called Zelan（泽蓝）and Shishou（豕首）. [According to] Agriculture God（神农）and Yellow Emperor（黄帝），[it is] sweet and pungent [in taste] and non-toxic [in property]，growing in Wanju（宛句）and to be collected in May.

[In the book entitled] *Ming Yi Bie Lu*（《名医别录》，*Special*

主治皮肤寒热病,胃中热邪症,寒湿邪所致痹证,能使筋骨强壮,能提高食欲。长期服用能使人身体轻盈。其花叶能祛除绦虫。又称为剧草,又称为三坚,又称为豕首。该物生长在山川河谷之中。

Record of Great Doctors）, [it] says [that Lishi（蠡实，seed of swordlike iris, Semen Iridis Ensatae）is also] called Lishi（荔实），growing in Hedong（河东）. [It can be] collected in May and dried in the shade.

[In] case [analysis in the book entitled] *Shuo Wen*（《说文》，*On Culture*）, [it] says [that] Li（荔），[another name of Lishi（蠡实，seed of swordlike iris, Semen Iridis Ensatae）] is a herb, similar to it but smaller [than it]. [Its] root can [be used] as a brush. [In the book entitled] *Guang Ya*（《广雅》，*The First Chinese Encyclopedic Dictionary*）, [it] says [that the so-called] Maxie（马薤）refers to Li（荔）.

Notes

1. Lishi（蠡实，seed of swordlike iris, Semen Iridis Ensatae）is a herbal medicinal, sweet in taste and mild in property, entering the liver meridian, the stomach meridian, the spleen meridian and the lung meridian, effective in clearing heat and resolving dampness, removing toxin and killing worms, stopping bleeding and relieving pain. Clinically it is used to treat jaundice, stranguria, dysuria, intestinal abscess, accumulation of worms, malaria, pain due to wind-dampness, throat impediment, toothache, hematemesis, nosebleed, hematochezia, flooding and spotting（metrostaxis and metrorrhagia），ulcer, scrofula, hernia, hemorrhoids, scald and bite of snake.

25. 瞿麦

【原文】

味苦,寒。

主关格,诸癃结,小便不通,出刺,决痈肿,明目去翳,破胎堕子,下闭血。一名巨句麦。生川谷。

【考据】

1.《名医》曰:一名大菊,一名大兰,生大山,立秋,采实,阴干。

2. 案《说文》云:蘧,蘧麦也。菊,大菊,蘧麦。《广雅》云:茈葳,陵苕,蘧麦也。《尔雅》云:大菊,蘧麦。郭璞云:一名麦句姜,即瞿麦。陶宏景云:子颇似麦,故名瞿麦。

【今译】

味苦,性寒。

25. Qumai（瞿麦，Chinese pink herb；rainbowpink herb，lilac pink herb，Herba Dianthi）[1]

[Original Text]

[Qumai（瞿麦，Chinese pink herb；rainbowpink herb，lilac pink herb，Herba Dianthi），] bitter in taste and cold [in property]，[is mainly used] to treat Guange[2] and retention of urine，to withdraw stab，to expel abscess，to improve vision and to eliminate nebula. [But it also can] damage fetus，cause abortion and obstruct the blood. [It is also] called Jujumai（巨句麦），growing in mountain valleys and river valleys.

[Textual Research]

[In the book entitled] *Ming Yi Bie Lu*（《名医别录》，*Special Record of Great Doctors*），[it] says [that Qumai（瞿麦，Chinese pink herb；rainbowpink herb，lilac pink herb，Herba Dianthi）is also] called Daju（大菊）and Dalan（大兰），growing in high mountains. [Its] fruit [can be] collected on the Autumn Solstice and dried in the shade.

Guo Pu（郭璞）said，"[Qumai（瞿麦，Chinese pink herb；rainbowpink herb，lilac pink herb，Herba Dianthi）[is also] called Maijujiang（麦句姜）."Tao Hongjing（陶宏景）said，"[Its] seeds are quite similar to [that of] wheat. That is why it is so named."

　　主治关格,各种癃闭结聚,小便不通,能拔出刺入人体之刺,能消解痈肿,能使眼睛明亮,能祛除翳膜,能破胎堕子,能停止下血。又称为巨句麦。该物生长在山川河谷之中。

神农本草经

Notes

1. Qumai (瞿麦, Chinese pink herb; rainbowpink herb, lilac pink herb, Herba Dianthi) is a herbal medicinal, bitter in taste and cold in property, entering the heart meridian, the kidney meridian, the small intestine meridian and the bladder meridian, effective in clearing dampness-heat, promoting urination, breaking blood stasis and unobstructing meridians. Clinically it is used to treat dysuria, stranguria, edema, amenorrhea, acute conjunctivitis, eczema and sore.

2. Guange (关格) means two things, one is dysuria, the other is rapid pulse in the Renying (人迎) and Cunkou (寸口) regions.

26. 元参

【原文】

味苦,微寒。

主腹中寒热积聚,女子产乳余疾,补肾气,令人目明。一名重台。生川谷。

【考据】

1.《吴普》曰:元参,一名鬼藏,一名正马,一名重台,一名鹿腹,一名端,一名元台,神农桐君黄帝雷公扁鹊苦无毒,岐伯咸,李氏寒,或生冤朐山阳,二月生叶如梅毛,四四相值似芍药,黑茎方高四五尺,华赤,生枝间,四月,实黑。(《御览》)

2.《名医》曰:一名元台,一名鹿肠,一名正马,一名减,一名端,生河间及冤句,三月四月采根,暴干。

3. 案《广雅》云:鹿肠,元参也。《范子计然》云:元参出三辅,青色者善。

26. Yuanshen（元参, root of Ningpo figwort, Radix Scrophulariae）[1]

[Original Text]

[Yuanshen（元参, root of Ningpo figwort, Radix Scrophulariae）,] bitter in taste and slightly cold [in property], [is mainly used] to resolve accumulation of cold and heat in the abdomen, to treat various diseases in women after delivery of baby, to tonify kidney-Qi and to improve vision. [It is also] called Zhongtai（重台）, growing in mountain valleys and river valleys.

[Textual Research]

[In the book entitled] *Wu Pu Ben Cao*（《吴普本草》, *Wu Pu's Studies of Materia Medica*）, [it] says [that] Yuanshen（元参, root of Ningpo figwort, Radix Scrophulariae）[is also] called Guizang（鬼藏）, Zhengma（正马）, Zhongtai（重台）, Lufu（鹿腹）, Duan（端）and Yuantai（元台）. [According to] Agriculture God（神农）, Tongjun（桐均）, Yellow Emperor（黄帝）, Leigong（雷公）and Bianque（扁鹊）, [it is] bitter [in taste] and non-toxic [in property]; [according to] Qibo（岐伯）, [it is] salty [in taste]; [according to] Li's（李氏）, [it is] cold [in property]. [It] may grow in the sunny side of the Yuanju（冤朐）mountain, sprouting in February with the leaves like [that of] plum. [Its] stalks are about 4 to 5 *Chi*（尺）in length; [it] blossoms between the branches; [its]

【今译】

味苦,性微寒。

主治腹中寒热积聚,女子产后所患的多种疾病,能滋补肾气,能使人视力清晰。又称为重台。该物生长在山川河谷之中。

fruits become black in April [according to the book entitled] *Tai Ping Yu Lan* (《太平御览》, *Imperial Studies in Taiping Times*).

[In the book entitled] *Ming Yi Bie Lu* (《名医别录》, *Special Record of Great Doctors*), [it] says [that Yuanshen (元参, root of Ningpo figwort, Radix Scrophulariae) is also] called Yuantai (元台), Luchang (鹿肠), Zhengma (正马), Jian (减) and Duan (端), growing in Hejian (河间) and Yuanju (冤句). [Its] root [can be] collected in March and April, and dried in the sun.

[In the book entitled] *Fan Zi Ji Ran* (《范子计然》, *Studies About Fan Li's Teacher*), [it] says [that] Yuanshen (元参, root of Ningpo figwort, Radix Scrophulariae) grows in three places. The green one is more effective.

Agriculture God's Canon of Materia Medica

Notes

1. Yuanshen （元 参, root of Ningpo figwort, Radix Scrophulariae) is a herbal medicinal, bitter and salty in taste, cold in property, entering the stomach meridian, the lung meridian and the kidney meridian, effective in clearing heat, enriching Yin, purging fire and removing toxin. Clinically it is used to treat damage of fluid by heat disease, vexing thirst, constipation due to intestinal dryness, bone steaming due to Yin deficiency, hemoptysis, nosebleed, swelling and pain of the throat, redness and pain of the eyes and scrofula.

27. 秦艽

【原文】

味苦,平。

主寒热邪气,寒湿,风痹,肢节痛,下水,利小便。生山谷。

【考据】

1.《名医》曰:生飞乌山,二月八月,采根,暴干。

2. 案《说文》云:萛草之相芁者,玉篇作芁,居包切。云秦芁,药芁同。萧炳云:本经名秦瓜,然则今本经名,亦有《名医》改之者。

27. Qinjiao（秦艽，root of largeleaf gentian，root of thickstemen gentian，root of straw-coloured gentian，root of dahuria gentian，Radix Gentianae Macrophyllae）[1]

[Original Text]

[Qinjiao（秦艽，root of largeleaf gentian，root of thickstemen gentian，root of straw coloured gentian，root of dahuria gentian，Radix Gentianae Macrophyllae），] bitter in taste and mild [in property], [is mainly used to] treat [syndrome/pattern caused by] cold-heat and evil-Qi，cold-dampness [disease]，wind impediment and pain of limbs and joints，and to promote urination. [It] grows in mountains and valleys.

[Textual Research]

[In the book entitled] *Ming Yi Bie Lu* （《名医别录》，*Special Record of Great Doctors*），[it] says [that Qinjiao（秦艽，root of largeleaf gentian，root of thickstemen gentian，root of straw-coloured gentian，root of dahuria gentian，Radix Gentianae Macrophyllae）] grows in Feiwu（飞乌）mountain. [Its] root [can be] collected in February and August，and dried in the sun.

[In] case [analysis in the book entitled] *Shuo Wen* （《说文》，*On Culture*），[it] says [that] Qinjiao（秦艽，root of largeleaf gentian，root of thickstemen gentian，root of straw-coloured

【今译】

味苦,性平。

主治寒热邪气所致病症,寒湿证,风痹证,肢节疼痛,能祛除水湿,能使小便通畅。该物生长在山谷之中。

gentian, root of dahuria gentian, Radix Gentianae Macrophyllae) is the same as root of largeleaf gentian.

Notes

1. Qinjiao (秦艽, root of largeleaf gentian, root of thickstemen gentian, root of straw-coloured gentian, root of dahuria gentian, Radix Gentianae Macrophyllae) is a herbal medicinal, bitter and pungent in taste, mild in property, entering the stomach meridian, the liver meridian and the gallbladder meridian, effective in expelling wind-dampness and clearing deficiency-heat. Clinically it is used to treat wind-dampness impediment and pain, spasm of sinews and bones, jaundice due to dampness-heat, hematochezia due to intestinal wind, bone steaming with tidal fever, infantile malnutrition and constipation due to intestinal dryness.

28. 百合

【原文】

味甘,平。

主邪气腹张心痛,利大小便,补中益气。生川谷。

【考据】

1.《吴普》曰:百合一名重迈,一名中庭,生冠朐及荆山。(艺文类聚引云:一名重匡)

2.《名医》曰:一名重箱,一名摩罗,一名中逢花,一名强瞿,生荆州,二月八月,采根,暴干。

3. 案玉篇云:蹯,百合蒜也。

28. Baihe（百合，lily bulb，Bulbus Lilii）[1]

[Original Text]

[Baihe（百合，lily bulb，Bulbus Lilii），] sweet in taste [and] mild [in property], [is mainly used] to treat abdonminal distension and heart pain [due to] evil-Qi, to promote defecation and urination, to tonify the middle (the internal organs) and to replenish Qi. [It] grows in mountain valleys and river valleys.

[Textual Research]

[In the book entitled] *Wu Pu Ben Cao*（《吴普本草》，*Wu Pu's Studies of Materia Medica*），[it] says [that] Baihe（百合，lily bulb，Bulbus Lilii）[is also] called Chongmai（重迈）and Zhongting（中庭），growing in Guanqu（冠朐）and Jingshan（荆山）.

[In the book entitled] *Ming Yi Bie Lu*（《名医别录》，*Special Record of Great Doctors*），[it] says [that Baihe（百合，lily bulb，Bulbus Lilii）is also] called Zhongxiang（重箱），Moluo（摩罗），Zhongfenghua（中逢花）and Jiangqu（强瞿），growing in Jingzhou（荆州）. [Its] root [can be] collected in February and August，and dried in the sun.

Notes

1. Baihe（百合，lily bulb，Bulbus Lilii）is a herbal medicinal，sweet and bitter in taste，slightly cold in property，entering the lung

619

【今译】

味甘,性平。

主治邪气所致病症,腹胀,心痛,能通利大小便,能充实人体内脏,能补益精气。该物生长在山川河谷之中。

神农本草经

meridian and the heart meridian, effective in moistening the lung and stopping cough, clearing the heart and pacifying the spirit, fortifying the spleen and stomach, and strengthening kidney-Yin. Clinically it is used to treat cough due to tuberculosis, hemoptysis due to blood deficiency, remnant heat after heat disease, vexation with deficiency, fright with palpitation and dispiritedness.

29. 知母

【原文】

味苦,寒。

主消渴,热中,除邪气,肢体浮肿,下水,补不足,益气。

【考据】

1. 一名蚔母,一名连母,一名野蓼,一名地参,一名水参,一名水浚,一名货母,一名蜇母。生川谷。

2.《吴普》曰:知母,神农桐君无毒,补不足益气。(《御览》引云:一名提母)

3.《名医》曰:一名女雷,一名女理,一名儿草,一名鹿列,一名韭蓬,一名儿踵草,一名东根,一名水须,一名沈燔,一名薅,生河内,二月八月,采根暴干。

4. 案《说文》云:芪,芪母也。荨,苨藩也,或从爻作薅。《广雅》云:芪母儿踵,东根也。《尔雅》云:薅,茂藩。郭璞云:生山上,叶如韭,一日蜇母。《范子计然》云:蜇母,出三辅,黄白者善。玉篇作莐母。

29. Zhimu（知母，rhizome of common anemarrhena，Rhizoma Anemarrhenae）[1]

［Original Text］

［Zhimu（知母，rhizome of common anemarrhena，Rhizoma Anemarrhenae），］bitter in taste and cold［in property］，［is mainly used］to treat wasting-thirst and heat attack[2]，to eliminate evil-Qi，to relieve dropsy of limbs，to promote urination，to improve insufficiency and to replenish Qi.

［Textual Research］

［It is also］called Chimu（蚳母），Lianmu（连母），Yeliao（野蓼），Dishen（地参），Shuishen（水参），Shuijun（水浚），Huomu（货母）and Dimu（蝭母），growing in mountains and valleys.

［In the book entitled］*Wu Pu Ben Cao*（《吴普本草》，*Wu Pu's Studies of Materia Medica*），［it］says［that］Zhimu（知母，rhizome of common anemarrhena，Rhizoma Anemarrhenae），［according to］Agriculture God（神农）and Tongjun（桐均），［is］non-toxic［in property］and［can be used］to tonify insufficiency and replenish Qi.

［In the book entitled］*Ming Yi Bie Lu*（《名医别录》，*Special Record of Great Doctors*），［it］says［that Zhimu（知母，rhizome of common anemarrhena，Rhizoma Anemarrhenae）is also］called Nǔlei（女雷），Nǔli（女理），Ercao（儿草），Lulie（鹿列），Jiupeng

【今译】

味苦,性寒。

主治消渴症,能消除内脏中的热邪,能清除邪气,能治疗肢体浮肿,能使水泻下,能补充精气不足,能补益精气。

（韭蓬），Zhongcao（踵草），Donggen（东根），Shuixu（水须），Shenfan（沈燔）and Hao（薅），growing in Henei（河内）. [Its] root [can be] collected in February and August，and dried in the sun.

[In the book entitled] *Fan Zi Ji Ran*（《范子计然》，*Studies About Fan Li's Teacher*），[it] says [that] Dimu（蝭母）grows in three places. The yellow and white one is more effective.

Notes

1. Zhimu（知母，rhizome of common anemarrhena，Rhizoma Anemarrhenae）is a herbal medicinal，bitter in taste and cold in property，entering the stomach meridian，the lung meridian and the kidney meridian，effective in clearing heat and reducing fire，enriching Yin and moistening dryness. Clinically it is used to treat heat disease with high fever，thirst with vexation，lung heat with cough，diabetes and constipation due to dryness of stool.

30. 贝母

【原文】

味辛,平。

主伤寒烦热,淋沥邪气,疝瘕,喉痹,乳难,金疮,风痉。一名空草。

【考据】

1.《名医》曰:一名药实,一名苦花,一名苦菜,一名商(茼字)草,一名勤母,生晋地,十月采根暴干。

2. 案《说文》云:茼,贝母也。《广雅》云:贝父,药实也。《尔雅》云:茼,贝母。郭璞云:根如小贝,圆而白华,叶似韭。《毛诗》云:言采其虻。《传》云:虻,贝母也。陆玑云:其叶如括楼而细小,其子在根下如芋子,正白,四方连累相着有分解也。

30. Beimu（贝母，fritillaria，Bulbus Fritillariae Thunbergii）[1]

［Original Text］

［Beimu（贝母，fritillaria，Bulbus Fritillariae Thunbergii），］pungent in taste and mild［in property］，［is mainly used］to treat cold damage with vexing fever，dribbling urine［due to］evil-Qi，hernia，abdominal mass，throat impediment，dystocia，injury［caused by］metal and tetanus.［It is also］called Kongcao（空草）.

［Textual Research］

［In the book entitled］*Ming Yi Bie Lu*（《名医别录》，*Special Record of Great Doctors*），［it］says［that Beimu（贝母，fritillaria，Bulbus Fritillariae Thunbergii）is also］called Yaoshi（药实），Kuhua（苦花），Kucai（苦菜），Mengcao（茵草）and Qinmu（勤母），growing in Jindi（晋地）.［Its］root［can be］collected in October and dried in the sun.

［In］case［analysis in the book entitled］*Shuo Wen*（《说文》，*On Culture*），［it］says［that the so-called］Meng（茵）refers to Beimu（贝母，fritillaria，Bulbus Fritillariae Thunbergii）. Guo Pu（郭璞云）said，"［Its］root is like a shellfish，round with white flower.［Its］leaf is similar to Chinese chives."

【今译】

味辛,性平。

主治伤寒病,烦热症,淋沥邪气,疝瘕病,喉痹证,分娩困难,因金属创伤而导致的痈疮及破伤风。又称为空草。

Notes

1. Beimu（贝母，fritillaria，Bulbus Fritillariae Thunbergii），a herbal medicinal，is divided into three major categories，Chuanbeimu（川贝母，tendrilleaf fritillary bulb，Bulbus Frityllariae Cirrhosae），Zhebeimu（浙贝母，bulb of thunberg fritillary，Bulbus Fritillariae Thunbergii）and Tubeimu（土贝母，rhizome of paniculate bolbostemma，Rhizoma Bolbostemmae）．

Chuanbeimu （川贝母，tendrilleaf fritillary bulb，Bulbus Frityllariae Cirrhosae）is bitter and sweet in taste，cool in property，entering the lung meridian，effective in moistening the lung，stopping cough，resolving phlegm and dispersing bind. Clinically it is used to treat lung heat with cough，hemoptysis，flaccidity of the lung，and abscess in the lung.

Zhebeimu （浙贝母，bulb of thunberg fritillary，Bulbus Fritillariae Thunbergii）is bitter in taste and cold in property，entering the lung meridian，the stomach meridian and the heart meridian，effective in clearing heat and resolving phlegm，dispersing bind and removing toxin. Clinically it is used to treat common cold due to wind-heat，swelling and pain of the throat，cough with excessive sputum due to lung heat，abscess with pus，ulceration of the digestive tract，oppression and pain of the chest and heart，scrofula and scabies.

Tubeimu （土贝母，rhizome of paniculate bolbostemma，Rhizoma Bolbostemmae）is what mentioned in this part in Agriculture God's Canon of Materia Medica.

31. 白芷

【原文】

味辛,温。

主女人漏下赤白,血闭,阴肿,寒热,风头,侵目,泪出,长肌肤、润泽,可作面脂。一名芳香。生川谷。

【考据】

1.《吴普》曰:白芷,一名虈,一名符离,一名泽芬,一名晞(《御览》)。

2.《名医》曰:一名白茝,一名虈,一名莞,一名符离,一名泽芬,叶一名蒚麻,可作浴汤,生河东下泽,二月八月,采根,暴干。

3. 案《说文》云:茝,虈也。虈,楚谓之蓠。晋谓之虈,齐谓之茝。《广雅》云:白芷,其叶谓之药。《西山经》云:号山,其草多药虈。郭璞云:药,白芷,别名虈,香草也。《淮南子》修务训云:身苦秋药被风。高诱云:药,白芷,香草也。王逸注《楚词》云:药,白芷,按《名医》一名莞云云,似即《尔雅》莞,符离,其上蒚,而《说文》别有,夫离也。蒚,夫蓠上也,是非一草。舍人云:白蒲一名符离,楚谓之莞,岂蒲与芷相似,而《名

31．Baizhi（白芷，root of dahurian angelica，root of Taiwan angelica，Radix Angelicae Dahuricae）[1]

[Original Text]

［Baizhi（白芷，root of dahurian angelica，root of Taiwan angelica，Radix Angelicae Dahuricae），］pungent in taste and warm ［in property］，［is mainly used］to treat vaginal bleeding with red and white leucorrhea，blood stasis with vulva swelling，cold-heat ［disease］，［headache due to invasion of］wind into the head and eyes with tearing，to promote and moisten muscles.［It can be］used to luster the face.［It is also］called Fangxiang（芳香），growing in mountain valleys and river valleys.

［Textual Research］

［In the book entitled］*Wu Pu Ben Cao*（《吴普本草》，*Wu Pu's Studies of Materia Medica*），［it］says［that］Baizhi（白芷，root of dahurian angelica，root of Taiwan angelica，Radix Angelicae Dahuricae）［is also］called Qi(蕲)，Fuli（苻离），Zefen（泽芬）and Wan（蒝）［according to the book entitled］*Tai Ping Yu Lan*（《太平御览》，*Imperial Studies in Taiping Times*）.

［In the book entitled］*Ming Yi Bie Lu*（《名医别录》，*Special Record of Great Doctors*），［it］says［that］Baizhi（白芷，root of dahurian angelica，root of Taiwan angelica，Radix Angelicae Dahuricae）［is also］called Qi（蕲），Guan（莞），Fuli（苻离）and

医》误合为一乎。或《说文》云：楚谓之蓠，即夫篱也，未可得详，旧作
芷，非。

【今译】

味辛，性温。

主治女子阴道出血淋漓不断，赤白带下，经闭，阴肿，寒热病，风邪
侵袭头部和眼睛，泪流不止，能促进肌肤生长，能滋润面部光泽，可作面
脂。又称为芳香。该物生长在山川河谷之中。

Zefen (泽芬). [Its] leaf is called Lima (蔄麻) and can be boiled for bath. [It] grows in the pool below Hedong (河东). [Its] root [can be] collected in February and August, and dried in the sun.

[In the book entitled] *Guang Ya* (《广雅》, *The First Chinese Encyclopedic Dictionary*), [it] says [that] the leave of Baizhi (白芷, root of dahurian angelica, root of Taiwan angelica, Radix Angelicae Dahuricae) is taken as medicinal. Guo Pu (郭璞) said, "Baizhi (白芷, root of dahurian angelica, root of Taiwan angelica, Radix Angelicae Dahuricae) is a fragrant herb."

Notes

1. Baizhi (白芷, root of dahurian angelica, root of Taiwan angelica, Radix Angelicae Dahuricae) is a herbal medicinal, pungent in taste and warm in property, entering the lung meridian and the stomach meridian, effective in expelling wind and relieving superficies, dispersing dampness and ceasing pain. Clinically it is used to treat common cold due to wind-cold attack, headache, toothache, pain in crista superciliaris, nasosinusitis, hematochezia due to intestinal wind, hemorrhoids and reddish white leucorrhea.

神农本草经

32. 淫羊藿

【原文】

味辛,寒。

主阴痿绝伤,茎中痛,利小便,益气力,强志。一名刚前。生山谷。

【考据】

1.《吴普》曰:淫羊藿,神农雷公辛,李氏小寒,坚骨(《御览》)。

2.《名医》曰:生上山郡阳山。

32.　Yinyanghuo（淫羊藿，shorthorned epimedium herb，sagittate epimedium herb，pubescent epimedium herb，Korean epimedium herb，Herba Epimedii）[1]

[Original Text]

[Yinyanghuo（淫羊藿，shorthorned epimedium herb，sagittate epimedium herb，pubescent epimedium herb，Korean epimedium herb，Herba Epimedii），] pungent in taste and cold [in property]，[is mainly used] to treat impotence with flaccidity and pain in the penis，to promote urination，to replenish Qi and energy，and to strengthen memory. [It is also] called Gangqian（刚前），growing in mountains and valleys.

[Textual Research]

[In the book entitled] *Wu Pu Ben Cao*（《吴普本草》，*Wu Pu's Studies of Materia Medica*），[it] says [that] Yinyanghuo（淫羊藿，shorthorned epimedium herb，sagittate epimedium herb，pubescent epimedium herb，Korean epimedium herb，Herba Epimedii），[according to] Agriculture God（神农）and Leigong（雷公），[is] pungent [in taste]；[according to] Li's（李氏），[it is] slightly cold [in property]. [It is effective in] strengthening the bones [according to the book entitled] *Tai Ping Yu Lan*（《太平御览》，*Imperial Studies in Taiping Times*）.

[In the book entitled] *Ming Yi Bie Lu*（《名医别录》，*Special*

【今译】

味辛,性寒。

主治阳痿绝伤,阴茎疼痛,能使小便通畅,能补益气力,能增强记忆力。又称为刚前。该物生长在山谷之中。

Record of Great Doctors），［it］says［that Yinyanghuo（淫羊藿，shorthorned epimedium herb，sagittate epimedium herb，pubescent epimedium herb，Korean epimedium herb，Herba Epimedii)］grows in the sunny side of the Shangshanjun（上山郡）mountain.

Notes

1. Yinyanghuo（淫羊藿，shorthorned epimedium herb，sagittate epimedium herb，pubescent epimedium herb，Korean epimedium herb，Herba Epimedii) is a herbal medicinal，pungent and sweet in taste，warm in property，entering the liver meridian and the kidney meridian，effective in warming the kidney and assisting Yang，expelling wind and eliminating dampness. Clinically it is used to treat impotence，premature ejaculation，chronic bronchitis，wind-dampness impediment and pain，and hypertension during menopause.

33. 黄芩

【原文】

味苦,平。

主诸热黄疸,肠澼,泄利,逐水,下血闭,恶疮疽蚀,火疡。一名腐肠。生川谷。

【考据】

1.《吴普》曰:黄芩,一名黄文,一名妒妇,一名虹胜,一名经芩,一名印头,一名内虚,神农桐君黄帝雷公扁鹊苦无毒。李氏小温,二月生赤黄叶,两两四四相值,茎空中,或方员,高三四尺,四月花紫红赤,五月实黑根黄,二月至九月采。(《御览》)

2.《名医》曰:一名空肠,一名内虚,一名黄文,一名经芩,一名妒妇,生秭归及冤句,三月三日,采根阴干。

3. 案《说文》云:菳,黄菳也。《广雅》云:菳葿,黄文,内虚,黄芩也。《范子计然》云:黄芩出三辅,色黄者,善。

33. Huangqin（黄芩，scutellaria，Radix Scutellariae）[1]

[Original Text]

［Huangqin（黄芩，scutellaria，Radix Scutellariae），］bitter in taste and mild［in property］，［is mainly used］to treat various heat ［syndromes/patterns］，jaundice and bloody stool，to expel water，to relieve amenorrhea，and to cure severe sore，ulcer and scald.［It is also］called Fuchang（腐肠），growing in mountain valleys and river valleys.

[Textual Research]

［In the book entitled］*Wu Pu Ben Cao*（《吴普本草》，*Wu Pu's Studies of Materia Medica*），［it］says［that］Huangqin（黄芩，scutellaria，Radix Scutellariae）［is also］called Huangwen（黄文），Jifu（妒妇），Hongsheng（虹胜），Hongqin（红芩），Yintou（印头）and Neixu（内虚）.［According to］Agriculture God（神农），Tongjun（桐均），Yellow Emperor（黄帝），Leigong（雷公）and Bianque（扁鹊），［it is］bitter［in taste］and non-toxic［in property］；［according to］Li's（李氏），［it is］slightly warm［in property］.［In］February，［it］sprouts with yellow leaves gathering with each other；［its］stalks are hollow and about 3 to 4 *Chi*（尺）in length；［in］April，［it begins］to blossom in purple and red［color］；［in］May，［its］fruit［becomes］black and［its］root［turns］yellow；［in］February and September，［it can be］collected［according to

【今译】

味苦,性平。

主治各种热证,黄疸病,泄泻,痢疾,能祛除水湿,能消解经闭,能治疗恶性疮疽溃烂以及因烧伤所致的疮疡。又称为腐肠。该物生长在山川河谷之中。

神农本草经

the book entitled] *Tai Ping Yu Lan* (《太平御览》, *Imperial Studies in Taiping Times*).

[In the book entitled] *Ming Yi Bie Lu* (《名医别录》, *Special Record of Great Doctors*), [it] says [that Huangqin （黄芩, scutellaria，Radix Scutellariae) is also] called Kongchang （空肠）, Neixu（内虚），Huangwen（黄文），Jingqin（经芩）and Jifu（妒妇）, growing in Zigui（秭归）and Yuanju（冤句）. [On] March 3, [its] root [can be] collected and dried in the shade.

[In the book entitled] *Fan Zi Ji Ran* （《范子计然》, *Studies About Fan Li's Teacher*), [it] says [that] Huangqin （黄芩, scutellaria，Radix Scutellariae) grows in the three places. The yellow [one is] more effective.

Notes

1. Huangqin （黄芩, scutellaria，Radix Scutellariae) is a herbal medicinal，bitter in taste and cold in property，entering the heart meridian，the lung meridian，the gallbladder meridian and the large intestine meridian，effective in clearing heat and drying dampness，purging fire and removing toxin. Clinically it is used to treat warm disease with fever，vexing thirst，cough due to heat in the lung，diarrhea due to dampness-heat，dysentery， jaundice， heat stranguria，hypertension，hematemesis，nosebleed，hematochezia and flooding and spotting（metrostaxis and metrorrhagia）.

34. 狗脊

【原文】

味苦,平。

主腰背强,关机缓急,周痹,寒湿,膝痛,颇利老人。一名百枝。生川谷。

【考据】

1.《吴普》曰:狗脊一名狗青,一名赤节,神农苦,桐君黄帝岐伯雷公扁鹊甘无毒李氏小温,如草薢,茎节如竹,有刺,叶圆赤,根黄白,亦如竹根,毛有刺。岐伯经云:茎长节,叶端员青赤,皮白有赤脉。

2.《名医》曰:一名强膂,一名扶盖,一名扶筋,生常山,二月八月,采根暴干。

3. 案《广雅》云:菝洁,狗脊也。玉篇云:菝菰狗脊根也。《名医》别出菝契条,非。

【今译】

味苦,性平。

34. Gouji（狗脊，east Asian tree ferm rhizome，Rhizoma Cibotii）[1]

[Original Text]

[Gouji（狗脊，east Asian tree ferm rhizome，Rhizoma Cibotii），] bitter in taste and mild [in property]，[is mainly used] to resolve stiffness of the waist and back，to relieve spasm of the spine，and to treat generalized impediment [due to] cold-dampness and pain of knees. [It is] beneficial to old people. [It is also] called Baizhi（百枝），growing in mountain valleys and river valleys.

[Textual Research]

[In the book entitled] *Wu Pu Ben Cao*（《吴普本草》，*Wu Pu's Studies of Materia Medica*），[it] says [that] Gouji（狗脊，east Asian tree ferm rhizome，Rhizoma Cibotii）[is also] called Gouqing（狗青）and Chijie（赤节）. [According to] Agriculture God（神农），[it is] bitter [in taste]；[according to] Tongjun（桐均），Yellow Emperor（黄帝），Qibo（岐伯），Leigong（雷公）and Bianque（扁鹊），[it is] sweet [in taste] and non-toxic [in property]；[according to] Li's（李氏），[it is] slightly warm [in property]. [It is] similar to Bixie（萆薢，rhizome of hypoglaucous collett yam，rhizome of collett yam，rhizome of mountain yam，rhizome of thinnest yam，Rhizoma Dioscoreae Hypoglaucae）with stalks like bamboo，stabs，round and red leaves，yellow and white roots like roots of bamboo with stabs.

643

　　主治腰部背部强硬,能使关节舒缓,能使筋脉舒畅,能治疗全身流窜性疼痛,寒湿证,膝部疼痛。对老年人的健康非常有利。又称为百枝。该物生长在山川河谷之中。

[According to] the Canon of Qibo（岐伯）, [its] stalks are long, [its] leaves are yellow and red, [its] bark is white with red vessels.

[In the book entitled] *Ming Yi Bie Lu*（《名医别录》, *Special Record of Great Doctors*）, [it] says [that Gouji（狗脊, east Asian tree ferm rhizome, Rhizoma Cibotii) is also] called Qianglǔ（强膂）, Fugai（扶盖）and Fujin（扶筋）, growing in Changshan（常山）. [Its] root [can be] collected in February and August, and dried in the sun.

[In the book entitled] *Guang Ya*（《广雅》, *The First Chinese Encyclopedic Dictionary*）, [it] says [that the so-called] Jie（洁）refers to Gouji（狗脊, east Asian tree ferm rhizome, Rhizoma Cibotii）.

Notes

1. Gouji（狗脊, east Asian tree ferm rhizome, Rhizoma Cibotii）is a herbal medicinal, bitter and sweet in taste, warm in property, entering the liver meridian and the kidney meridian, effective in tonifying the liver and kidney, strengthening the sinews and bones, eliminating wind and dampness, relieving impediment and pain. Clinically it is used to treat ache and flaccidity of the waist and spine, weakness of the legs and feet, frequent urination, enuresis, leucorrhea, and impediment and pain due to wind-dampness.

35. 石龙芮

【原文】

味苦,平。

主风寒湿痹,心腹邪气,利关节,止烦满。久服,轻身明目,不老。一名鲁果能(《御览》作食果),一名地椹,生川泽石边。

【考据】

1.《吴普》曰:龙芮一名姜苔,一名天豆,神农苦平岐伯酸,扁鹊李氏大寒,雷公咸无毒,五月五日采。(《御览》)

2.《名医》曰:一名石能,一名彭根,一名天豆,生太山,五月五日采子,二月八月采皮,阴干。

3. 案《范子计然》云:石龙芮,出三辅,色黄者善。

【今译】

味苦,性平。

35. Shilongrui（石龙芮，poisonous buttercup herb，Herba Ranunculi Scelerati）[1]

[Original Text]

[Shilongrui （石龙芮，poisonous buttercup herb，Herba Ranunculi Scelerati），] bitter in taste and mild [in property]，[is mainly used] to treat wind-cold dampness impediment and evil-Qi in the abdomen，to disinhibit joints，and to resolve vexation and fullness. Long-term taking [of it will] relax the body，improve vision and prevent aging. [It is also] called Luguoneng（鲁果能）and Dizhen（地椹），growing in the areas with stones in the valleys and swamps.

647

[Textual Research]

[In the book entitled] *Wu Pu Ben Cao*（《吴普本草》，*Wu Pu's Studies of Materia Medica*），[it] says [that] Shilongrui（石龙芮，poisonous buttercup herb，Herba Ranunculi Scelerati）[is also] called Jiangtai（姜苔）and Tiandou（天豆）. [According to] Agriculture God（神农），[it is] bitter [in taste]；[according to] Qibo（岐伯），[it is] sour [in taste]；[according to] Bianque（扁鹊）and Li's（李氏），[it is] severely cold [in property]；[according to] Leigong（雷公），[it is] salty [in taste] and non-toxic [in property]；[it can be] collected on May 5 [according to the book entitled] *Tai Ping Yu Lan*（《太平御览》，*Imperial Studies in Taiping Times*）.

　　主治风寒湿邪所致痹证，心腹中因邪气所致之症，能使关节通畅，

能消除烦躁和郁闷。长期服用，能使人身体轻盈，眼睛明亮，长寿不老。

又称为鲁果能，又称为地椹，该物生长在山川和平泽的石边。

[In the book entitled] *Ming Yi Bie Lu* (《名医别录》, *Special Record of Great Doctors*), [it] says [that Shilongrui (石龙芮, poisonous buttercup herb, Herba Ranunculi Scelerati) is also called] Shineng (石能), Penggen (彭根) and Tiandou (天豆), growing in Taishan (太山). [Its] seeds [can be] collected on May 5, [its] bark [can be] collected in February and August, [which should be] dried in the shade.

[In the book entitled] *Fan Zi Ji Ran* (《范子计然》, *Studies About Fan Li's Teacher*), [it] says [that] Shilongrui (石龙芮, poisonous buttercup herb, Herba Ranunculi Scelerati) grows in the three places. The yellow one is more effective.

Notes

1. Shilongrui (石龙芮, poisonous buttercup herb, Herba Ranunculi Scelerati) is a herbal medicinal, bitter and pungent in taste, cold and toxic in property, entering the lung meridian and the heart meridian, effective in removing toxin, dispersing bind, dispersing wind and dampness, tonifying the kidney and improving vision. Clinically it is used to treat rheumatic arthritis, scrofula, ulceration of the shanks, blood stasis, abscess and malaria.

36. 茅根

【原文】

味甘,寒。

主劳伤虚羸,补中益气,除瘀血,血闭寒热,利小便。

其苗,主下水。一名兰根,一名茹根。生山谷田野。

【考据】

1.《名医》曰:一名地管,一名地筋,一名兼杜,生楚地,六月采根。

2. 案《说文》云:茅,菅也。菅,茅也。《广雅》云:菅,茅也。《尔雅》云:白华野菅。郭璞云:菅,茅属。诗云:白华菅兮,白茅束兮。《传》云:白华,野菅也,已沤,为菅。

【今译】

味甘,性寒。

主治劳伤所致的虚弱消瘦,能充实人体内脏,能补益精气,能消除

36. Maogen（茅根，rhizome of lalang grass，Rhizoma Imperatae）[1]

[Original Text]

［Maogen （茅根，rhizome of lalang grass，Rhizoma Imperatae），］sweet in taste and cold ［in property］，［is mainly used］ to treat deficiency and emaciation ［caused by］ overstrain，to tonify the middle （the internal organs），to replenish Qi，to eliminate blood stasis，［to relieve］ block of the blood and cold-heat ［disease］，and to promote urination. Its seedling can reduce water. ［It is also］ called Langen（兰根）and Rugen（茹根），growing in mountains，valleys and lands.

［Textual Research］

［In the book entitled］ *Ming Yi Bie Lu* （《名医别录》，*Special Record of Great Doctors*），［it］ says ［that Maogen（茅根，rhizome of lalang grass，Rhizoma Imperatae）is also］ called Diguan（地管），Dijin（地筋）and Jiandu（兼杜），growing in Chudi（楚地）. ［Its］ root ［can be］ collected in June.

Notes

1. Maogen（茅根，rhizome of lalang grass，Rhizoma Imperatae）is a herbal medicinal，sweet in taste and cold in property，entering the lung meridian，the stomach meridian and the bladder meridian，

瘀血,能治疗经闭和寒热病,能使小便通畅。

其苗,能祛除水湿。又称为兰根,又称为茹根。该物生长在山谷之中和田野里。

effective in clearing heat, cooling the blood, ceasing bleeding and promoting urination. Clinically it is used to treat vexing thirst [caused by] heat disease, vomiting [due to] stomach heat, hematemesis, nosebleed, hemoptysis, hematuria, acute nephritis, edema and jaundice.

37. 紫菀

【原文】

味苦,温。

主咳逆上气,胸中寒热结气,去蛊毒痿蹶,安五脏。生山谷。

【考据】

1.《吴普》曰:紫菀,一名青菀。(《御览》)

2.《名医》曰:一名紫茜,一名青菀,生房陵及真定邯郸,二月三月,采根,阴干。

3. 案《说文》云:菀,茈菀,出汉中,房陵。陶宏景云:白者名白菀。《唐本》注云:白菀,即女菀也。

【今译】

味苦,性温。

主治咳嗽及呼吸困难,胸中寒热,气结,能祛除虫毒,能治疗足部痿瘸,能安静五脏。该物生长在山谷之中。

37. Ziwan（紫菀，aster，Radix Asteris）[1]

[Original Text]

［Ziwan（紫菀，aster，Radix Asteris），］bitter in taste and warm ［in property］，［is mainly used］ to treat cough with dyspnea and upward counterflow of Qi，cold-heat ［disease］ in the chest and ［disease caused by］ Qi binding，to eliminate worm toxin and flaccidity of legs，and to harmonize the five Zang-organs. ［It］ grows in mountains and valleys.

[Textual Research]

［In the book entitled］ *Wu Pu Ben Cao*（《吴普本草》，*Wu Pu's Studies of Materia Medica*），［it］ says ［that］ Ziwan（紫菀，aster，Radix Asteris）［is also］ called Qingyuan（青苑）［according to the book entitled］ *Tai Ping Yu Lan*（《太平御览》，*Imperial Studies in Taiping Times*）.

［In the book entitled］ *Ming Yi Bie Lu*（《名医别录》，*Special Record of Great Doctors*），［it］ says ［that Ziwan（紫菀，aster，Radix Asteris）is also］ called Ziqian（紫茜）and Qingyuan（青苑），growing in Fangling（房陵），Zhending（真定）and Handan（邯郸）. ［Its］ root ［can be］ collected in February and March，and dried in the shade.

655

Notes

1. Ziwan（紫菀，aster，Radix Asteris）is a herbal medicinal，bitter in taste and warm in property，entering the lung meridian，effective in warming the lung and descending Qi，resolving phlegm and stopping cough. Clinically it is used to treat cough with inhibited phlegm，lung deficiency with overstrain，hemoptysis，throat impediment and dysuria.

38. 紫草

【原文】

味苦,寒。

主心腹邪气,五疸,补中益气,利九窍,通水道。一名紫丹,一名紫芙(《御览》引云:一名地血,《大观本》,无文)。生山谷。

【考据】

1.《吴普》曰:紫草节赤,二月花。(《御览》)

2.《名医》曰:生砀山及楚地,三月采根,阴干。

3. 案《说文》云:茈,草也,藐,茈草也,茛草也,可以染留黄。《广雅》云:茈,草也。《山海经》云:劳山多茈草。郭璞云:一名紫茋,中染紫也。《尔雅》云:藐,茈草。郭璞云:可以染紫。

【今译】

味苦,性寒。

38. Zicao（紫草，root of Sinkiang-Tibet arnebia，root of redroot gromwell，Radix Arnebiae seu Lithospermi）[1]

[Original Text]

[Zicao（紫草，root of Sinkiang-Tibet arnebia，root of redroot gromwell，Radix Arnebiae seu Lithospermi），] bitter in taste and cold [in property]，[is mainly used] to treat [disease caused by] evil-Qi in the heart and abdomen and five [kinds of] jaundice，to tonify the middle（the internal organs），to replenish Qi，to disinhibit the nine orifices and to unobstruct waterway [in the body]. [It is also] called Zidan（紫丹）and Zifu（紫芙）. [It] grows in mountains and valleys.

[Textual Research]

[In the book entitled] *Wu Pu Ben Cao*（《吴普本草》，*Wu Pu's Studies of Materia Medica*），[it] says [that] the branches of Zicao（紫草，root of Sinkiang-Tibet arnebia，root of redroot gromwell，Radix Arnebiae seu Lithospermi）are red [and can be] collected in February [according to the book entitled] *Tai Ping Yu Lan*（《太平御览》，*Imperial Studies in Taiping Times*）.

[In the book entitled] *Ming Yi Bie Lu*（《名医别录》，*Special Record of Great Doctors*），[it] says [that Zicao（紫草，root of Sinkiang-Tibet arnebia，root of redroot gromwell，Radix Arnebiae seu Lithospermi）] grows in Dangshan（砀山）and Chudi（楚地）.

　　主治心腹中因邪气所致病症,五种黄疸症,能充实人体内脏,能补益精气,能使九窍通畅,能通利水道。又称为紫丹,又称为紫芙。该物生长在山谷之中。

[Its] root [can be] collected in March and dried in the shade.

Notes

1. Zicao (紫草, root of Sinkiang-Tibet arnebia, root of redroot gromwell, Radix Arnebiae seu Lithospermi) is a herbal medicinal, bitter in taste and cold in property, entering the heart meridian and the liver meridian, effective in cooling the blood, removing toxin and smoothing the intestines. Clinically it is used to treat macula in warm disease, jaundice caused by dampness-heat, purpura, hematemesis, nosebleed, hematuria, bloody dysentery, stranguria and constipation.

39. 败酱

【原文】

味苦,平。

主暴热,火疮赤气,疥搔,疽痔,马鞍热气。一名鹿肠。生川谷。

【考据】

1.《名医》曰:"一名鹿首,一名马草,一名泽败,生江夏,八月采根曝干。

2. 案《范子计然》云:败酱出三辅。陶宏景云:气如败酱。故以为名。

【今译】

味苦,性平。

主治暴热之症,能治疗因火烧所致之疮疡和毒热之气,疥疮瘙痒,疽痔以及马鞍热邪所致之病。又称为鹿肠。该物生长在山川河谷之中。

39. Baijiang（败酱，patrinia，Herba Patriniae）[1]

[Original Text]

[Baijiang（败酱，patrinia，Herba Patriniae），] bitter in taste and mild [in property], [is mainly used] to treat sudden fever, scald with heat-Qi, scabies, itching, jaundice, hemorrhoids and heat-Qi [in the skin due to] riding horse. [It is also] called Luchang（鹿肠）and grows in mountain valleys and river valleys.

[Textual Research]

[In the book entitled] *Ming Yi Bie Lu*（《名医别录》，*Special Record of Great Doctors*），[it] says [that Baijiang（败酱，patrinia, Herba Patriniae) is also] called Lushou（鹿首），Macao（马草）and Zebai（泽败），growing in Jiangxia（江夏）. [Its] root [can be] collected in August and dried in the sun.

[In the book entitled] *Fan Zi Ji Ran*（《范子计然》，*Studies About Fan Li's Teacher*），[it] says [that] Baijiang（败酱，patrinia，Herba Patriniae) grows in the three places. Tao Hongjing（陶宏景）said, "[Its] effect is similar to [that of] Baijiang（败酱）. That is why it is so named."

Notes

1. Baijiang（败酱，patrinia，Herba Patriniae) is a herbal medicinal, pungent and bitter in taste, slightly cold in property, entering the stomach meridian, the large intestine meridian and the liver meridian, effective in clearing heat and removing toxin, eliminating stasis and expelling pus. Clinically it is used to treat appendicitis, pulmonary ulcer, hepatitis, enteritis, dysentery, cervicitis, abdominal pain with blood stasis after delivery of baby, abscess and conjunctivitis.

40. 白鲜

【原文】

味苦,寒。

主头风,黄疸,咳逆,淋沥,女子阴中肿痛,湿痹死肌,不可屈伸,起止行步。生川谷。

【考据】

1.《名医》曰:生上谷及冤句,四月五月,采根阴干。

2. 案陶宏景云:俗呼为白羊鲜,气息正似羊膻或名白膻。

【今译】

味苦,性寒。

主治风邪袭头,黄疸症,咳嗽气逆,淋沥病,女子阴中肿痛,湿邪所致痹证,肌肉坏死,不能弯曲直伸,不能起止行步。该物生长在山川河谷之中。

40. Baixian（白鲜，root bark of densefruit pittany Cortex Dictamni）[1]

［Original Text］

［Baixian （白 鲜，root bark of densefruit pittany Cortex Dictamni），］bitter in taste and cold ［in property］, ［is mainly used］ to treat ［headache caused by invasion of］ wind into the head, jaundice, cough with dyspnea, stranguria, vulva swelling and pain, dampness impediment, necrotic muscles and difficulty to stretch and walk. ［It］ grows in mountain valleys and river valleys.

［Textual Research］

［In the book entitled］ *Ming Yi Bie Lu* （《名医别录》, *Special Record of Great Doctors*）, ［it］ says ［that Baixian （白鲜，root bark of densefruit pittany Cortex Dictamni)］ grows in Shanggu （上谷） and Yuanju （冤句）. ［Its］ root ［can be］ collected in April and May, and dried in the shadel.

Tao Hongjing （陶 宏 景） said, "［It is］ popularly called Baiyangxian（白羊鲜）because it smells like mutton."

Notes

1. Baixian （白鲜，root bark of densefruit pittany Cortex Dictamni） is a herbal medicinal, bitter in taste and cold in property, entering the spleen meridian and the stomach meridian, effective in expelling wind, drying dampness, clearing heat and removing toxin. Clinically it is used to treat pruritus, urticaria, eczema, scabies and impetigo.

41. 酸酱

【原文】

味酸,平。

主热烦满,定志益气,利水道,产难。吞其实立产。一名醋酱。生川泽。

【考据】

1.《吴普》曰:酸酱,一名酢酱。(《御览》)

2.《名医》曰:生荆楚,及人家田园中,五月采,阴干。

3. 案《尔雅》云:葴,寒酱。郭璞云:今酸酱草,江东呼曰苦葴。

【今译】

味酸,性平。

主治发热,烦躁,郁闷,能提高记忆力,能补益精气,能通利水道,能治疗难产。食用其果实能使胎儿产出。又称为醋酱。该物生长在山川和平泽之中。

41. Suanjiang (酸酱, root of franchet groundcherry, Radix Physalis Franchetii) [1]

[Original Text]

[Suanjiang (酸酱, root of franchet groundcherry, Radix Physalis Franchetii),] sour in taste and mild [in property], [is mainly used] to treat fever, vexation and fullness, to strengthen memory, to replenish Qi, to disinhibit waterway [in the body] and to relieve infertility. Taking the fruit [will enable people] to conceive baby. [It is also] called Cujiang (醋酱) and grows in valleys and swamps.

[Textual Research]

[In the book entitled] *Wu Pu Ben Cao* (《吴普本草》, *Wu Pu's Studies of Materia Medica*), [it] says [that] Suanjiang (酸酱, root of franchet groundcherry, Radix Physalis Franchetii) [is also] called Zuojiang (酢酱) [according to the book entitled] *Tai Ping Yu Lan* (《太平御览》, *Imperial Studies in Taiping Times*).

[In the book entitled] *Ming Yi Bie Lu* (《名医别录》, *Special Record of Great Doctors*), [it] says [that Suanjiang (酸酱, root of franchet groundcherry, Radix Physalis Franchetii)] grows in the private land in Jingchu (荆楚). [It can be] collected in May and dried in the shade.

Notes

1. Suanjiang (酸酱, root of franchet groundcherry, Radix Physalis Franchetii) is a herbal medicinal, bitter in taste and cold in property, entering the lung meridian and the spleen meridian, effective in clearing heat, relieving cough and promoting urination. Clinically it is used to treat malaria, acute bronchitis, tonsillitis, sore-throat, jaundice and hernia.

42. 紫参

【原文】

味苦,辛寒。

主心腹积聚,寒热邪气。通九窍,利大小便。一名牡蒙。生山谷。

【考据】

1.《吴普》曰:伏蒙,一名紫参,一名泉戎,一名音腹,一名伏菟,一名重伤。神农黄帝苦,李氏小寒,生河西山谷或宛句商山,圆聚生,根黄赤有文,皮黑中紫,五月花紫,赤实黑,大如豆,三月采根。(《御览》《大观本》节文)

2.《名医》曰:一名众戎,一名童肠:一名马行,生河西及宛句,三月采根,火炙使紫色。

3. 案《范子计然》云:紫参出三辅,赤青色者善。

42. Zishen（紫参，Chinese sage herb，Herba Salviae Chinesnsis）[1]

[**Original Text**]

［Zishen（紫参，Chinese sage herb，Herba Salviae Chinesnsis），］bitter and pungent in taste，cold［in property］，［is mainly used］to treat［disease marked by］accumulation［of pathogenic factors as well as］cold-heat and evil-Qi，to unobstruct the nine orifices and to promote urination and defecation.［It is also］called Mumeng（牡蒙），growing in mountains and valleys.

[**Textual Research**]

［In the book entitled］*Wu Pu Ben Cao*（《吴普本草》，*Wu Pu's Studies of Materia Medica*），［it］says［that Zishen（紫参，Chinese sage herb，Herba Salviae Chinesnsis）is also］called Fumeng（伏蒙），Quanrong（泉戎），Yinfu（音腹），Futu（伏菟）and Zhongshang（重伤）.［According to］Agriculture God（神农）and Yellow Emperor（黄帝），［it is］bitter［in taste］；［according to］Li's（李氏），［it is］slightly cold［in property］.［It］grows in the mountains and valleys in Hexi（河西）or Shangshan（商山）mountain in Wanju（宛句）.［Its］root is yellow and red with texture，［its］bark is black and purple.［In］May［its］flower is purple，［its］fruit is black like soybean.［Its］root［can be］collected in March.

［In the book entitled］*Ming Yi Bie Lu*（《名医别录》，*Special*

【今译】

味苦,性辛寒。

主治心腹积聚,寒热病邪。能使九窍畅通,能通利大小便。又称为牡蒙。该物生长在山谷之中。

Record of Great Doctors）, ［it］says ［that Zishen（紫参, Chinese sage herb, Herba Salviae Chinesnsis) is also］called Zhongrong（众戎）, Tongchang（童肠）and Maxing（马行）, growing in Hexi（河西）and Yuanju（冤句）.［Its］root［can be］collected in March.［When］broiled,［it］becomes purple.

［In the book entitled］*Fan Zi Ji Ran*（《范子计然》, *Studies About Fan Li's Teacher*）,［it］says［that］Zishen（紫参, Chinese sage herb, Herba Salviae Chinesnsis) grows in the three places. The red and green one is more effective.

Notes

1. Zishen（紫参, Chinese sage herb, Herba Salviae Chinesnsis) is a herbal medicinal, bitter and pungent in taste, cold and non-toxic in property, effective in clearing heat and removing toxin, activating the blood and regulating Qi, unobstructing the nine orifices and promoting urination and defecation. Clinically it is used to treat severe heat in the intestines and stomach, nosebleed, stagnation of the blood in the intestines, abdominal hardness and distension, amenorrhea, malaria, chronic hepatitis, mastitis, ulcer and scabies.

神农本草经

43. 藁本

【原文】

味辛,温。

主妇人疝瘕,阴中寒肿痛,腹中急,除风头痛,长肌肤:悦颜色。一名鬼卿,一名地新。生山谷。

【考据】

1.《名医》曰:一名微茎,生崇山,正月二月采根暴干,三十日成。

2. 案《广雅》云:山芷蔚香,藁本也。《管子·地员篇》云:五臭畴生藁本。《荀子·大略篇》云:兰芷藁本,渐于蜜醴,一佩易之。樊光注《尔雅》云:藁本一名麋芜,根名靳芷,归作藁,非。

【今译】

味辛,性温。

43. Gaoben（藁本，rhizome of Chinese ligusticum，rhizome of jehol ligusticum，Rhizoma Ligustici）[1]

［Original Text］

［Gaoben（藁本，rhizome of Chinese ligusticum，rhizome of jehol ligusticum，Rhizoma Ligustici），］pungent in taste and warm ［in property］，［is mainly used］to treat hernia and abdominal mass in women，genital coldness，swelling and pain，abdominal contracture and spasm and headache［caused by invasion of］wind into the head，to promote［growth of］muscles and to luster facial expression.［It is also］called Guiqing（鬼卿）and Dixin（地新），growing in mountains and valleys.

［Textual Research］

［In the book entitled］*Ming Yi Bie Lu*（《名医别录》，*Special Record of Great Doctors*），［it］says［that Gaoben（藁本，rhizome of Chinese ligusticum，rhizome of jehol ligusticum，Rhizoma Ligustici）is also］called Weijing（微茎）and grows in Chongshan（崇山）.［Its］root［can be］collected in January and February，and dried in the sun for thirty days.

［In the book entitled］*Guang Ya*（《广雅》，*The First Chinese Encyclopedic Dictionary*），［it］says［that the so-called］Shanzhi Weixiang（山芷蔚香）refers to Gaoben（藁本，rhizome of Chinese ligusticum，rhizome of jehol ligusticum，Rhizoma Ligustici）.

主治妇人疝瘕,阴器受寒而肿痛,腹中挛急,能解除因风邪侵袭而头痛,能促进肌肤生长,能使面部色彩艳丽。又称为鬼卿,又称为地新。该物生长在山谷之中。

神农本草经

Notes

1. Gaoben（藁本，rhizome of Chinese ligusticum，rhizome of jehol ligusticum，Rhizoma Ligustici）is a herbal medicinal，pungent in taste and warm in property，entering the bladder meridian，effective in expelling wind，dispersing dampness and stopping pain，Clinically it is used to treat common cold，headache，migraine，ostalgia due to wind-dampness and abdominal pain due to cold-dampness.

44. 石韦

【原文】

味苦,平。

主劳热邪气,五癃闭不通,利小便水道。一名石蘇。生山谷石上。

【考据】

1.《名医》曰:一名石皮,生华阴山谷,不闻水及人声者,良,二月采叶,阴干。

44. Shiwei（石韦，frond of Japanese felt fern，shearers pyrrosia frond，petioled pyrrosia frond，Folium Pyrrosiae）[1]

[Original Text]

[Shiwei（石韦，frond of Japanese felt fern，shearers pyrrosia frond，petioled pyrrosia frond，Folium Pyrrosiae），] bitter in taste and mild [in property]，[is mainly used] to treat overstrained heat [caused by] evil-Qi and five [kinds of] dysuria[2]，to promote urination and to unobstruct waterway [in the body]. [It is also] called Shizhe（石韄），growing over the stones in mountains and valleys.

675

[Textual Research]

[In the book entitled] *Ming Yi Bie Lu*（《名医别录》，*Special Record of Great Doctors*），[it] says [that Shiwei（石韦，frond of Japanese felt fern，shearers pyrrosia frond，petioled pyrrosia frond，Folium Pyrrosiae）is also] called Shipi（石皮），growing in the mountains and valleys in Huayin（华阴）.[If] not touched by water and man [in growing]，[it is] more effective. [Its] leaves [can be] collected in February and dried in the shade.

Notes

1. Shiwei（石韦，frond of Japanese felt fern，shearers pyrrosia

【今译】

味苦,性平。

主治虚劳发热,邪气所致之症,五种淋证,能使小便通畅,能通利水道。又称为石韀。该物生长在山谷之中石上。

frond, petioled pyrrosia frond, Folium Pyrrosiae) is a herbal medicinal, bitter and sweet in taste, slightly cold in property, entering the lung meridian and the bladder meridian, effective in promoting urination, unobstructing waterway [in the body], clearing the lung, purging heat and stopping bleeding. Clinically it is used to treat nephritis, edema, cystitis, urethritis, lung heat [disease] with cough, bronchial asthma, hematemesis, hemoptysis, nosebleed, hematuria, flooding and spotting (metrostaxis and metrorrhagia).

2. Five kinds of dysuria may include stony stranguria, Qi stranguria, paste stranguria, overstrained stranguria and heat stranguria, or refer to bloody stranguria.

45. 萆薢

【原文】

味苦,平。

主腰背痛,强骨节,风寒湿,周痹,恶疮不瘳,热气。生山谷。

【考据】

1.《名医》曰:一名赤节,生真定,八月采根曝干。

2. 案《博物志》云:菝葜与萆薢相乱。

45. Bixie（萆薢，rhizome of hypoglaucous collett yam，rhizome of collett yam，rhizome of mountain yam，rhizome of thinnest yam，Rhizoma Dioscoreae Hypoglaucae）[1]

[Original Text]

［Bixie（萆薢，rhizome of hypoglaucous collett yam，rhizome of collett yam，rhizome of mountain yam，rhizome of thinnest yam，Rhizoma Dioscoreae Hypoglaucae），］ bitter in taste and mild ［in property］，［is mainly used］ to treat pain of the waist and back，stiffness of joints，wind-cold dampness ［disease］，generalized impediment，severe sore difficult to heal and ［disease caused by］ heat-Qi.［It］ grows in mountains and valleys.

[Textual Research]

［In the book entitled］ *Ming Yi Bie Lu*（《名医别录》，*Special Record of Great Doctors*），［it］ says ［that Bixie（萆薢，rhizome of hypoglaucous collett yam，rhizome of collett yam，rhizome of mountain yam，rhizome of thinnest yam，Rhizoma Dioscoreae Hypoglaucae）is also］ called Chijie（赤节）and grows in Zhending（真定）.［Its］ root ［can be］ collected in August and dried in the sun.

［In the book entitled］ *Bo Wu Zhi*（《博物志》，*History of All Plants*），［it］ says ［that］ Bixie（萆薢，rhizome of hypoglaucous collett yam，rhizome of collett yam，rhizome of mountain yam，

【今译】

味苦,性平。

主治腰部背部疼痛,能强壮骨节,能治疗风寒湿之症,全身流窜性疼痛,恶性痈疮不愈以及热邪所致之病。该物生长在山谷之中。

rhizome of thinnest yam, Rhizoma Dioscoreae Hypoglaucae) is confused with Youqia (芨葜).

Notes

1. Bixie (萆薢, rhizome of hypoglaucous collett yam, rhizome of collett yam, rhizome of mountain yam, rhizome of thinnest yam, Rhizoma Dioscoreae Hypoglaucae) is a herbal medicinal, bitter in taste and mild in property, entering the liver meridian, the stomach meridian and the bladder meridian, effective in expelling wind and eliminating dampness. Clinically it is used to treat wind-dampness impediment and pain, ache of the waist and knees, dysuria, stranguria, leucorrhea and turbid urine.

46. 白薇

【原文】

味苦,平。

主暴中风,身热肢满,忽忽不知人,狂惑,邪气,寒热酸疼,温疟、洗洗发作有时。生川谷。

【考据】

1.《名医》曰:一名白幕,一名薇草,一名春草,一名骨美,生平原,三月三日,采根阴干。

46. Baiwei（白薇，root of blackend swallowwort， root of versicolorous swallowwort， Radix Cynanchi Atrati）[1]

[Original Text]

[Baiwei（白薇，root of blackend swallowwort， root of versicolorous swallowwort，Radix Cynanchi Atrati），] bitter in taste and mild ［in property］, ［is mainly used］ to treat sudden wind stroke， fever， distension of limbs， unconsciousness， manic confusion， cold-heat ［disease caused by］ evil-Qi， aching ［muscles］ and warm malaria with shivering and regular onset. ［It］ grows in mountain valleys and river valleys.

[Textual Research]

［In the book entitled］ *Ming Yi Bie Lu*（《名医别录》，*Special Record of Great Doctors*），［it］ says ［that Baiwei（白薇，root of blackend swallowwort， root of versicolorous swallowwort， Radix Cynanchi Atrati）is also］ called Baimu（白幕），Weicao（薇草），Chuncao（春草）and Gumei（骨美），growing in plain. ［Its］ root ［can be］ collected on March 3rd ［in the Chinese lunar calender］ and dried in the shade.

Notes

1. Baiwei（白薇，root of blackend swallowwort， root of versicolorous swallowwort， Radix Cynanchi Atrati）is a herbal

【今译】

味苦,性平。

主治突然中风,身体发热,四肢胀满,迷惑不省人事,疯狂性的迷惑,邪气所引起的寒热病,酸痛,温疟,时时瑟瑟颤栗。该物生长在山川河谷之中。

medicinal, bitter and salty in taste, cold in property, entering the liver meridian and the stomach meridian, effective in clearing deficiency-fire, eliminating blood-heat and promoting urination. Clinically it is used to treat internal heat due to Yin deficiency, remnant fever after illness, vexation and vomiting after delivery of baby, scorching heat due to wind-warmth, hemoptysis due to lung heat and malaria.

47. 水萍

【原文】

味辛,寒。

主暴热身痒(艺文类聚初学记痒,此是),下水气胜酒,长须发(艺文类聚作乌发),消渴。久服轻身。一名水华(艺文类聚引云:一名水廉)。生池泽。

神农本草经

【考据】

1.《吴普》曰:水萍一名水廉,生泽水上,叶员小,一茎,一叶,根入水,五月华白,三月采,日干。(《御览》)

2.《名医》曰:一始水白,一名水苏,生雷泽,三月采,曝干。

3. 案《说文》云:萍,苹也,无根,浮水而生者。萍,苹也,蓱,大萍也。《广雅》云:藻,萍也。《夏小正》云:七月湟潦生苹。《尔雅》云:萍苹。郭璞云:水中浮萍,江东谓之藻.又其大者苹。《毛诗》云:于以采苹。《传》云:苹,大萍也。

《范子计然》曰:水萍出三辅,色青者善。《淮南子·原道训》云:萍树根于水。高诱云:萍,大苹也。

47. Shuiping（水萍，common ducksmeat herb，Herba Spirodelae）[1]

［Original Text］

［Shuiping （水 萍， common ducksmeat herb， Herba Spirodelae），］pungent in taste and cold ［in property］，［is mainly used］to treat itching ［caused by］sudden heat，to promote urination，［to eliminate］wine ［toxin］，to invigorate hair and to relieve thirst. Long-term taking ［of it will］relax the body. ［It is also］called Shuihua（水华），growing in lakes and swamps.

［Textual Research］

687

［In the book entitled］*Wu Pu Ben Cao*（《吴普本草》，*Wu Pu's Studies of Materia Medica*），［it］says ［that］Shuiping （水 萍，common ducksmeat herb， Herba Spirodelae）［is also］called Shuilian（水廉），growing in pools with round and small leaf，just one stalk and one leaf. The root is inside water. ［In］May，the flower is white. ［It can be］collected in March and dried in the sun ［according to the book entitled］*Tai Ping Yu Lan*（《太平御览》，*Imperial Studies in Taiping Times*）.

［In the book entitled］*Ming Yi Bie Lu*（《名医别录》，*Special Record of Great Doctors*），［it］says ［that Shuiping（水萍，common ducksmeat herb，Herba Spirodelae）is also］called Shishuibai（始水白）and Shuisu（水苏），growing in Leize（雷泽）. ［It can be］

【今译】

味辛,性寒。

主治突然感受热邪引发身痒,能使水湿流下,能消除酒毒,能使须发生长,能治疗消渴症。长期服用能使人身体轻盈。又称为水华。该物生长在池泽中。

collected in March and dried in the sun.

［In the book entitled］ *Fan Zi Ji Ran* （《范子计然》, *Studies About Fan Li's Teacher*）, ［it］ says ［that］ Shuiping （水萍, common ducksmeat herb, Herba Spirodelae） grows in the three places. The green one is the best. ［In the book entitled］ *Huai Nan Zi* （《淮南子》, *A Philosophy Book Compiled by Liu An , King in Huainan*）, ［it］ says ［that］ Shuiping （水萍, common ducksmeat herb, Herba Spirodelae） grows in water.

Notes

1. Shuiping （水萍, common ducksmeat herb, Herba Spirodelae） is herbal medicinal, pungent in taste and cold in property, entering the lung meridian and the bladder meridian, effective in inducing sweating, expelling wind, promoting urination and cooling the blood. Clinically it is used to treat common cold with fever and no sweating, measles, urticaria, skin itching, dropsy, dysuria and oral ulcer.

48. 王瓜

【原文】

味苦,寒。

主消渴内痹瘀血,月闭,寒热,酸疼,益气,俞聋。一名土瓜。生平泽。

【考据】

1.《名医》曰:生鲁地田野,及人家垣墙间,三月采根,阴干。

2. 案《说文》云:菳,王菳也。《广雅》云:葵菇,瓜瓤,王瓜也。《夏小正》云:四月王菳秀。《尔雅》云:钩葵菇。郭璞云:钩,瓟也。一名王瓜,实如胞瓜,正赤,味苦,月令,王瓜生。郑元云:月令云,王菳生,孔颖连云:疑王菳,则王瓜也。《管子·地员篇》,剽土之次,曰:五沙:其种大菳细菳,白茎青秀以蔓。本草图经云:大菳,即王菳也。菳亦谓之土瓜,自别是一物。

48. Wanggua（王瓜，fruit of Japanese snakegourd，Fructus Trichosanthis Cucumeroidis）[1]

[Original Text]

[Wanggua （王瓜，fruit of Japanese snakegourd，Fructus Trichosanthis Cucumeroidis），] bitter in taste and cold ［in property］，［is mainly used］ to treat wasting-thirst，internal impediment with blood stasis，amenorrhea，cold-heat ［disease］ and ache ［of limbs］，to replenish Qi and to resolve deafness. ［It is also］ called Tugua（土瓜），growing in plains and swamps.

[Textual Research]

［In the book entitled］ *Ming Yi Bie Lu* （《名医别录》，*Special Record of Great Doctors*），［it］ says ［that Wanggua（王瓜，fruit of Japanese snakegourd，Fructus Trichosanthis Cucumeroidis）］ grows in the lands in Ludi（鲁地）and in between the walls in people's homes. ［Its］ root ［can be］ collected in March and dried in the shade.

691

Notes

1. Wanggua （王瓜，fruit of Japanese snakegourd，Fructus Trichosanthis Cucumeroidis） is a herbal medicinal，bitter in taste and cold in property，entering the heart meridian and the kidney

【今译】

　　味苦,性寒。

　　主治消渴病,内痹证,因瘀血所致的经闭,寒热病,酸疼症,能补益精气,能治愈耳聋。又称为土瓜。该物生长在平川水泽之中。

meridian, effective in clearing heat, producing fluid and promoting lactation. Clinically it is used to treat wasting-thirst, jaundice, nausea and agalactia.

49. 地榆

【原文】

味苦,微寒。

主妇人乳痓痛,七伤带下病,止痛。除恶肉,止汗,疗金疮(《御览》引云:主消酒,又云明目,《大观本草》,消酒作黑字,而无明目)。生山谷。

【考据】

1.《名医》曰:生桐柏及冤句,二月八月,采根,暴干。

2. 案《广雅》云:菗蒢,地榆也。陶宏景云:叶似榆而长,初生布地,而花子紫黑色如豉,故中玉豉。

【今译】

味苦,性微寒。

49. Diyu（地榆，root of garden burnet，Radix Sanguisorbae）[1]

［Original Text］

［Diyu（地榆，root of garden burnet，Radix Sanguisorbae），］ bitter in taste and slightly cold［in property］，［is mainly used］to treat convulsion and pain of the breast in women，seven［kinds of］ damage[2] and leucorrhea，to cease pain，to eliminate necrotic muscles，to stop sweating and to cure injury［caused by］metal.［It］ grows in mountains and valleys.

［Textual Research］

［In the book entitled］*Ming Yi Bie Lu*（《名医别录》，*Special Record of Great Doctors*），［it］says［that Diyu（地榆，root of garden burnet，Radix Sanguisorbae）］grows in Tongbai（桐柏）and Yuanju （冤句）.［Its］root［can be］collected in February and August，and dried in the sun.

［In the book entitled］*Guang Ya*（《广雅》，*The First Chinese Encyclopedic Dictionary*），［it］says［that the so-called］Chouchu（菗 蒢） refers to Diyu（地榆，root of garden burnet，Radix Sanguisorbae）. Tao Hongjing（陶宏景）said，"The leaves are as long as［that of］elm. Initially［it］grows all over the land. The flowers are purple and black like fermented soybean."

主治妇女乳房抽搐性疼痛,七种损伤性疾病,能消除疼痛,能祛除坏死肌肉,能止汗,能治疗因金属创伤而导致的疮疡。该物生长在山谷之中。

Notes

1. Diyu (地榆, root of garden burnet, Radix Sanguisorbae) is a herbal medicinal, bitter and sour in taste, cold in property, entering the liver meridian and the large intestine meridian, effective in cooling the blood and stopping bleeding, purging fire and relieving sore. Clinically it is used to treat hematochezia due to intestinal wind, bloody dysentery, hematuria, flooding and spotting (metrostaxis and metrorrhagia), hemorrhoids with bleeding, hematemesis, nosebleed and leucorrhea.

2. Seven kinds of damage refer to damage caused by food, anxiety, drinking, sexual activity, hunger, overstrain and meridians.

50. 海藻

【原文】

味苦,寒。

主瘿瘤气,颈下核,破散结气,痈肿症瘕坚气,腹中上下鸣,下水十二肿。一名落首。生池泽。

【考据】

1.《名医》曰:一名薄,生东海,七月七日采,暴干。

2. 案《说文》云:藻,水草也,或作藻。《广雅》云:海萝,海藻也。《尔雅》云:薅,海藻也。郭璞云:药草也。一名海萝,如乱发,生海中。本草云:又藻石衣。郭璞云:水苔也,一名石发,江东食之,或曰薄,叶似莛而大,生水底也,亦可食。

【今译】

味苦,性寒。

50. Haizao（海藻，pale sargassum，Sargassum；fusiform sargassum）[1]

[Original Text]

[Haizao （海藻，pale sargassum，Sargassum；fusiform sargassum），] bitter in taste and cold [in property], [is mainly used] to treat goiter，tumor and lump in the neck，to disperse bind of Qi，borborygum in the upper and lower abdomen，and to resolve twelve [kinds of] swelling[2]. [It is also] called Luoshou（落首），growing in lakes and swamps.

[Textual Research]

[In the book entitled] *Ming Yi Bie Lu* （《名医别录》，*Special Record of Great Doctors*），[it] says [that Haizao （海藻，pale sargassum，Sargassum；fusiform sargassum） is also] called Tan（薄），growing in Donghai（东海，East Sea）. [It can be] collected on July 7th [in the chinese lunar calender] and dried in the sun.

[In the book entitled] *Guang Ya* （《广雅》，*The First Chinese Encyclopedic Dictionary*），[it] says [that the so-called] Hailuo（海萝）refers to Haizao （海藻，pale sargassum，Sargassum；fusiform sargassum）.

Notes

1. Haizao （海藻，pale sargassum，Sargassum；fusiform

主治颈部瘿瘤邪气,颈部之下的肿块,能破散气结,能祛除痈肿,症痕,积气,腹中上下回鸣,能治疗多种水肿之症。又称为落首。该物生长在池泽中。

sargassum) is a herbal medicinal, bitter and salty in taste, cold in property, entering the liver meridian, the stomach meridian and the kidney meridian, effective in resolving phlegm, softening hardness, dispersing binding, promoting urination and purging heat. Clinically it is used to treat thyroid tumor, abdominal mass, edema, beriberi, swelling and pain of testicle.

51. 泽兰

【原文】

味苦,微温。

主乳妇内(《御览》作衄衄血),中风余疾,大腹水肿,身面四肢浮肿,骨节中水,金疮痈肿疮脓。一名虎兰,一名龙枣。生大泽傍。

【考据】

1.《吴普》曰:泽兰,一名水香,神农黄帝岐伯桐君酸无毒,李氏温,生下地水傍,叶如兰,二月生,香,赤节,四叶相值枝节间。

2.《名医》曰:一名虎蒲,生汝南,三月三日采,阴干。

3. 案《广雅》云:虎兰,泽兰也。

【今译】

味苦,性微温。

主治乳妇女产后因出血而导致瘀血,因感受风邪而导致的疾病,

51. Zelan（泽兰，hirsute shiny bugleweed herb，Herba Lycopi）[1]

[Original Text]

[Zelan（泽兰，hirsute shiny bugleweed herb，Herba Lycopi），] bitter in taste and slightly warm [in property], [is mainly used] to treat internal bleeding after delivery of baby，remnant disease after wind stroke，dropsy of the body，face and limbs，retention of water in the joints，injury [caused by] metal，abscess and ulcer. [It is also] called Hulan（虎兰）and Longzao（龙枣），growing beside the large swamps.

[Textual Research]

[In the book entitled] *Wu Pu Ben Cao*（《吴普本草》，*Wu Pu's Studies of Materia Medica*），[it] says [that] Zelan（泽兰，hirsute shiny bugleweed herb，Herba Lycopi）[is also] called Shuixiang（水香）. [According to] Agriculture God（神农），Yellow Emperor（黄帝），Qibo（岐伯）and Tongjun（桐均），[it is] sour [in taste] and non-toxic [in property]；[according to] Li's（李氏），[it is] warm [in property]. [It] grows in water and beside water with the leaves like orchid. [It begins] to grow in February with fragrance，red joints and four leaves among the branches.

[In the book entitled] *Ming Yi Bie Lu*（《名医别录》，*Special Record of Great Doctors*），[it] says [that Zelan（泽兰，hirsute shiny

腹部因水肿而凸起，身体、面部和四肢浮肿，骨节积聚水邪，因金属创伤而导致的痈疮，痈肿和脓疮。又称为虎兰，又称为龙枣。生在大泽旁边。

bugleweed herb，Herba Lycopi）is also］called Hupu （虎蒲），growing in Runan（汝南）.［It can be］collected on March 3rd ［in the chinese lunar calender］and dried in the shade.

［In the book entitled］ *Guang Ya* （《广雅》，*The First Chinese Encyclopedic Dictionary*），［it］says ［that the so-called］ Hulan（虎兰）refers to Zelan （泽兰，hirsute shiny bugleweed herb，Herba Lycopi）.

Notes

1. Zelan（泽兰，hirsute shiny bugleweed herb，Herba Lycopi）is a herbal medicinal，bitter and pungent in taste，warm in property，entering the spleen meridian and the liver meridian，effective in activating the blood，expelling stasis and moving water. Clinically it is used to treat amenorrhea，dysmenorrhea，lumps in the abdomen，abdominal pain after delivery of baby due to blood stasis，dropsy of the body and face，traumatic injury，abscess，ulcer and snake bite.

52. 防己

【原文】

味辛,平。

主风寒,温疟,热气,诸痫,除邪,利大小便。一名解离(《御览》作石

解引云:通凑理,利九窍,《大观本》,六字黑)。生川谷。

【考据】

1.《吴普》曰:木防己,一名解离,一名解燕,神农辛,黄帝岐伯桐君

苦无毒,李氏大寒,如芳,茎蔓延,如艽,白根外黄似桔梗,内黑又如车辐

解,二月八月十月,采根。(《御览》)

2.《名医》曰,生汉中,二月八月,采根阴干。

3. 案《范子计然》云:防已出汉中旬阳。

52. Fangji（防己，root of fourstamen stephania，Radix Stephaniae Tetrandrae）[1]

[Original Text]

[Fangji（防己，root of fourstamen stephania，Radix Stephaniae Tetrandrae），] pungent in taste and mild [in property]，[is mainly used] to treat wind-cold [disease]，warm malaria and [disease caused by] heat-Qi，to eliminate evil and to promote defecation and urination. [It is also] called Jieli（解离），growing in mountain valleys and river valleys.

[Textual Research]

[In the book entitled] *Wu Pu Ben Cao*（《吴普本草》，*Wu Pu's Studies of Materia Medica*），[it] says [that] Mufangji（防己，root of fourstamen stephania，Radix Stephaniae Tetrandrae）[is also] called Jieli（解离）and Jieyan（解燕）. [According to] Agriculture God（神农），[it is] pungent [in taste]；[according to] Yellow Emperor（黄帝），Qibo（岐伯）and Tongjun（桐均），[it is] bitter [in taste] and non-toxic [in property]；[according to] Li's（李氏），[it is] severely cold [in property]. [It looks] like taro and spreads like large-leaved gentian. [Its] root is white；[its] external is as yellow as Jiegeng（桔梗，platycodon grandiflorum，Radix Platycodi）；[its] internal is as black as spokes；[its] root [can be] collected in February，August and October [according to the book entitled] *Tai*

707

【今译】

　　味辛,性平。

　　主治外感风寒,温疟,热邪所致各种痈疮,清除病邪,通利大小便。

又称为解离。该物生长在山川河谷之中。

Ping Yu Lan (《太平御览》, *Imperial Studies in Taiping Times*).

［In the book entitled］*Ming Yi Bie Lu* (《名医别录》, *Special Record of Great Doctors*), ［it］says ［that Fangji (防己, root of fourstamen stephania, Radix Stephaniae Tetrandrae)］grows in Hanzhong (汉中). ［Its］root ［can be］collected in February and August, and dried in the shade

［In the book entitled］*Fan Zi Ji Ran* (《范子计然》, *Studies About Fan Li's Teacher*), ［it］says ［that］Fangji (防己, root of fourstamen stephania, Radix Stephaniae Tetrandrae) grows in Hanzhong (汉中) and Xunyang (旬阳).

Notes

1. Fangji (防己, root of fourstamen stephania, Radix Stephaniae Tetrandrae) is a herbal medicinal, bitter and pungent in taste, cold in property, entering the bladder meridian and the lung meridian, effective in promoting urination and resolving swelling, expelling wind and eliminating dampness, reducing blood pressure and relieving abscess. Clinically it is used to treat edema, beriberi, panting and cough due to retention of fluid, dysuria, arthritis due to wind-dampness, hypertension, eczema, ulceration of the shanks, abscess and ulcer.

53. 款冬花

【原文】

味辛,温。

主咳逆上气,善喘,喉痹,诸惊痫,寒热邪气。一名橐吾(《御览》作石),一名颗东(《御览》作颗冬),一名虎须,一名兔奚。生山谷。

【考据】

1.《吴普》曰:款冬十二月,花黄白。(艺文类聚)

2.《名医》曰:一名氏冬,生常山及上党水傍,十一月,采花阴干。

3. 案《广雅》云:苦萃款东也。《尔雅》云:菟奚颗东。郭璞云:款冬也。紫赤华生水中。西京杂记云:款冬,华于严冬。传咸款冬赋序曰:仲冬之月,冰凌积雪,款冬独敷华艳。

【今译】

味辛,性温。

53. Kuandonghua（款冬花，immature flower of common coltsfoot，Flos Farfarae）[1]

[Original Text]

[Kuandonghua（款冬花，immature flower of common coltsfoot，Flos Farfarae），] pungent in taste and warm [in property], [is mainly used] to treat cough with dyspnea and upward counterflow of Qi，frequent panting，throat impediment，various epilepsy，cold-heat [disease caused by] evil-Qi. [It is also] called Tuowu（橐吾），Huxu（虎须）and Mianxi（兔奚），growing in mountains and valleys.

[Textual Research]

[In the book entitled] *Wu Pu Ben Cao*（《吴普本草》，*Wu Pu's Studies of Materia Medica*），[it] says [that] Kuandonghua（款冬花，immature flower of common coltsfoot，Flos Farfarae）blossoms in December with yellow and white flowers.

[In the book entitled] *Ming Yi Bie Lu*（《名医别录》，*Special Record of Great Doctors*），[it] says [that Kuandonghua（款冬花，immature flower of common coltsfoot，Flos Farfarae）is also] called Shidong（氏冬），growing in Changshan（常山）and beside water in Shangdang（上党）. [Its] flowers [can be] collected in November and dried in the shade.

Guo Pu（郭璞）said，"Kuandonghua（款冬花，immature flower of common coltsfoot，Flos Farfarae）blossoms in water with purple

　　主治咳嗽及呼吸困难,时常气喘,治疗喉痹,各种惊恐,心悸,癫痫,寒热病,祛除邪气。又称为囊吾,又称为虎须,又称为免奚。该物生长在山谷之中。

and red flowers." [In the book entitled] Chuan Xian Kuan Dong Fu Xu (传咸款冬赋序), (*Foreword of Prose about Kuandonghua*), [it] says, "In cold winter, water is frozen and snow covers all the earth. But Kuandonghua (款冬花, immature flower of common coltsfoot, Flos Farfarae) blossoms gorgeously."

Notes

1. Kuandonghua (款冬花, immature flower of common coltsfoot, Flos Farfarae) is a herbal medicinal, pungent in taste and warm in property, entering the lung meridian, effective in moistening the lung to descend Qi, stopping cough and resolving phlegm. Clinically it is used to treat cough, panting, lung abscess and throat impediment.

54. 牡丹

【原文】

味苦,辛寒。

主寒热,中风,瘈疭,痉,惊痫,邪气,除症坚,瘀血留舍肠胃,安五脏,疗痈疮。一名鹿韭,一名鼠姑。生山谷。

【考据】

1.《吴普》曰:牡丹,神农岐伯辛,李氏小寒,雷公桐君苦无毒,黄帝苦有毒,叶如蓬相植,根如柏,黑中有核,二月采,八月采,日干,人食之,轻身益寿。(《御览》)

2.《名医》曰:生巴郡及汉中,二月八月,采根阴干。

3. 案《广雅》云:白术,牡丹也。《范子计然》云:牡丹出汉中河内,赤色者亦善。

【今译】

味苦,性辛寒。

主治寒热病,因感受风邪而导致的疾病,抽搐,痉挛,惊恐,心悸,

54. Mudan（牡丹，moutan，Cortex Moutan Radicis）[1]

[Original Text]

[Mudan（牡丹，moutan，Cortex Moutan Radicis），] bitter and pungent in taste and cold [in property], [is mainly used] to treat cold-heat [disease], wind stroke, convulsion, spasm and epilepsy [caused by] evil-Qi, to eliminate hard syndrome/pattern, to relieve blood stasis in the intestines and stomach, to harmonize the five Zang-organs and to cure abscess. [It is also] called Lujiu（鹿韭）and Shugu（鼠姑），growing in mountains and valleys.

[Textual Research]

[In the book entitled] *Wu Pu Ben Cao*（《吴普本草》，*Wu Pu's Studies of Materia Medica*），[it] says [that] Mudan（牡丹，moutan，Cortex Moutan Radicis），[according to] Agriculture God（神农）and Qibo（岐伯），[is] pungent [in taste]; [according to] Li's（李氏），[is] slightly cold [in taste]; [according to] Leigong（雷公）and Tongjun（桐均），[is] bitter [in taste] and non-toxic [in property]; [according to] Yellow Emperor（黄帝），[is] bitter [in taste] and toxic [in property]. [Its] leaves look like that of bitter fleabane，[its] root looks like cypress. [It can be] collected in February and August，and dried in the sun. Taking of it will relax the body and prolong life [according to the book entitled] *Tai Ping Yu Lan*（《太平御览》，*Imperial Studies in Taiping Times*）.

癫痫,清除邪气,能祛除坚固痹症,能消除滞留在肠胃中的瘀血,能安静五脏,能治疗痈疮。又称为鹿韭,又称为鼠姑。该物生长在山谷之中。

[In the book entitled] *Ming Yi Bie Lu* (《名医别录》, *Special Record of Great Doctors*), [it] says [that Mudan (牡丹, moutan, Cortex Moutan Radicis)] grows in Bajun (巴郡) and Hanzhong (汉中). [Its] root [can be] collected in February and August, and dried in the shade.

[In the book entitled] *Guang Ya* (《广雅》, *The First Chinese Encyclopedic Dictionary*), [it] says [that the so-called] Baizhu (白术) refers to Mudan (牡丹, moutan, Cortex Moutan Radicis). [In the book entitled] *Fan Zi Ji Ran* (《范子计然》, *Studies About Fan Li's Teacher*), [it] says [that] Mudan (牡丹, moutan, Cortex Moutan Radicis) grows in Hanzhong (汉中) and Henei (河内). The red one is more effective.

Notes

1. Mudan (牡丹, moutan, Cortex Moutan Radicis) is a herbal medicinal, pungent and bitter in taste, cold in property, entering the heart meridian, the liver meridian and the kidney meridian, effective in clearing heat and cooling the blood, activating the blood and dispersing stasis. Clinically it is used to treat heat disease with spots, hematemesis, nosebleed, bone steaming without sweating, epilepsy, amenorrhea, dysmenorrhea, abdominal mass, traumatic injury, intestinal abscess, carbuncle and hypertension.

55．马先蒿

【原文】

味平。

主寒热，鬼注，中风湿痹，女子带下病，无子。一名马尿蒿。生川泽。

【考据】

1.《名医》曰：生南阳。

2. 案《说文》云：蔚，牡蒿也。《广雅》云：因尘，马先也。《尔雅》云：蔚，牡菣。

3. 郭璞云：无子者。《毛诗》云：匪莪伊蔚。《传》云：菣，牡菣也。陆玑云：三月始生，七月华，华似胡麻华而紫赤，八月为角，角似小豆，角锐而长，一名马新蒿，案新先声相近。

【今译】

味平。

55. Maxianhao（马先蒿，leaf or root of resupinate woodbetony，Folium seu Radix Pedicularidis Resupinatae）[1]

[Original Text]

［Maxianhao（马先蒿，leaf or root of resupinate woodbetony，Folium seu Radix Pedicularidis Resupinatae），］ bitter in taste and mild［in property］，［is mainly used］ to treat cold-heat［disease］，［disease like］ ghost attack[2]，wind stroke，dampness impediment，leukorrheal disease and infertility.［It is also］ called Maniaohao（马尿蒿），growing in valleys and swamps.

[Textual Research]

［In the book entitled］ *Ming Yi Bie Lu*《名医别录》，*Special Record of Great Doctors*），［it］ says［that Maxianhao（马先蒿，leaf or root of resupinate woodbetony，Folium seu Radix Pedicularidis Resupinatae）］grows in Nanyang（南阳）.

Lu Ji（陆玑）said，"［Maxianhao（马先蒿，leaf or root of resupinate woodbetony，Folium seu Radix Pedicularidis Resupinatae）］begins to grow in March and blossom in July.［Its］ flowers look like that of flax，purple and red.［In］August，［it begins］to bear beans like red beans，sharp and long.［It is also］called Mxinhao（马新蒿）."

719

　　主治寒热病,鬼怪之邪所致之症,因感受风邪而导致的疾病,湿邪所致痹证,女子带下病,不孕之症。又称为马尿蒿。该物生长在山川和平泽之中。

Notes

1. Maxianhao (马先蒿, leaf or root of resupinate woodbetony, Folium seu Radix Pedicularidis Resupinatae) is a herbal medicinal, bitter in taste and mild in property, effective in expelling wind, removing dampness and promoting urination. Clinically it is used to treat arthritis, arthralgia, dysuria, urethral infection and swelling.

56. 积雪草

【原文】

味苦,寒。

主大热,恶疮痈疽,浸淫,赤㮛,皮肤赤,身热。生川谷。

【考据】

1.《名医》曰:生荆州。

2. 案陶宏景云:荆楚人以叶如钱,谓为地钱草,徐仪药图名连钱草。本草图经云:咸洛二京亦有,或名胡薄荷。

【今译】

味苦,性寒。

主治身体高热,恶性疮,痈疽,浸淫疮,赤㮛火丹,皮肤发红,身体发热。该物生长在山川河谷之中。

56. Jixuecao（积雪草，Asiatic pennywort herb，Herba Centellae）[1]

[Original Text]

[Jixuecao （积雪草，Asiatic pennywort herb，Herba Centellae），] bitter in taste and cold [in property], [is mainly used] to treat [disease caused by] severe heat，severe sore，abscess，eczema with itching，red erysipelas，febrile skin and fever. [It] grows in mountain valleys and river valleys.

[Textual Research]

[In the book entitled] *Ming Yi Bie Lu* （《名医别录》，*Special Record of Great Doctors*），[it] says [that Jixuecao （积雪草，Asiatic pennywort herb，Herba Centellae）] grows in Jingzhou （荆州）.

Notes

1. Jixuecao （积雪草，Asiatic pennywort herb，Herba Centellae） is a herbal medicinal，bitter and pungent in taste，cool in property，entering the liver meridian，the spleen meridian and the kidney meridian，effective in clearing heat，relieving dampness，dispersing stasis and removing toxin. Clinically it is used to treat common cold with fever，heatstroke，redness of eyes due to wind-fire attack，tonsillitis，sore-throat，urethral infection，infectious hepatitis，enteritis，dysentery，hemoptysis，nosebleed，abscess，eczema and erysipelas.

神农本草经

57. 女菀

【原文】

味辛,温。

主风,洗洗,霍乱,泄利,肠鸣上下无常处,惊痫,寒热百疾。生川谷,或山阳。

【考据】

1.《吴普》曰:女菀,一名白菀,一名识女苑。(《御览》)

2.《名医》曰:一名白菀,一名织女菀,一名茆,生汉中,正月二月采,阴干。

3. 案《广雅》云:女肠,女菀也。

【今译】

味辛,性温。

57．Nǚwan（女菀，Common turczanionowia herb，Herba Turczaninowiae Fastigiatae）[1]

［Original Text］

［Nǚwan （女菀，Common turczanionowia herb， Herba Turczaninowiae Fastigiatae），］ pungent in taste and warm ［in property］，［is mainly used］ to treat ［disease caused by］ wind ［-cold and marked by］ chilliness and shivering，Huoluan （simultaneous vomiting and diarrhea），diarrhea，dysentery，borborygmu in the upper and lower ［abdomen］ without fixed position，epilepsy，cold-heat ［disease］ and various other diseases．［It］ grows in mountain valleys and river valleys or the sunny sides of mountains.

［Textual Research］

［In the book entitled］ *Wu Pu Ben Cao* （《吴普本草》，*Wu Pu's Studies of Materia Medica*），［it］ says ［that］ Nǚwan （女菀，Common turczanionowia herb，Herba Turczaninowiae Fastigiatae） ［is also］ called Baiwan （白菀） and Shinǚwan （识女菀） ［according to the book entitled］ *Tai Ping Yu Lan* （《太平御览》，*Imperial Studies in Taiping Times*）.

［In the book entitled］ *Ming Yi Bie Lu* （《名医别录》，*Special Record of Great Doctors*），［it］ says ［that Nǚwan （女菀，Common turczanionowia herb，Herba Turczaninowiae Fastigiatae） is also］ called Baiwan （白菀），Zhinǚwan （织女菀） and Mao （茆），growing

主治外感风寒而颤栗,霍乱,泄泻,痢疾,上下肠鸣无定处,惊恐,心悸,癫痫,寒热病以及各种各样的疾病。该物生长在山川河谷之中,或山阳。

in Hanzhong (汉中). [It can be] collected in January and February, and dried in the shade.

[In the book entitled] *Guang Ya* (《广雅》, *The First Chinese Encyclopedic Dictionary*), [it] says [that the so-called] Nǚchang (女肠) refers to Nǚwan (女菀, Common turczanionowia herb, Herba Turczaninowiae Fastigiatae).

Notes

1. Nǚwan (女菀, Common turczanionowia herb, Herba Turczaninowiae Fastigiatae) is a herbal medicinal, pungent in taste and warm in property, effective in warming the lung and resolving phlegm, harmonizing the middle (the internal organs) and promoting urination. Clinically it is used to treat cough with panting, borborygmus, diarrhea and dysuria.

58. 王孙

【原文】

味苦,平。

主五臧邪气,寒湿痹,四肢疼酸,膝冷痛。生川谷。

【考据】

1.《吴普》曰:黄孙一名王孙,一名蔓延,一名公草,一名海孙,神农雷公苦无毒。黄帝甘无毒,生西海山谷,及汝南城郭垣下,蔓延,赤文,茎叶相当。(《御览》)

2.《名医》曰:吴名白功草,楚名王孙,齐名长孙,一名黄孙,一名黄昏,一名海孙,一名蔓延,生海西及汝南城郭下。

3. 案陶宏景云:今方家皆呼王昏,又云壮蒙。

58. Wangsun（王孙，rhizome of tetraphyllous paris，Rhizoma Paris Tetraphyllae）[1]

[Original Text]

[Wangsun（王孙，rhizome of tetraphyllous paris，Rhizoma Paris Tetraphyllae），] bitter in taste and mild [in property]，[is mainly used] to treat [disease in] the five Zang-organs [caused by] evil-Qi，cold-dampness impediment，ache of the four limbs，coldness and pain of the knees. [It] grows in mountain valleys and river valleys.

[Textual Research]

[In the book entitled] *Wu Pu Ben Cao*（《吴普本草》，*Wu Pu's Studies of Materia Medica*），[it] says [that] Huangsun（黄孙）[is also] called Wangsun（王孙），Manyan（蔓延），Gongcao（公草）and Haisun（海孙）. [according to] Agriculture God（神农）and Leigong（雷公），[it is] bitter [in taste] and non-toxic [in property]；[according to] Yellow Emperor（黄帝），[it is] sweet [in taste] and toxic [in property]. [It] grows in the mountains and valleys in Xihai（西海，West Sea）and below the cities in Runan（汝南）. [It] spreads [in growing] with red texture and stalks and leaves of certain length [according to the book entitled] *Tai Ping Yu Lan*（《太平御览》，*Imperial Studies in Taiping Times*）.

[In the book entitled] *Ming Yi Bie Lu*（《名医别录》，*Special Record of Great Doctors*），[it] says [that Wangsun（王孙，rhizome

【今译】

味苦,性平。

主治五脏中的邪气,寒湿邪所致痹证,四肢疼酸,膝部冷痛。该物生长在山川河谷之中。

of tetraphyllous paris, Rhizoma Paris Tetraphyllae) is] called Baigongcao (白功草) in Wu (吴) State, Wangsun (王孙) in Chu (楚) State, Changsun (长孙) in Qi (齐) State. [It is also] called Huangsun (黄孙), Huanghun (黄昏), Haisun (海孙) and Manyan (蔓延), growing in the Haixi (海西) and below the cities in Runan (汝南).

Notes

1. Wangsun (王孙, rhizome of tetraphyllous paris, Rhizoma Paris Tetraphyllae) is a herbal meidicinal, bitter in taste, mild and non-toxic in property, effective in replenishing Qi, resolving cold and dampness, relieving pain and regulating internal organs. Clinically it is used to treat visceral disease, cold-dampness impediment, coldness and pain of limbs and various other diseases.

59. 蜀羊泉

【原文】

味苦,微寒。

主头秃恶疮,热气,疥搔,痂癣虫,疗齲齿。生川谷。

【考据】

1. 《名医》曰:一名羊泉,一名饴,生蜀郡。

2. 案《广雅》云:陵姑,艾但鹿何,泽翱也。《唐本》注云:此草,一名漆姑。

【今译】

味苦,性微寒。

主治头部秃疮,恶性疮,热邪所致之病,疥疮,瘙痒,皮癣,祛除寄生虫,治疗齲齿。该物生长在山川河谷之中。

59. Shuyangquan（蜀羊泉，solanum herb，Herba Solanum Septemlobum）[1]

[Original Text]

[Shuyangquan （蜀羊泉, solanum herb, Herba Solanum Septemlobum）,] bitter in taste and slightly cold [in property], [is mainly used] to treat falvus of the scalp, severe sore, heat-Qi, scabies with itching, ringworm and caries. [It] grows in mountain valleys and river valleys.

[Textual Research]

[In the book entitled] *Ming Yi Bie Lu* （《名医别录》, *Special Record of Great Doctors*）, [it] says [that Shuyangquan （蜀羊泉, solanum herb, Herba Solanum Septemlobum) is also] called Yangquan （羊泉）and Yi （饴）, growing in Shujun （蜀郡）.

[In the book entitled] *Tang Ben* （《唐本》, *Cannon of Materia Medica in the Tang Dynasty*）, [it] says [that] Shuyangquan（蜀羊泉，solanum herb，Herba Solanum Septemlobum）[is also] called Qigu （漆姑）.

Notes

1. Shuyangquan （蜀羊泉, solanum herb, Herba Solanum Septemlobum）is a herbal medicinal, bitter in taste, slightly cold and non-toxic in property, entering the liver meridian and the lung meridian, effective in clearing heat and removing toxin. Clinically it is used to treat sore-throat, blurred vision, mastitis, mumps, scabies, ringworm, itching and caries.

60. 爵床

【原文】

味咸,寒。

主腰脊痛,不得着床,俯仰艰难,除热,可作浴汤。生川谷及田野。

【考据】

1.《吴普》曰:爵床,一名爵卿。(《御览》)

2.《名医》曰:生汉中。

3. 案别本注云:今人名为香苏。

60. Juechuang（爵床，creeping rostellularia herb，Herba Rostellulariae Procumbentis）[1]

[Original Text]

[Juechuang （爵床，creeping rostellularia herb，Herba Rostellulariae Procumbentis），] salty in taste and cold [in property]，[is mainly used] to treat pain of the waist and spine，inability to lie on bed and difficulty in raising and lowering [the head]，and to eliminate heat. [It] can be boiled for bathing. [It] grows in mountain valleys，river valleys and fields.

[Textual Research]

[In the book entitled] *Wu Pu Ben Cao* （《吴普本草》，*Wu Pu's Studies of Materia Medica*），[it] says [that] Juechuang（爵床，creeping rostellularia herb，Herba Rostellulariae Procumbentis）[is also] called Jueqing（爵卿）[according to the book entitled] *Tai Ping Yu Lan* （《太平御览》，*Imperial Studies in Taiping Times*）.

[In the book entitled] *Ming Yi Bie Lu* （《名医别录》，*Special Record of Great Doctors*），[it] says [that Juechuang（爵床，creeping rostellularia herb，Herba Rostellulariae Procumbentis）] grows in Hanzhong（汉中）.

People nowadays call it Xiangsu（香苏）.

【今译】

味咸,性寒。

主治腰脊部疼痛,不能躺床,抬头低头艰难,能消除热邪所致之病,可煎煮成洗浴用的汤剂。该物生长在山川河谷之中及田野。

Notes

1. Juechuang （爵 床，creeping rostellularia herb，Herba Rostellulariae Procumbentis） is a herbal medicinal，salty and pungent in taste，cold in property，entering the lung meridian，the liver meridian and the bladder meridian，effective in clearing heat and removing toxin，promoting urination and resolving swelling. Clinically it is used to treat common cold with fever，malaria，sorethroat，infantile malnutrition，enteritis，nephritis with edema，infection of urinary system，scabies，sores and traumatic injury.

61. 假苏

【原文】

味辛,温。

主寒热,鼠瘘,瘰疬,生疮,破结聚气,下瘀血,除湿痹,一名鼠蓂,生川泽。(旧在菜部,今移)

【考据】

1.《吴普》曰:假苏一名鼠实,一名姜芥也。(《御览》)名荆芥,叶似落藜而细,蜀中生啖之。(蜀本注)

2.《名医》曰:一名姜芥,生汉中。

3. 案陶宏景云:即荆芥也,姜荆声讹耳,先居草部中,令人食之,录在菜部中也。

【今译】

味辛,性温。

61. Jiasu（假苏，fineleaf schizonepeta herb，Herba Schizonepetae）[1]

[**Original Text**]

[Jiasu （ 假 苏， fineleaf schizonepeta herb， Herba Schizonepetae），] pungent in taste and warm [in property]，[is mainly used] to treat cold-heat [disease]，mouse scrofula[2] and ulcer [caused by] scrofula，to relieve blood stasis，and to eliminate dampness impediment. [It is also] called Shuming （鼠莫），growing in valleys and swamps.

[**Textual Research**]

[In the book entitled] *Wu Pu Ben Cao* （《吴普本草》，*Wu Pu's Studies of Materia Medica*)，[it] says [that] Jiasu （假苏，fineleaf schizonepeta herb，Herba Schizonepetae）[is also] called Shushi （鼠实）and Jiangjie （姜芥）. [According to the book entitled] *Tai Ping Yu Lan* （《太平御览》，*Imperial Studies in Taiping Times*)，[it is also] called Jingjie （荆芥）with thin leaves.

[In the book entitled] *Ming Yi Bie Lu* （《名医别录》，*Special Record of Great Doctors*)，[it] says [that Jiasu （假苏，fineleaf schizonepeta herb，Herba Schizonepetae）is also] called Jiangjie （姜芥），growing in Hanzhong （汉中）

739

　　主治寒热病，鼠瘘，瘰疬，长疮，能破除结聚邪气，能祛除瘀血，能治疗湿邪所致痹证，又称为鼠莫，该物生长在山川和平泽之中。

Notes

1. Jiasu （假 苏, fineleaf schizonepeta herb, Herba Schizonepetae) is a herbal medicinal, pungent in taste and warm in property, entering the lung meridian and the liver meridian, effective in relieving the superficies, expelling wind, ceasing bleeding and resolving sores. Clinically it is used to treat common cold with fever, headache, cough, sore-throat, measles, urticaria, hemoptysis, nosebleed, hematochezia, flooding and spotting (metrostaxis and metrorrhagia), and unconsciousness after delivery of baby.

62. 翘根

【原文】

味甘,寒平(《御览》作味苦平)。

主下热气,益阴精,令人面悦好,明目。久服轻身耐老。生平泽。

(旧在《唐本》退中,今移)

【考据】

1.《吴普》曰:翘根,神农雷公甘有毒,三月八月采,以作蒸,饮酒病人。(《御览》)

2.《名医》曰:生嵩高,二月八月采。

3. 案陶宏景云:方药不复用,俗无识者。

上草中品四十九种,旧四十六种,考菜部假苏,及《唐本》退中,翘根,宜入此。

62. Qiaogen（翘根，root of weeping forsythia，Radix Forsythiae）[1]

【Original Text】

［Qiaogen （翘根，root of weeping forsythia，Radix Forsythiae），］sweet in taste and cold and mild ［in property］，［is mainly used］ to relieve heat-Qi，to replenish Yin and essence，to luster the face and to improve vision. Long-term taking ［of it will］ relax the body and prevent aging. ［It］ grows in plains and swamps.

【Textual Research】

［In the book entitled］ *Wu Pu Ben Cao*（《吴普本草》，*Wu Pu's Studies of Materia Medica*），［it］ says ［that］ Qiaogen（翘根，root of weeping forsythia，Radix Forsythiae），［according to Agriculture God（神农）and Leigong（雷公），［is］ sweet ［in taste］ and toxic ［in property］. ［It can be］ collected in March and August and steamed. ［If taken with］ wine，［it will］ cause disease ［according to the book entitled］ *Tai Ping Yu Lan*（《太平御览》，*Imperial Studies in Taiping Times*）.

［In the book entitled］ *Ming Yi Bie Lu*（《名医别录》，*Special Record of Great Doctors*），［it］ says ［that Qiaogen（翘根，root of weeping forsythia，Radix Forsythiae）］ grows in Haogao（蒿高）and ［can be］ collected in February and August.

Tao Hongjing （陶宏景） said，"［It is］ no longer used in

【今译】

味甘,性寒平。

主治清热泻火,补益阴精,能使人面荣美好,能使眼睛明亮。长期
服用能使人身体轻盈,不易衰老。该物生长在平川水泽之中。

formulae, [and therefore] ordinary people do not know it."

Notes

1. Qiaogen (翘根, root of weeping forsythia, Radix Forsythiae) is a herbal medicinal, sweet in taste, cold, mild and slightly toxic in property, entering the stomach meridian and the lung meridian, effective in purging heat, reducing fire and replenishing Yin and essence. Clinically it is used to treat jaundice due to cold damage and stagnation of heat, scabies, sore and fever.

63. 桑根白皮

【原文】

味甘,寒。

主伤中,五劳六极,羸瘦,崩中,脉绝,补虚益气。

叶主除寒热出汗。

桑耳黑者,主女子漏下,赤白汁,血病,症瘕积聚,阴痛,阴阳寒热无子。

五木耳名檽,益气不饥,轻身强志。生山谷。

【考据】

1.《名医》曰:桑耳一名桑菌,一名木麦,生犍为,六月多雨时采,即暴干。

2. 案《说文》云:桑,蚕所食叶,木薆,木耳也。蕈,桑薆。《尔雅》云:桑瓣有葚栀。舍人云:桑树一半有葚,半无葚,名栀也。郭璞云:瓣,半也,又女桑,荑桑。郭璞云:今俗呼桑树小而条长者,为女桑树,又檿山桑。郭璞云:似桑材中作弓及车辕,又桑柳槐条。郭璞云:阿那垂条。

63. Sanggen Baipi（桑根白皮，bark of white mulberry，Cortex Mori）[1]

[Original Text]

[Sanggen Baipi（桑根白皮，bark of white mulberry，Cortex Mori），] sweet in taste and cold [in property]，[is mainly used] to treat damage of the middle（internal organs），five [kinds of] overstrain[2] and six [kinds of] extreme [syndrome/pattern]，weakness and emaciation，profuse vaginal bleeding and no pulsation，to improve deficiency and to replenish Qi.

[Its] leaves [are used to] treat cold-heat [disease] and induce sweating.

The black fungus on mulberry can treat vaginal bleeding with red and white fluid，blood disease，abdominal mass，genital pain，cold-heat [disease] in man and woman with sterility and infertility.

[There are] five [kinds of] wood fungus known as Ru（檽），[effective in] replenishing Qi，[making people feel] no hunger，relaxing the body and strengthening memory.

[It] grows in mountains and valleys.

[Textual Research]

[In the book entitled] *Ming Yi Bie Lu*（《名医别录》，*Special Record of Great Doctors*），[it] says [that Sanggen Baipi（桑根白皮，bark of white mulberry，Cortex Mori）is also] called Sang'er（桑

【今译】

味甘,性寒。

主治内脏损伤,五种劳症,六种极度损伤,能治疗身体瘦弱,妇女暴下经血,脉搏断绝,能补充虚弱,能补益精气。

桑叶,主治寒热病,令人发汗。

黑的桑木耳,主治女子阴道出血淋漓不断,赤白带下,血分病,症瘕积聚,阴部疼痛,能治疗男女寒热病及不孕症。

五种木耳,名为檽,能补益精气,能使人减少饥饿感,能使身体轻盈,能增强记忆力。该物生长在山谷之中。

耳）, Sangjun（桑菌）and Mumai（木麦）, growing in Jianwei（犍为）. [It can be] collected in June [when there is] excessive rain, and dried in the sun.

Notes

1. Sanggen Baipi（桑根白皮, bark of white mulberry, Cortex Mori）is a herbal medicinal, sweet in taste and cold in property, entering the lung meridian and the spleen meridian, effective in purging the lung, relieving panting, promoting urination and reducing blood pressure. Clinically it is used to treat lung heat with cough, edema, beriberi, dysuria, hypertension and jaundice.

2. Five kinds of overstrain refer to either seeing, walking, standing, sitting and sleeping for a long time, or damage of the heart, liver, spleen, lung and kidney, or damage of sinews, muscles, bones, Qi and blood.

3. Six kinds of extreme syndromes/patterns include extreme disorders of Qi, blood, sinews, bones, muscles and essence.

749

神农本草经

64. 竹叶

【原文】

味苦,平。

主咳逆上气溢筋急,恶疡,杀小虫。

根,作汤,益气止渴,补虚下气。

汁,主风痉。

实,通神明,轻身益气。

750

【考据】

《名医》曰:生益州。

案《说文》云:竹,冬生草也,象形,下垂者,箈,箬也。

【今译】

味苦,性平。

主治咳嗽及呼吸困难,能治疗筋脉拘急,恶性疮,能杀除小虫。

竹根,煎煮成汤剂,能补益精气,能止渴,能补充虚弱,能使气下行

64. Zhuye（竹叶，leaf of henon bamboo，Folium Phyllostachydis Henonis）[1]

[Original Text]

[Zhuye（竹叶，leaf of henon bamboo，Folium Phyllostachydis Henonis），] bitter in taste and mild [in property]，[is mainly used] to treat cough with dyspnea and upward counterflow of Qi，spasm of sinews and severe sores，and to kill small worms.

[Its] root [can be] decocted into decoction to replenish Qi，relieve thirst，tonify deficiency and descend Qi.

[Its] juice [can be used] to treat wind convulsion[2].

[Its] fruit [can be used] to invigorate the spirit and mentality，relax the body and replenish Qi.

751

[Textual Research]

[In the book entitled] *Ming Yi Bie Lu*（《名医别录》，*Special Record of Great Doctors*），[it] says [that Zhuye（竹叶，leaf of henon bamboo，Folium Phyllostachydis Henonis）] grows in Yizhou（益州）.

Notes

1. Zhuye（竹叶，leaf of henon bamboo，Folium Phyllostachydis Henonis）is a herbal medicinal，sweet and bland in taste，cold in property，entering the heart meridian and the stomach meridian，

以降逆。

竹沥汁，主治风邪所致抽搐。

竹子果实，能使神志清晰，精神旺盛，身体轻盈，能补益精气。

effective in clearing heat and relieving vexation, cooling the blood and stopping fright. Clinically it is used to treat heat disease with vexing thirst, oral ulcer, infantile epilepsy, heat stranguria and pain of the penis.

2. Wind convulsion here means stiffness of the neck, or wind stroke after delivery of baby, or convulsion before delivery of baby.

65. 吴茱萸（《御览》引：无吴字，是）

【原文】

味辛，温。

主温中，下气，止痛，咳逆，寒热，除湿血痹，逐风邪，开凑（旧作腠，《御览》作涛，是）理。

根杀三虫。一名藙。生山谷。

【考据】

1.《名医》曰：生冤句，九月九日采，阴干。

2. 案《说文》云：茱，茱萸，属，萸，茱萸也。煎茱萸，汉律，会稽献藙一斗。

3.《广雅》云：枕，榝，档，樧，茱萸也。三苍云：莍，茱萸也。（《御览》）《尔雅》云：椒、榝，丑莍.郭璞云：茱萸子，聚生成房貌，今江东亦呼榝，似茱萸而小，赤色。礼记云：三牲用藙。郑云：藙煎茱萸也。汉律会稽献焉，《尔雅》谓之榝.《范子计然》云：茱萸，出三辅。陶宏景云：礼记名藙而作俗中呼为藙子，当是不识藙字似杂字，仍以相传。

65. Wuzhuyu（吴茱萸，evodia，Fructus Evodiae）[1]

[Original Text]

[Wuzhuyu（吴茱萸，evodia，Fructus Evodiae），] pungent in taste and warm [in property], [is mainly used] to warm the middle (internal organs), to descend Qi, cease pain, to treat cough with dyspnea and cold-heat [disease], to eliminate dampness and blood impediment, to expel wind-evil and to open the grain of skin.

[Its] root can kill three worms. [It is also] called Yi（藙），growing in mountains and valleys.

[Textual Research]

[In the book entitled] *Ming Yi Bie Lu*（《名医别录》，*Special Record of Great Doctors*），[it] says [that Wuzhuyu（吴茱萸，evodia，Fructus Evodiae）] grows in Yuanju（冤句）. [It can be] collected on September 9 and dried in the shade.

Notes

1. Wuzhuyu（吴茱萸，evodia，Fructus Evodiae）is a herbal medicinal, pungent and bitter in taste, warm and slightly toxic in property, entering the liver meridian, the stomach meridian, the spleen meridian and the kidney meridian, effective in warming the middle (the internal organs) and stopping pain, preventing counterflow and ceasing vomiting. Clinically it is used to treat cold

【今译】

味辛，性温。

能温煦人体脏器，能使气下行以降逆，能治疗疼痛，咳嗽，气逆，寒热病，能消除湿气，能治疗血虚所致痹证，能祛除风邪，能通开腠理。

吴茱萸的根能杀死三种寄生虫。又称为藙。该物生长在山谷之中。

pain in the abdomen and gastric region, abdominal pain due to hernia, beriberi with swelling and pain, vomiting and dyspnea, indigestion and diarrhea.

66. 卮子（旧作栀，艺文类聚及《御览》引，作支，是）

【原文】

味苦,寒。

主五内邪气,胃中热气面赤,酒炮皶鼻,白赖,赤癞,疮疡。一名木丹。生川谷。

【考据】

1.《名医》曰:一名樾桃,生南阳,九月采实,暴干。

2. 案《说文》云:栀,黄木可染者。《广雅》云:栀子,楮桃也。《史记·货殖传》云:巴蜀地饶卮。集解云:徐广曰音支,烟支也。紫,赤色也,据《说文》当为栀。

【今译】

味苦,性寒。

主治邪伤五脏,胃中热邪所致面赤,酒皶鼻,白皮病,赤皮病,疮疡。又称为木丹。该物生长在山川河谷之中。

66. Zhizi（卮子，fruit of cape jasmine，
Fructus Gardeniae） [1]

［Original Text］

［Zhizi（卮子，fruit of cape jasmine，Fructus Gardeniae），］bitter in taste and cold ［in property］，［is mainly used］ to treat ［disease in］ the five Zang-organs ［caused by］ evil-Qi，severe heat in the stomach with red face，rosacea，white leprosy and ulcer ［caused by］ injury. ［It is also］ called Mudan（木丹），growing in mountain valleys and river valleys.

［Textual Research］

［In the book entitled］ *Ming Yi Bie Lu*（《名医别录》，*Special Record of Great Doctors*），［it］ says ［that Zhizi（卮子，fruit of cape jasmine，Fructus Gardeniae）is also］ called Yuetao（樾桃），growing in Nanyang（南阳）. ［Its］ fruit ［can be］ collected in September and dried in the sun.

Notes

1. Zhizi（卮子，fruit of cape jasmine，Fructus Gardeniae），now called Zhizi（栀子），also called Shanzhizi（山栀子）and Shanzhi（山枝），is a herbal medicinal，bitter in taste and cold in property，entering the liver meridian，the heart meridian，the lung meridian，the stomach meridian and the triple energizer meridian，effective in purging fire and eliminating vexation，clearing heat and relieving dampness，cooling the blood and removing toxin，resolving swelling and stopping pain. Clinically it is used to treat heat disease with vexation and depression，jaundice due to heat-dampness，unconsciousness with delirium，hypertension，hematemesis and nosebleed.

67. 芜荑

【原文】

味辛,平。

主五内邪气,散皮肤,骨节中淫淫温行毒,去三虫,化食。一名无姑,一名殿塘(《御览》引云:逐寸白,散腄中,温温喘息,《大观本》作黑字)。生川谷。

【考据】

1. 《名医》曰:一名殿塘,生晋山,三月采实,阴干。

2. 案《说文》云:梗,山枌榆,有束荑可为芜荑者。《广雅》云:山榆,母估也。

3. 《尔雅》云:莁荑蔱蘠。郭璞云:一名白蒉,又无姑,其实夷。郭璞云:无姑,姑榆也。生山中,叶圆而厚,剥取皮合渍之,其味辛香,所谓芜荑。《范子计然》云:芜荑在地,赤心者善。

【今译】

味辛,性平。

67. Wuyi（芜荑，great elm seed，Semen Ulmus Macrocarpa）^[1]

[Original Text]

[Wuyi（芜荑，great elm seed，Semen Ulmus Macrocarpa），] pungent in taste and mild [in property], [is mainly used] to treat [disease in] the five Zang-organs [caused by] evil-Qi, to disperse [retention of pathogenic factors in] the skin, to move [pathogenic wind and] febrile and toxic [elements] in the joints, to expel three worms and to digest food. [It is also] called Wugu（无姑）and Diantang（殿塘），growing in mountains and valleys.

[Textual Research]

[In the book entitled] *Ming Yi Bie Lu*（《名医别录》，*Special Record of Great Doctors*），[it] says [that Wuyi（芜荑，great elm seed，Semen Ulmus Macrocarpa) is also] called Diantang（殿塘） and grows in Jinshan（晋山）. [Its] fruit [can be] collected in March and dried in the shade.

Guo Pu（郭璞）said，"[Wuyi（芜荑，great elm seed，Semen Ulmus Macrocarpa) is also called] Wugu（无姑）and Guyu（姑榆）. [It] grows in mountains with round and thick leaves. [When] the bark is peeled，[it] smells fragrant and pungent. That is why it is called Wuyi（芜荑）."

[In the book entitled] *Fan Zi Ji Ran*（《范子计然》，*Studies*

主治邪伤五脏，能消散积聚在皮肤和骨节中的邪气和温热毒气，能祛除三种虫子，能消化食物。又称为无姑，又称为殿塘。该物生长在山川河谷之中。

About Fan Li's Teacher), [it] says [that] Wuyi (芜荑, great elm seed, Semen Ulmus Macrocarpa) grows in the soil. The red kernel is more effective.

Notes

1. Wuyi (芜荑, great elm seed, Semen Ulmus Macrocarpa) is a herbal medicinal, pungent and bitter in taste, mild in property, entering the lung meridian and the stomach meridian, effective in killing worms and promoting digestion. Clinically it is used to treat infantile malnutrition, ascaridiasis and oxyuriasis.

神农本草经

68. 枳实

【原文】

味苦,寒。

主大风在皮肤中,如麻豆苦痒(《御览》作痰,非),除寒热结,止利(旧作痢,《御览》作利,是),长肌肉,利五脏,益气轻身。生川泽。

【考据】

1.《吴普》曰:枳实苦,雷公酸无毒,李氏大寒,九月十月采,阴干。(《御览》)

2.《名医》曰:生河内,九月十月采,阴干。

3. 案《说文》云:枳木似橘。《周礼》云:橘逾淮而化为枳。沈括《补笔谈》云:六朝以前,医方,唯有枳实,无枳壳,后人用枳之小嫩者为枳实,大者为枳壳。

【今译】

味苦,性寒。

68. Zhishi（枳实，processed unripe bitter orange，Fructus Aurantii Immaturus）[1]

〔Original Text〕

〔Zhishi（枳实，processed unripe bitter orange，Fructus Aurantii Immaturus），〕bitter in taste and cold〔in property〕，〔is mainly used〕to treat〔disease marked by〕pain and itching〔caused by invasion of〕severe wind into the skin like sesame and soybean〔in the skin〕，to eliminate retention of cold and heat，to cease dysentery，to promote〔growth of〕muscles，to harmonize the five Zang-organs，to replenish Qi and to relax the body. 〔It〕grows in valleys and swamps.

〔Textual Research〕

〔In the book entitled〕*Wu Pu Ben Cao*（《吴普本草》，*Wu Pu's Studies of Materia Medica*），〔it〕says〔that〕Zhishi（枳实，processed unripe bitter orange，Fructus Aurantii Immaturus）〔is〕bitter〔in taste〕；〔according to〕Leigong（雷公），〔it is〕sour〔in taste〕and non-toxic〔in property〕；〔according to〕Li's（李氏），〔it is〕severely cold〔in property〕. 〔It can be〕collected in September and October，and dried in the shade〔according to the book entitled〕*Tai Ping Yu Lan*（《太平御览》，*Imperial Studies in Taiping Times*）.

〔In the book entitled〕*Ming Yi Bie Lu*（《名医别录》，*Special Record of Great Doctors*），〔it〕says〔that Zhishi（枳实，processed unripe bitter orange，Fructus Aurantii Immaturus）〕grows in Henei

主治皮肤中的重风之邪，身体上有如芝麻大豆般的疥疮，极为瘙痒，能清除寒热气聚结，能停止泄泻痢疾，能增长肌肉，能调理五脏，能补益精气，能使人身体轻盈。该物生长在山川和平泽之中。

（河内）. [It can be] collected in September and October, and dried in the shade.

[In] case [analysis in the book entitled] *Shuo Wen* (《说文》, *On Culture*), [it] says [that] Zhishi（枳实, processed unripe bitter orange, Fructus Aurantii Immaturus）looks like tangerine. [In the book entitled] *Zhou Li* (《周礼》, *Canon of Rites*), [it says that when] tangerine is planted far away from Huai（淮）region, [it] changes into Zhishi（枳实, processed unripe bitter orange, Fructus Aurantii Immaturus）.

Shen Kuo（沈括）said, "Before the Six Dynasties (222 AD – 589 AD), there was only Zhishi（枳实, processed unripe bitter orange, Fructus Aurantii Immaturus）in the formulae, no Zhike（枳壳 bitter orange, Fructus Aurantii）. Later on, the small and tender one is regarded as Zhishi（枳实, processed unripe bitter orange, Fructus Aurantii Immaturus）[while] the large one is regarded as Zhike（枳壳 bitter orange, Fructus Aurantii）."

Notes

1. Zhishi（枳实, processed unripe bitter orange, Fructus Aurantii Immaturus）is a herbal medicinal, bitter in taste, slightly cold in property, entering the spleen meridian and the stomach meridian, effective in breaking Qi, expelling phlegm and resolving accumulation. Clinically it is used to treat lumps, fullness, distension and pain of the abdomen and chest, retention of phlegm, indigestion, constipation, heaviness of the stomach, prolapse of uterus and anus.

69. 厚朴

【原文】

味苦,温。

主中风,伤寒,头痛,寒热,惊悸,气血痹,死肌,去三虫。

【考据】

1.《吴普》曰:厚朴,神农岐伯雷公苦无毒,李氏小温。(《御览》引云,一名厚皮,生交址)

2.《名医》曰:一名厚皮,一名赤朴,其树名榛,其子名逐,生交址冤句,九月十月采皮。阴干。

3. 案《说文》云:朴,木皮也,榛木也。《广雅》云:重皮,厚朴也。《范子计然》云:厚朴出宏农,按今俗以榛为亲,不知是厚朴,《说文》榛栗,字作亲。

69. Houpu（厚朴，magnolia bark，Cortex Magnoliae Officinalis）[1]

［Original Text］

［Houpu（厚朴，magnolia bark，Cortex Magnoliae Officinalis），］bitter in taste and warm ［in property］, ［is mainly used］ to treat wind stroke，cold damage，headache，cold-heat ［disease］，fright，palpitation，Qi and blood impediment and necrotic muscles，and to eliminate three worms.

［Textual Research］

［In the book entitled］ *Wu Pu Ben Cao* （《吴普本草》，*Wu Pu's Studies of Materia Medica*），［it］ says ［that］ Houpu（厚朴，magnolia bark，Cortex Magnoliae Officinalis），［according to］ Agriculture God（神农），Qibo（岐伯）and Leigong（雷公），［is］ bitter ［in taste］ and non-toxic ［in property］; ［according to］ Li's（李氏），［it is］ slightly warm ［in property］.

［In the book entitled］ *Ming Yi Bie Lu* （《名医别录》，*Special Record of Great Doctors*），［it］ says ［that Houpu （厚朴，magnolia bark，Cortex Magnoliae Officinalis） is also］ called Houpi（厚皮）and Chipu（赤朴）. Its tree is called Qin（榛）and its seed is called Zhu（逐）. ［It］ grows in Jiaozhi（交址）and Yuanju（冤句）. ［Its］ bark ［can be］ collected in September and October，and dried in the shade.

【今译】

味苦,性温。

主治中风,伤寒,头痛,寒热病,惊恐,心悸,气血痹阻,肌肉坏死,能祛除三种虫子。

［In］case［analysis in the book entitled］ *Shuo Wen* （《说文》， *On Culture*），［it］says［that］its bark is called Pu（朴）and its wood is called Qin（榛）.［In the book entitled］ *Guang Ya* （《广雅》，*The First Chinese Encyclopedic Dictionary*），［it］says［that］the thick bark is called Houpu（厚朴，magnolia bark，Cortex Magnoliae Officinalis）.［In the book entitled］ *Fan Zi Ji Ran* （《范子计然》， *Studies About Fan Li's Teacher*），［it］says［that］Houpu（厚朴， magnolia bark，Cortex Magnoliae Officinalis）is produced in Hongnong（宏农）. Now people only care about Qin（榛）and are unclear about Houpu（厚朴，magnolia bark，Cortex Magnoliae Officinalis）.

Notes

1. Houpu（厚朴，magnolia bark，Cortex Magnoliae Officinalis） is a herbal medicinal，bitter and pungent in taste，warm in property，entering the spleen meridian，the stomach meridian and the large intestine meridian，effective in warming the middle（the internal organs）and descending Qi，drying dampness and resolving phlegm. Clinically it is used to treat lumps，fullness，distension and pain of the chest and abdomen，vomiting，diarrhea，dysentery， indigestion，cough and panting with retention of phlegm.

70. 秦皮

【原文】

味苦,微寒。

主风寒湿痹,洗洗寒气,除热,目中青翳,白膜。久服,头不白,轻身。生川谷。

【考据】

1.《吴普》曰:岑皮,一名秦皮,神农雷公黄帝岐伯酸无毒,李氏小寒,或生冤句水边,二月八日采。(《御览》)

2.《名医》曰:一名岑皮,一名石檀,生庐江及冤句,二月八月采皮,阴干。

3. 案《说文》云:梣、青皮木,或作檔。《淮南子》俶真训云:梣木,色青翳。高诱云:梣木,苦历木也,生于山,剥取其皮,以水浸之,正青,用洗眼,愈人目中肤翳。据《吴普》云:岑皮,名秦皮,本经作秦皮者,后人以俗称改之,当为岑皮。

70. Qinpi（秦皮，ash，Cortex Fraxini）[1]

[Original Text]

[Qinpi（秦皮，ash，Cortex Fraxini），] bitter in taste and slightly cold [in property], [is mainly used] to treat wind-cold and dampness impediment with chilliness and shivering [due to] cold-Qi, to eliminate heat, and to relieve nebula and albuginea in the eyes. Long-term taking [of it will] prevent white hair and relax the body. [It] grows in mountain valleys and river valleys.

[Textual Research]

[In the book entitled] *Wu Pu Ben Cao*（《吴普本草》，*Wu Pu's Studies of Materia Medica*）, [it] says [that] Qinpi（秦皮，ash，Cortex Fraxini）[is also] called Qinpi（岑皮）. [According to] Agriculture God（神农）, Leigong（雷公）, Yellow Emperor（黄帝）and Qibo（岐伯）, [it is] sour [in taste] and non-toxic [in property]; [according to] Li's（李氏）, [it is] slightly cold [in property]. [It] may grow beside water in Yuanju（冤句）and [can be] collected on February 8th [according to the book entitled] *Tai Ping Yu Lan*（《太平御览》，*Imperial Studies in Taiping Times*）.

[In the book entitled] *Ming Yi Bie Lu*（《名医别录》，*Special Record of Great Doctors*）, [it] says [that Qinpi（秦皮，ash，Cortex Fraxini）is also] called Qinpi（岑皮）and Shitan（石檀）, growing in Lujiang（庐江）and Yuanju（冤句）. [Its] bark [can be] collected in

【今译】

味苦,性微寒。

主治风寒湿邪所致痹证,身体瑟瑟发抖,能消除热邪以及眼睛中的青翳和白膜。长期服用,能使人头发不变白,身体轻盈。该物生长在山川河谷之中。

February and August, and dried in the shade.

Gao You (高诱) said, "Qinpi (秦皮, ash, Cortex Fraxini) is a bitter wood. [It] grows in mountains. Its bark can be peeled and soaked in water to wash the eyes in order to relieve nebula."

Notes

1. Qinpi (秦皮, ash, Cortex Fraxini) is a herbal medicinal, bitter in taste, astringent and cold in property, entering the large intestine meridian, the liver meridian and the gallbladder meridian, effective in clearing heat and drying dampness, stopping cough and expelling phlegm, cooling the liver and improving vision. Clinically it is used to treat bacterial dysentery, enteritis, leucorrhea, chronic bronchitis, redness and pain of eyes and psoriasis.

71. 秦菽

【原文】

味辛,温。

主风邪气,温中,除寒痹,坚齿发,明目。久服,轻身,好颜色,耐老增年,通神。生川谷。

【考据】

1.《名医》曰:生太山及秦岭上,或琅邪,八月九月采实。

2. 案《说文》云:菽,菽萸.莍菽橵实菉裹如裘者,橵似茱萸,出淮南。《广雅》云:橵朹,茱萸也。北山经云:景山多秦椒。郭璞云,子似椒面细叶草也。

3.《尔雅》云:橵,大椒。郭璞云:今椒树丛生实大者,名为橵,又椒橵丑莍.郭璞云:裹萸子聚成房貌,今江东亦呼莍橵,似茱萸而小,赤色。《毛诗》云:椒聊之实。《传》云:椒卿,椒也。陆玑云:椒树似茱萸,有针刺,叶坚而滑泽,蜀人作茶,吴人作茗,皆合煮其叶以为香。《范子计然》云:秦椒出天水陇西,细者善。《淮南子》人间训云:申椒杜茝,美人之所怀服,旧作椒,非,据《山海经》,有秦椒,生闻喜景山,则秦非秦地之

71. Qinjiao（秦菽，Qin pepper，Qin Xanthoxylum Piperitum）[1]

［Original Text］

［Qinjiao（秦菽，Qin pepper，Qin Xanthoxylum Piperitum），］pungent in taste and warm［in property］，［is mainly used］to treat［disease caused by pathogenic］wind and evil-Qi，to warm the middle（the internal organs），to eliminate cold impediment，to strengthen teeth and hair，and to improve vision. Long-term taking［of it will］relax the body，luster the facial expression，prevent aging，prolong life and invigorate spirit.［It］grows in mountain valleys and river valleys.

［Textual Research］

［In the book entitled］*Ming Yi Bie Lu*（《名医别录》，*Special Record of Great Doctors*），［it］says［that Qinjiao（秦菽，Qin pepper，Qin Xanthoxylum Piperitum）］grows in Taishan（太山）and Qinling（秦岭）or Langxie（琅邪）.［Its］fruit［can be］collected in August and September.

［In the book entitled］*Fan Zi Ji Ran*（《范子计然》，*Studies About Fan Li's Teacher*），［it］says［that］Qinjiao（秦菽，Qin pepper，Qin Xanthoxylum Piperitum）is produced in Longxi（陇西）in Tianshui（天水）. The thin one is better.［In the book entitled］*Shan Hai Jing*（《山海经》，*Canon of Mountains and Seas*），［it］says

秦也。

【今译】

味辛,性温。

主治风邪所致之症,能温煦人体脏器,能消除寒痹证,能使牙齿和头发坚固,能使眼睛明亮。长期服用,能使身体轻盈,面部色彩美丽,能使人不易衰老,能延长寿命,能通畅神气。该物生长在山川河谷之中。

[that] Qinjiao（秦菽，Qin pepper，Qin Xanthoxylum Piperitum）actually grows in Jingshan（景山），not in [the State named] Qin（秦）.

Notes

1. Qinjiao（秦菽，Qin pepper，Qin Xanthoxylum Piperitum）is a herbal medicinal，effective in tonifying the kidney and warming Yang，expelling wind and harmonizing the blood，strengthening the teeth and improving vision. Clinically it is used to treat throat impediment，hernia，abdominal mass，abdominal pain after delivery of baby，sweating，cough，wind-dampness impediment，numbness of the limbs，amenorrhea，chronic dysentery and oral dropsy.

72. 山茱萸

【原文】

味酸,平。

主心下邪气,寒热,温中,逐寒湿痹,去三虫。久服轻身。一名蜀
枣。生山谷。

【考据】

1.《吴普》曰,山茱萸,一名魃实,一名鼠矢,一名鸡足,神农黄帝
雷公扁鹊酸无毒,岐伯辛,一经酸,或生冤句琅邪,或东海承县,叶
如梅,有刺毛,二月,华如杏四月实如酸枣,赤,五月采实。(《御
览》)

2.《名医》曰,一名鸡足,一名魃实,生汉中及琅邪冤句,东海承县,
九月十月采实,阴干。

【今译】

味酸,性平。

72. Shanzhuyu（山茱萸，cornus，Fructus Corni） [1]

[Original Text]

[Shanzhuyu（山茱萸，cornus，Fructus Corni），] sour in taste and mild [in property]，[is mainly used] to treat [disease caused by] evil-Qi in the region below the heart and cold-heart [disease]，to warm the middle（the internal organs），to eliminate cold-dampness impediment and to kill three worms. Long-term taking [of it will] relax the body. [It is also] called Shuzao（蜀枣），growing in mountains and valleys.

[Textual Research]

[In the book entitled] *Wu Pu Ben Cao*（《吴普本草》，*Wu Pu's Studies of Materia Medica*），[it] says [that] Shanzhuyu（山茱萸，cornus，Fructus Corni）[is also] called Jishi（魃实），Shuishi（鼠矢）and Jizu（鸡足）. [According to] Agriculture God（神农），Yellow Emperor（黄帝），Leigong（雷公）and Bianque（扁鹊），[it is] sour [in taste] and non-toxic [in property]；[according to] Qibo（岐伯），[it is] pungent [in taste]. [It may be] sour [in taste] in some literature. [It] may grow in Yuanju（冤句），Langxie（琅邪）or Chengxian（承县）in Donghai（东海，East Sea）. [Its] leaf is like [that of] plum with bristle. [In] February，[it] blossoms like [the flower of] apricot；[in] April，[it] bears fruit like red spiny jujube；[in] May，[its] fruit [can be] collected [according to the book

Agriculture
God's Canon of
Materia Medica

主治消除心下邪气，能治疗寒热病，能温煦人体脏器，能消除寒湿邪所致痹证，能祛除三种虫子。长期服用，能使人身体轻盈。又称为蜀枣。该物生长在山谷之中。

entitled] *Tai Ping Yu Lan* (《太平御览》, *Imperial Studies in Taiping Times*).

[In the book entitled] *Ming Yi Bie Lu* (《名医别录》, *Special Record of Great Doctors*), [it] says [that Shanzhuyu (山茱萸, cornus, Fructus Corni) is also] called Jizu (鸡足) and Jishi (魃实), growing in Hanzhong (汉中), Liangxie (琅邪), Yuanju (宛句) and Chengxian (承县) in Donghai (东海, East Sea). [Its] fruit [can be] collected in September and October, and dried in the shade.

Notes

1. Shanzhuyu (山茱萸, cornus, Fructus Corni) is a herbal medicinal, sour in taste, slightly warm in property, entering the liver meridian and the kidney meridian, effective in tonifying and replenishing the liver and kidney, enriching essence and inducing sweating. Clinically it is used to treat vertigo, tinnitus, ache and flaccidity of the waist and knees, seminal emission, frequent urination and frequent sweating.

73. 紫葳

【原文】

味酸,(《御览》作咸)微寒。

主妇人产乳余疾,崩中,症瘕,血闭,寒热,羸瘦,养胎。生川谷。

【考据】

1.《吴普》曰,紫葳一名武威,一名瞿麦,一名陵居腹,一名鬼目,一名茏华,神农雷公酸,岐伯辛,扁鹊苦咸,黄帝甘无毒,如麦根黑,正月八月采,或生真定(《御览》)。

2.《名医》曰,一名陵苕,一名茏华,生西海及山阳。

3. 案《广雅》云:茈葳,陵苕,蘧麦也。《尔雅》云:苕。陵苕,郭璞云:一名陵时。本草云:又黄华蒵,白华茏。郭璞云:苕、华、色异,名亦不同。《毛诗》云:苕之华。《传》云:苕,陵苕也。《范子计然》云:紫葳出三辅。李当之云:是瞿麦根据李说与《广雅》合,而《唐本》注引《尔雅》注,有一名陵霄四字,谓即陵霄花,陆玑以为鼠尾,疑皆非,故不采之。

73. Ziwei（紫葳, root of Chinese trumpetcreeper, Radix Campsis Grandiflorae）[1]

[Original Text]

[Ziwei（紫葳, root of Chinese trumpetcreeper, Radix Campsis Grandiflorae）,] sour taste and slightly cold [in property], [is mainly used] to treat remnant disease after delivery of baby, sudden uterine bleeding, abdominal mass, amenorrhea, cold-heat [disease], weakness and emaciation, and to cultivate fetus. [It] grows in mountain valleys and river valleys.

[Textual Research]

[In the book entitled] *Wu Pu Ben Cao* (《吴普本草》, *Wu Pu's Studies of Materia Medica*), [it] says [that] Ziwei（紫葳, root of Chinese trumpetcreeper, Radix Campsis Grandiflorae）[is also] called Wuwei（武威）, Qumai（瞿麦）, Lingjufu（陵居腹）, Guimu（鬼目）and Longhua（茏华）. [According to] Agriculture God（神农）and Leigong（雷公）, [it is] sour [in taste]; [according to] Qibo（岐伯）, [it is] pungent [in taste]; [according to] Bianque（扁鹊）, [it is] bitter and salty [in taste]; [according to] Yellow Emperor（黄帝）, [it is] sweet [in taste] and non-toxic [in property]. [It looks] like the black root of wheat. [It can be] collected in January and August. [It] may grow in Zhending（真定）[according to the book entitled] *Tai Ping Yu Lan* (《太平御览》, *Imperial Studies in*

【今译】

味酸,微寒。

主治女子生育后瘀血疼痛,子宫突然出血,症瘕,经闭,寒热病,能治疗身体瘦弱,能养胎保胎。该物生长在山川河谷之中。

Taiping Times).

［In the book entitled］*Ming Yi Bie Lu*（《名医别录》, *Special Record of Great Doctors*), ［it］ says ［that Ziwei（紫葳, root of Chinese trumpetcreeper, Radix Campsis Grandiflorae) is also］ called Lingzhao（陵苕) and Longhua（茏华), growing in Xihai（西海, West Sea) and Shanyang（山阳).

Notes

1. Ziwei（紫葳, root of Chinese trumpetcreeper, Radix Campsis Grandiflorae) is a herbal medicinal, pungent and sour in taste, cold in property, entering the liver meridian and the pericardium meridian, effective in breaking blood stasis, expelling wind and cooling the blood. Clinically it is used to treat amenorrhea due to blood stasis, dysmenorhea, abdominal mass, blood heat, scabies with itching, eczema and ulcer.

74. 猪苓

【原文】

味甘,平。

主痎疟,解毒,蛊注(《御览》作蛀)不祥,利水道。久服轻身耐老。(《御览》作能老)一名豭猪尿。生山谷。

【考据】

1.《吴普》曰:猪苓,神农甘,雷公苦无毒。(《御览》引云,如茯苓,或生冤句,八月采。)

2.《名医》曰:生衡山及济阴冤句,二月八月采,阴干。

3. 案庄子云:豕零,司马彪注,作豕橐云,一名猪苓,根似猪卵,可以治渴。

【今译】

味甘,性平。

74. Zhuling（猪苓，polyporus，Polyporus Umbellatus）[1]

[Original Text]

[Zhuling（猪苓，polyporus，Polyporus Umbellatus），] sweet in taste and mild [in property], [is mainly used] to treat malaria, to relieve worm toxin and manifestations [that are] not auspicious, and to disinhibit waterway [in the body]. Long-term taking [of it will] relax the body and prevent aging. [It is also] called Jiazhushi（豭猪尿），growing in mountains and valleys.

[Textual Research]

[In the book entitled] *Wu Pu Ben Cao*（《吴普本草》，*Wu Pu's Studies of Materia Medica*），[it] says [that] Zhuling（猪苓，polyporus，Polyporus Umbellatus），[according to] Agriculture God（神农），[is] sweet [in taste]；[according to] Leigong（雷公），[is] bitter [in taste] and non-toxic [in property]. [In the book entitled] *Tai Ping Yu Lan*（《太平御览》，*Imperial Studies in Taiping Times*），[it] says [that] Zhuling（猪苓，polyporus，Polyporus Umbellatus）may grow in Yuanju（冤句）and [can be] collected in August.

[In the book entitled] *Ming Yi Bie Lu*（《名医别录》，*Special Record of Great Doctors*），[it] says [that Zhuling（猪苓，polyporus，Polyporus Umbellatus）] grows in Hengshan（衡山），Jiyin（济阴）and Yuanju（冤句）. [It can be] collected in February and August，

主治疟疾，能解毒，能治疗虫毒所致的不祥病症，能通利水道。长期服用能使人身体轻盈，不易衰老。又称为豭猪屎。该物生长在山谷之中。

and dried in the shade.

Notes

1. Zhuling (猪苓, polyporus, Polyporus Umbellatus) is a herbal medicinal, sweet and bland in taste, mild in property, entering the spleen meridian, the kidney meridian and the bladder meridian, effective in promoting urination and relieving dampness. Clinically it is used to treat dysuria, edema with distension and fullness, diarrhea, stranguria and leucorrhea.

75. 白棘

【原文】

味辛,寒。

主心腹痛,痈肿溃脓,止痛。一名棘针。生川谷。

【考据】

1.《名医》曰:一名棘刺,生雍州。

2. 案《说文》云:棘,小枣丛生者。《尔雅》云:髦颠棘。孙炎云:一名白棘。李当之云:此是酸枣树针,今人用天门冬苗代之,非是真也。案经云:天门冬一名颠勒,勒棘声相近,则今人用此,亦非无因也。

【今译】

味辛,性寒。

主治心腹部疼痛,痈肿,溃破流脓,能消除疼痛。又称为棘针。该物生长在山川河谷之中。

75. Baiji（白棘，spine of common jujube，Spina Jujubae）[1]

[Original Text]

［Baiji（白棘，spine of common jujube，Spina Jujubae），］pungent in taste and cold [in property]，［is mainly used］to treat abdominal pain and abscess with ulcer and pus，and to cease pain. ［It is also］called Jizhen（棘针），growing in mountain valleys and river valleys.

[Textual Research]

［In the book entitled］*Ming Yi Bie Lu*（《名医别录》，*Special Record of Great Doctors*），［it］says［that Baiji（白棘，spine of common jujube，Spina Jujubae）is also］called Jici（棘刺），growing in Yongzhou（雍州）.

［In］case［analysis in the book entitled］*Shuo Wen*（《说文》，*On Culture*），［it］says［that］Ji（棘）refers to the twigs［which］bear wild jujubes.

Notes

1. Baiji（白棘，spine of common jujube，Spina Jujubae）is a herbal medicinal，pungent in taste and cold in property，effective in resolving swelling，dispersing pus and stopping pain. Clinically it is used to treat abscess with pus，abdominal pain，lumbago，throat impediment，hypertension，coronary disease，angina and hematuria.

76. 龙眼

【原文】

味甘,平。

主五脏邪气,安志厌食。久服,强魂聪明,轻身,不老,通神明。一名益智。生山谷。

【考据】

1.《吴普》曰:龙眼一名益智,要术一名比目。(《御览》)

2.《名医》曰:其大者似槟榔,生南海松树上,五月采,阴干。

3. 案《广雅》云:益智,龙眼也。刘达注吴都赋云:龙眼,如荔枝而小,圆如弹丸,味甘,胜荔枝,苍梧,交址,南海,合浦皆献之,山中人家亦种之。

【今译】

味甘,性平。

76. Longyan（龙眼，longan aril，Arillus Longan）[1]

［Original Text］

［Longyan（龙眼，longan aril，Arillus Longan），］sweet in taste ［and］mild［in property］，［is mainly used］to treat［disease in］the five Zang-organs［caused by］evil-Qi，to balance mentality and to relieve anorexia. Long-term taking［of it will］strengthen the ethereal soul，improve hearing and vision，relax the body，prevent aging and invigorate spirit and mentality.［It is also］called Yizhi（益智），growing in mountains and valleys.

［Textual Research］

［In the book entitled］*Wu Pu Ben Cao*（《吴普本草》，*Wu Pu's Studies of Materia Medica*），［it］says［that］Longyan（龙眼，longan aril，Arillus Longan）［is also］called Yizhi（益智）and Bimu（比目）［according to the book entitled］*Tai Ping Yu Lan*（《太平御览》，*Imperial Studies in Taiping Times*）》.

［In the book entitled］*Ming Yi Bie Lu*（《名医别录》，*Special Record of Great Doctors*），［it］says［that］the big［Longyan（龙眼，longan aril，Arillus Longan）］is like areca，growing on the pine tree in Nanhai（南海，Southern Sea）.［It can be］collected in May and dried in the shade.

［In the book entitled］*Guang Ya*（《广雅》，*The First Chinese Encyclopedic Dictionary*），［it］says［that the so-called］Yizhi（益智）

主治五脏中的邪气,能使心智安定,能治疗厌食症。长期服用,能强壮魂魄,能使听力清晰,目光明亮,能使人身体轻盈,长寿不老,能使神志清晰,精神旺盛。又称为益智。该物生长在山谷之中。

refers to Longyan（龙眼，longan aril，Arillus Longan）.［In］ explaining the *Prose about Wudu*（吴都），Liu Da（刘达）said，"Longyan（龙眼，longan aril，Arillus Longan）is like litchi，but smaller［than it］and round like pill，sweet［in taste］，better than litchi.［It can be］found in Cangwu（苍梧），Jiaozhi（交址），Nanhai（南海，Southern Sea）and Hepu（合浦）. People living in mountains also plant it."

Notes

1. Longyan（龙眼，longan aril，Arillus Longan）is a herbal medicinal，sweet in taste and warm in property，entering the heart meridian and the spleen meridian，effective in tonifying the heart and pacifying the spirit，nourishing the blood and replenishing the spleen. Clinically it is used to treat amnesia，insomnia，palpitation，insufficiency of Qi and blood，and weakness of the body.

77. 松罗

【原文】

味苦,平。

主瞋怒邪气,止虚汗头风,女子阴寒肿病。一名女萝。生山谷。

【考据】

1.《名医》曰:生熊耳山。

2. 案《广雅》云:女萝松萝也。《毛诗》云:茑与女萝。《传》云:女萝
菟丝,松萝也。

3. 陆玑云:松萝自蔓松上,枝正青,与兔丝异。

【今译】

味苦,性平。

主治极度愤怒,能消除邪气,能止虚汗,能治疗头风,女子阴冷肿
病。又称为女萝。该物生长在山谷之中。

77．Songluo（松罗，long usnea filament，Filum Usneae）[1]

[Original Text]

[Songluo（松罗，long usnea filament，Filum Usneae），] bitter in taste and mild [in property], [is mainly used] to treat dosa [caused by] evil-Qi，cease deficiency-sweating and head [disorder due to invasion of] wind，vulva coldness，swelling and pain．[It is also] called Nǔluo（女萝），growing in mountains and valleys．

[Textual Research]

[In the book entitled] *Ming Yi Bie Lu*（《名医别录》，*Special Record of Great Doctors*），[it] says [that Songluo（松罗，long usnea filament，Filum Usneae）] grows in Xiong'er（熊耳）mountain．

[In the book entitled] *Guang Ya*（《广雅》，*The First Chinese Encyclopedic Dictionary*），[it] says [that the so-called] Nǔluo（女萝）refers to Songluo（松萝，long usnea filament，Filum Usneae）．

Luji（陆玑）said，"Songluo（松萝，long usnea filament，Filum Usneae）naturally spreads over spine tree with normally green twigs，different from dodder．"

Notes

1．Songluo（松萝，long usnea filament，Filum Usneae）is a herbal medicinal，bitter and sweet in taste，mild and slightly toxic in property，effective in stopping cough and resolving phlegm，activating the blood and unobstructing the collaterals，clearing heat and removing toxin．Clinically it is used to treat scrofula，abscess，ulcer，bleeding due to traumatic injury and scald．

78. 卫矛

【原文】

味苦,寒。

主女子崩中下血,腹满汗出,除邪,杀鬼毒虫注。一名鬼箭。生山谷。

【考据】

1.《吴普》曰:鬼箭一名卫矛,神农黄帝桐君苦无毒,叶如桃如羽,正月二月七月采,阴干,或生野田(《御览》)。

2.《名医》曰:生霍山,八月采,阴干。

3. 案《广雅》云:鬼箭,神箭也。陶宏景云:其茎有三羽,状如箭羽。

【今译】

味苦,性寒。

78. Weimao（卫矛，branchlet of winged euonymus，Ramulus Euonymi Alati）[1]

[Original Text]

[Weimao（卫矛，branchlet of winged euonymus，Ramulus Euonymi Alati），] bitter in taste and cold [in property]，[is mainly used] to treat fulminant vaginal bleeding, abdominal fullness and sweating, to eliminate evil, and to expel [pathogenic factors like] ghost and worm toxin. [It is also] called Guijian（鬼箭），growing in mountains and valleys.

[Textual Research]

[In the book entitled] *Wu Pu Ben Cao*（《吴普本草》，*Wu Pu's Studies of Materia Medica*），[it] says [that] Weimao（卫矛，branchlet of winged euonymus，Ramulus Euonymi Alati）[is also] called Guijian（鬼箭）．[According to] Agriculture God（神农），Yellow Emperor（黄帝）and Tongjun（桐均），[it is] bitter [in taste] and non-toxic [in property]．[Its] leaves are like [that of] peach tree and feather. [It can be] collected in January，February and July，and dried in the shade. [It] may grow in fields [according to the book entitled] *Tai Ping Yu Lan*（《太平御览》，*Imperial Studies in Taiping Times*）．

[In the book entitled] *Ming Yi Bie Lu*（《名医别录》，*Special Record of Great Doctors*），[it] says [that Weimao（卫矛，branchlet

　　主治女子因崩漏而出血，腹部胀满，出汗，能消除邪气，能杀除鬼怪之病，能祛除毒虫所致之症。又称为鬼箭。该物生长在山谷之中。

of winged euonymus, Ramulus Euonymi Alati)] grows in Huoshan (霍山). [It can be] collected in August and dried in the shade.

[In the book entitled] *Guang Ya* (《广雅》, *The First Chinese Encyclopedic Dictionary*), [it] says [that] Weimao (卫矛, branchlet of winged euonymus, Ramulus Euonymi Alati) is like magic arrow. Tao Hongjing (陶宏景) said, "Its stalk bears three feathers, quite like arrow."

Notes

1. Weimao (卫矛, branchlet of winged euonymus, Ramulus Euonymi Alati), also called Guijianyu (鬼箭羽), is a herbal medicinal, bitter in taste and cold in property, entering the liver meridian, effective in breaking the blood and dispersing stasis, expelling wind and killing worms. Clinically it is used to treat amenorrhea, abdominal mass, abdominal pain due to blood stasis after delivery of baby, rheumatism, abdominal pain due to gathering of worms and traumatic injury.

79. 合欢

【原文】

味甘,平。

主安五脏,利心志,(艺文类聚作和心志,《御览》作和心气。)令人献
乐无忧。久服轻身明目得所欲。生山谷。

【考据】

1.《名医》曰:生益州。

2. 案《唐本》注云:或曰合昏,欢昏音相近。日华子云:夜合。

上木,中品一十七种,旧同。

【今译】

味甘,性平。

能安静五脏,能利顺心志,能令人欢乐无忧。长期服用能使人身体
轻盈,眼睛明亮,实现理想。该物生长在山谷之中。

79. Hehuan（合欢，immature flower and bark of silktree albizia，Flos et Cortex Albiziae）[1]

［Original Text］

［Hehuan（合欢，immature flower and bark of silktree albizia，Flos et Cortex Albiziae），］sweet in taste［and］mild［in property］，［is mainly used］to harmonize the five Zang-organs，to balance heart and mentality，and to make people happy without any anxiety. Long-term taking［of it will］relax the body，improve vision and achieve［what one］desires.［It］grows in mountains and valleys.

［Textual Research］

［In the book entitled］*Ming Yi Bie Lu*（《名医别录》，*Special Record of Great Doctors*），［it］says［that Hehuan（合欢，immature flower and bark of silktree albizia，Flos et Cortex Albiziae）］grows in Yizhou（益州）.

805

［In］the explanation［about the book entitled］*Tang Ben*（《唐本》，*Canon of Materia Medica in the Tang Dynasty*），［it］says，"［It］is also called Hehun（合昏）［because］the pronunciation［of the Chinese characters］Huan（欢）and Hun（昏）is similar to each other."

Notes

1. Hehuan（合欢，immature flower and bark of silktree albizia，Flos et Cortex Albiziae）is a herbal medicinal，sweet in taste and mild in property，entering the heart meridian and the liver meridian，effective in tranquilizing the heart，relieving stagnation，harmonizing the blood，resolving swelling and ceasing bleeding. Clinically it is used to treat distraction，insomnia，lung abscess，cough and vomiting with pus，blood and phlegm，scrofula and pain caused by external injury.

神农本草经

80. 白马茎

【原文】

味咸,平。

主伤中脉绝,阴不起,强志益气,长肌肉,肥健,生子。

眼,主惊痫,腹满,疟疾,当杀用之。

悬蹄,主惊邪,瘈疭,乳难,辟恶气鬼毒,蛊注不祥,生平泽。

【考据】

1.《名医》曰:生云中。

【今译】

味咸,性平。

主治内脏损伤,脉搏断绝,阳痿不举,能增强记忆力,能补益精气,能增长肌肉,能使身体康健,能使人生育子女。

马眼,主治惊恐,心悸,癫痫,腹部胀满,疟疾。白马龟头去掉就可

80. Baimajing（白马茎，stallion penis，Penis Equi）[1]

[Original Text]

[Baimajing（白马茎，stallion penis，Penis Equi），] salty in taste and mild [in property], [is mainly used] to treat no pulsation [caused by] injury of the middle (the internal organs) and inability of penis to erect, to strengthen memory, to replenish Qi, to promote [growth of] muscles, to cultivate health and [to enable people] to conceive baby.

The eyes [of stallion can] treat epilepsy, abdominal fullness and malaria. [Its eyes can be] used [when its glans is] cut off.

The suspended [part of stallion's] hoof [can be used] to treat fright [caused by] evil, convulsion and dystocia, and to eliminate filthy Qi, severe toxin like ghost and [severe syndrome/pattern cause by] worm toxin. [It] grows in plains and swamps.

[Textual Research]

[In the book entitled] *Ming Yi Bie Lu*（《名医别录》，*Special Record of Great Doctors*），[it] says [that Baimajing（白马茎，stallion penis，Penis Equi)] grows in Yunzhong（云中）.

Notes

1. Baimajing（白马茎，stallion penis，Penis Equi) is an animal medicinal, sweet and salty in taste, mild and non-toxic in property,

使用。

　　马悬蹄,主治惊风症,癫痫,难产,能祛除鬼怪似的邪恶毒气,能治疗虫毒所致的不祥之症,该物生长在平川水泽之中。

entering the kidney meridian, effective in tonifying the kidney and strengthening Yang, replenishing essence and Qi. Clinically it is used to treat impotence, injury of the five Zang-organs, infertility, weakness and emaciation.

81. 鹿茸

【原文】

味甘,温。

主漏下恶血,寒热,惊痫,益气强志,生齿不老。

角,主恶疮痈肿,逐邪恶气,留血在阴中。

【考据】

1.《名医》曰:茸,四月五月解角时取阴干使时躁,角七月采。

【今译】

味甘,性温。

主治阴道出血淋漓不断,因瘀滞所致的死血症,寒热病,惊恐,心悸,癫痫,能补益精气,能增强记忆力,能生长牙齿,能使人长寿不老。

鹿角,主治恶性疮和痈肿,能祛除导致发热的邪恶之气以及滞留在阴部的瘀血。

81. Lurong (鹿茸, hairy antler, Cornu Cervi Pantotrichum) [1]

[Original Text]

[Lurong (鹿茸, hairy antler, Cornu Cervi Pantotrichum),] sweet in taste [and] warm [in property], [is mainly used] to treat vaginal discharge of blood stasis, cold-heat [disease] and epilepsy, to replenish Qi, to increase memory, to invigorate teeth and to prevent aging.

[Its] buckhorn [can be used] to treat severe sore and abscess, and to eliminate evil, vicious Qi and retention of blood [stasis] in the genitals.

[Textual Research]

[In the book entitled] *Ming Yi Bie Lu* (《名医别录》, *Special Record of Great Doctors*), [it] says [that] Lurong (鹿茸, hairy antler, Cornu Cervi Pantotrichum) [can be] collected in April and May, and dried in the shade. [Its] buckhorn [can be] collected in July.

Agriculture God's Canon of Materia Medica

811

Notes

1. Lurong (鹿茸, hairy antler, Cornu Cervi Pantotrichum) is an animal medicinal, sweet in taste and warm in property, entering the liver meridian and the kidney meridian, effective in strengthening kidney-Yang, tonifying essence and blood, and strengthening sinews and bones. Clinically it is used to treat impotence, spontaneous spermatorrhea, premature ejaculation, ache and coldness of the waist and knees, deficiency of essence and blood, vertigo, deafness, flooding and spotting (metrostaxis and metrorrhagia) as well as leucorrhea.

82. 牛角䚡

【原文】

下闭血，瘀血，疼痛，女人带下血。

髓，补中填骨髓。久服增年。胆可丸药。

【考据】

1. 案《说文》云：䚡，角中骨也。

【今译】

能治疗阴部有瘀血，闭经，瘀血疼痛，带下出血。

牛骨髓，能充实人体内脏，能使骨髓充实。长期服用能使人延长寿命。

牛胆可制成丸药。

82. Niujiaosai（牛角䚡，ox horn pith，Bos Baurus Domesticus）[1]

[**Original Text**]

[Niujiaosai（牛角䚡，ox horn pith，Bos Baurus Domesticus），bitter in taste and warm in property]，[is mainly used] to amenorrhea，blood stasis，dysmenorrhea and bloody leucorrhea.

[Its] bone marrow [can be used] to tonify the middle (the internal organs) and enrich bone marrow. Long-term taking [of it will] prolong life.

[Its] gallbladder [can be used] to make pills.

[**Textual Research**]

[In] case [analysis in the book entitled] *Shuo Wen*（《说文》，*On Culture*），[it] says [that] Sai（䚡）refers to pith in the ox horn.

Notes

1. Niujiaosai（牛角䚡，ox horn pith，Bos Baurus Domesticus）is an animal medicinal，bitter in taste and warm in property，entering the heart meridian and the liver meridian，effective in resolving stasis and ceasing bleeding. Clinically it is used to treat amenorrhea，abdominal pain，flooding and spotting（metrostaxis and metrorrhagia），hematochezia，dysentery，nosebleed，leucorrhea and diarrhea.

83. 羖羊角

【原文】

味咸,温。

主青盲明目,杀疥虫,止寒泄,辟恶鬼虎狼,止惊悸。久服,安心益气,轻身。生川谷。

【考据】

1.《名医》曰:生河西,取无时。

2. 案《说文》云:羖夏羊,牝曰羖.《尔雅》云:羊牝,羖。郭璞云:今人便以牂,羖,为黑白羊名。

【今译】

味咸,性温。

主治青盲症,能使眼睛明亮,能杀除引发疥疮的毒虫,能停止因受寒而泄泻,能辟开恶鬼虎狼,能制止惊风和心悸。长期服用,能安心定志,能补益精气,能使人身体轻盈。该物生长在山川河谷之中。

83. Guyangjiao（羖羊角，male goat horn，Cornu Maris Caprinus）[1]

[Original Text]

[Guyangjiao（羖羊角，male goat horn，Cornu Maris Caprinus），] salty in taste and warm [in property]，[is mainly used] to treat blue nebula，to improve vision，to kill worm [that has caused] scabies，to cease cold diarrhea，to prevent [severe pathogenic factors like] ghost，tiger and wolf，and to relieve fright and palpitation. Long-term taking [of it will] tranquilize the heart，replenish Qi and relax the body. [It is] produced in mountain valleys and river valleys.

[Textual Research]

[In the book entitled] *Ming Yi Bie Lu*（《名医别录》，*Special Record of Great Doctors*），[it] says [that Guyangjiao（羖羊角，male goat horn，Cornu Maris Caprinus）is] produced in Hexi（河西）and can be collected at any time.

Notes

1. Guyangjiao（羖羊角，male goat horn，Cornu Maris Caprinus） is an animal medicinal，salty in taste and cool in property，entering the liver meridian and the heart meridian，effective in clearing heat，relieving fright，improving vision and removing toxin. Clinically it is used to treat infantile epilepsy，vexation and depression，hematemesis and glaucoma.

84. 牡狗阴茎

【原文】

味咸,平。

主伤中,阴痿不起,令强热大,生子,除女子带下十二疾。一名狗精。

胆主明目。

【考据】

1.《名医》曰,六月上伏,取阴干百日。

【今译】

味咸,性平。

主治内脏损伤及因阳痿而阴茎不能勃起,能使阴茎充盈而强大,能使人生育子女,能消除女子带下多种疾病。又称为狗精。

狗胆,能使眼睛明亮。

84. Mugou Yinjing（牡狗阴茎，dog penis， Penis Canis）[1]

[Original Text]

[Mugou Yinjing（牡狗阴茎，dog penis，Penis Canis），] salty in taste and mild [in property]，[is mainly used] to treat injury of the middle（the internal organs）and impotence，to enable [penis] to strongly erect and conceive baby，and to eliminate twelve diseases in women．[It is also] called Goujing（狗精）．

[Its] gallbladder [can be used] to improve vision．

[Textual Research]

[In the book entitled] *Ming Yi Bie Lu*（《名医别录》，*Special Record of Great Doctors*），[it] says [that Mugou Yinjing（牡狗阴茎，dog penis，Penis Canis）can be] cut in June and dried for one hundred days．

Notes

1. Mugou Yinjing（牡狗阴茎，dog penis，Penis Canis）is an animal medicinal，salty in taste and warm in property，entering the kidney meridian and the liver meridian，effective in enriching fire in the life gate，warming the thoroughfare vessel，conception vessel and governor vessel．Clinically it is used to treat impotence，sexual apathy in women，infertility due to uterine coldness，seminal emission and leucorrhea．

85. 羚羊角

【原文】

味咸,寒。

主明目,益气起阴,去恶血注下,辟蛊毒恶鬼不祥,安心气,常不厌寐。生川谷。

【考据】

1.《名医》曰:生石城及华阴山,采无时。

2.案《说文》云:羚大羊而细角。《广雅》云:美皮冷角。《尔雅》云:羚大羊。郭璞云:羚羊似羊而大,角园锐,好在山崖间。陶宏景云:《尔雅》名羱羊。据《说文》云:苋山羊细角也。《尔雅》云:羱如羊。郭璞云:羱似吴羊而大角,角椭,出西方,苋即羱正字,然本经羚字,实羚字俗写,当以羚为是《尔雅》释文,引本草作羚。

【今译】

味咸,性寒。

85. Lingyangjiao（羚羊角，antelope horn，Cornu Saigae Tataricae）[1]

[Original Text]

［Lingyangjiao （羚羊角，antelope horn，Cornu Saigae Tataricae），］salty in taste and cold ［in property］，［is mainly used］to improve vision，to replenish Qi to erect penis，to discharge blood stasis，to prevent worm toxin and severe auspicious ［pathogenic factors like］ghost，to tranquilize heart-Qi and ［to avoid］nightmare all the time. ［It is］produced in mountain valleys and river valleys.

[Textual Research]

［In the book entitled］*Ming Yi Bie Lu*（《名医别录》，*Special Record of Great Doctors*），［it］says ［that Lingyangjiao（羚羊角，antelope horn，Cornu Saigae Tataricae）is］produced in Shicheng（石城）and Huayin（华阴）Mountain. ［It can be］collected at any time.

［In］case ［analysis in the book entitled］*Shuo Wen*（《说文》，*On Culture*），［it］says ［that Lingyangjiao（羚羊角，antelope horn，Cornu Saigae Tataricae）refers to］the thin horn of anelop. Guo Pu（郭璞云）said，"Antelope is similar to sheep，but bigger ［than it］. ［Its］horn is round and sharp. ［It］usually stays in the cliffs of mountains."

能使眼睛明亮，能补益精气，能使阴茎勃起，能祛除因瘀滞所致的死血，能使瘀血下流，能避免虫毒恶气所致之不祥疾患，能安静心气，能使人避免噩梦惊醒。该物生长在山川河谷之中。

Notes

1. Lingyangjiao （羚羊角, antelope horn, Cornu Saigae Tataricae) is an animal medicinal, salty in taste and cold in property, entering the liver meridian and the heart meridian, effective in soothing the liver, extinguishing fire, clearing heat, relieving fright and removing toxin. Clinically it is used to treat coma, convulsion, mania, delirium, headache, vertigo, epilepsy, spasm of hands and feet, redness of the eyes and nebula.

86. 犀角

【原文】

味苦,寒。

主百毒虫注,邪鬼,障气杀钩吻鸩羽蛇毒,除不迷或厌寐。久服轻身。生山谷。

【考据】

1.《名医》曰:生永昌及益州。

2. 案《说文》云:犀南徼外牛,一角在鼻,一角在顶,似豕。《尔雅》云:犀似豕。

3. 郭璞云:形似水牛,猪头大腹,痹脚,脚有三蹄,黑色,三角,一在顶上,一在鼻上,一在额上,鼻上者,即食角也,小而不椭,好食棘,亦有一角者。

4.《山海经》云:琴鼓之山多白犀。郭璞云:此与辟寒,蠲忿,辟尘,辟暑,诸犀,皆异种也。《范子计然》云:犀角出南郡,上价八千,中三千,下一千。

上兽,中品七种,旧同。

86. Xijiao（犀角，horn of Asiatic rhinoceros，Cornu Rhinocerotis Asiatici）[1]

[Original Text]

[Xijiao（犀角，horn of Asiatic rhinoceros，Cornu Rhinocerotis Asiatici），] bitter in taste and cold [in property]，[is mainly used] to treat diseases [caused by] various worm toxin，[to eliminate pathogenic factors like] evil and ghost，[to expel] miasma，to eliminate toxin from Gouwen（钩吻，graceful jessamine herb，Herba Gelsemii Elegantis），Zhenyu（鸩羽，a legendary bird with poisonous feathers）and snake [in order] to avoid obnubilation or nightmare. Long-term taking [of it will] relax the body. [It is] produced in mountains and valleys.

[Textual Research]

[In the book entitled] *Ming Yi Bie Lu*（《名医别录》，*Special Record of Great Doctors*），[it] says [that Xijiao（犀角，horn of Asiatic rhinoceros，Cornu Rhinocerotis Asiatici）is] produced in Yongchang（永昌）and Yizhou（益州）.

[In] case [analysis in the book entitled] *Shuo Wen*（《说文》，*On Culture*），[it] says [that] in Asiatic rhinoceros，one horn is located on the nose and the other horn is located on the top of the head，like a pig.

Guo Pu（郭璞）said，"[Asiatic rhinoceros is] physically similar

【今译】

味苦,性寒。

主治各种毒气所致的中毒症,能消除鬼怪恶邪和障气,能杀除钩吻毒、鸩羽毒和蛇毒,能使人神志清晰,不做噩梦。长期服用能使人身体轻盈。该物生长在山谷之中。

to a cow. [But its] head is like [that of] a pig, [its] abdomen is large, [its] hoofs are rough and each hoof bears three toes. [It] has three horns, one is on the top, one is on the nose and one is on the forehead. The one on the nose is for taking food, [which is] small but not round. [Those that] like to eat thorn also have another horn."

In the book entitled] *Fan Zi Ji Ran* (《范子计然》, *Studies About Fan Li's Teacher*), [it] says [that] Xijiao (犀角, horn of Asiatic rhinoceros, Cornu Rhinocerotis Asiatici) [is] produced in Nanjun (南郡).

Notes

1. Xijiao (犀角, horn of Asiatic rhinoceros, Cornu Rhinocerotis Asiatici) is an animal medicinal, bitter, salty and sour in taste, cold in property, entering the heart meridian and the liver meridian, effective in clearing heat, cooling the blood, relieving fright and removing toxin. Clinically it is used to treat cold damage, heat transmitted to the blood phase in warm disease, coma due to high fever, delirium, vexation, convulsion, hematemesis, nosebleed, bleeding, acute jaundice and sore due to heat toxin.

87. 燕屎

【原文】

味辛,平。

主蛊毒鬼注,逐不详邪气,破五癃,利小便。生平谷。

【考据】

1.《名医》曰:生高山。

2. 案《说文》云:燕、元鸟也,尔口、布翅枝尾,象形作巢,避戊巳,乙元鸟也,齐鲁谓之乙,取其名自呼,象形或作乱。《尔雅》云:燕乱。《夏小正》云,二月来降,燕乃睇。《传》云:燕、乙也,九月陟元鸟,蛰,《传》云:元鸟者,燕也。

【今译】

味辛,性平。

主治虫毒所致之病及鬼怪之邪所致之症,能祛除不详邪气,能破除五种癃闭症,能使小便通畅。该物生长在平谷中。

87. Yanshi (燕屎, feces of swiftlet, Faeces Collocaliae) [1]

[Original Text]

[Yanshi (燕屎, feces of swiftlet, Faeces Collocaliae),] pungent in taste and mild [in property], [is mainly used] to treat [disease caused by] worm toxin, to expel evil-Qi [that is] not auspicious, to break five [kinds of] stranguria[2] and to promote urination. [It is] produced in plains and valleys.

[Textual Research]

[In the book entitled] *Ming Yi Bie Lu* (《名医别录》, *Special Record of Great Doctors*), [it] says [that Yanshi (燕屎, feces of swiftlet, Faeces Collocaliae) is] produced in high mountains.

Notes

1. Yanshi (燕屎, feces of swiftlet, Faeces Collocaliae) is a bird medicinal, pungent in taste, mild and toxic in property, effective in relieving worm toxin and promoting urination. Clinically it is used to treat infantile epilepsy.

2. The five kinds of stranguria include heat stranguria, stony stranguria, paste stranguria, bloody stranguria and Qi stranguria.

88. 天鼠屎

【原文】

味辛,寒。

主面痈肿,皮肤洗洗,时痛,肠中血气,破寒热积聚,除惊悸。一名鼠沄,一名石肝。生山谷。

【考据】

1.《名医》曰:生合浦,十月十二月取。

2. 案李当之云:即伏翼屎也。李云:天鼠,方言,一名仙鼠。

3. 案今本方言云:或谓之老鼠,当为天字之误也。

上禽,中品二种,旧同。

【今译】

味辛,性寒。

主治面痈肿,皮肤寒冷,时常疼痛,肠中有血气,能破解寒热积聚,能消除惊恐心悸。又称为鼠沄,又称为石肝。该物生长在山谷之中。

88. Tianshushi（天鼠屎，bat dung， Faeces Vespertilionis）[1]

[Original Text]

[Tianshushi（天鼠屎，bat dung，Faeces Vespertilionis），] pungent in taste and cold [in property]，[is mainly used] to treat facial abscess and swelling，chilliness and shivering of skin with occasional pain and [disease caused by] bloody Qi in the intestines，to expel cold-heat [disease] and accumulation [of pathogenic factors in the internal organs]，and to eliminate fright and palpitation. [It is also] called Shuyun（鼠沄）and Shigan（石肝），produced in mountains and valleys.

[Textual Research]

[In the book entitled] *Ming Yi Bie Lu*（《名医别录》，*Special Record of Great Doctors*），[it] says [that Tianshushi（天鼠屎，bat dung，Faeces Vespertilionis) is] produced in Hepu（合浦）and [can be] collected in October and December.

Notes

1. Tianshushi（天鼠屎，bat dung，Faeces Vespertilionis）is an animal medicinal，pungent in taste and cold in property，entering the liver meridian，effective in clearing the liver and improving vision，dispersing blood stasis and resolving accumulation of pathogenic factors. Clinically it is used to treat heat in the liver and redness of the eyes，nebula，night blindness，cataract，malnutrition and traumatic injury.

89. 猬皮

【原文】

味苦,平。

主五痔阴蚀下血,赤白五色,血汁不止,阴肿痛引要背,酒煮杀之。生川谷。

【考据】

1.《名医》曰:生楚山田野,取无时。

2. 案《说文》云:帚似豪猪者,或作猬。《广雅》云:虎王,猬也。《尔雅》云:汇毛刺。郭璞云:今谓状似鼠。《淮南子》说山训云:鹊矢中猬。

【今译】

味苦,性平。

89. Weipi（猬皮，hedgehog hide，Corium Erinacei seu Hemiechini）[1]

[Original Text]

[Weipi（猬皮，hedgehog hide，Corium Erinacei seu Hemiechini），] bitter in taste and mild [in property], [is mainly used] to treat five [kinds of] hemorrhoids，genital ulcer，vaginal bleeding with five colors and difficult to cease，genital swelling and pain extending to the back. [It can be] boiled in wine to cure such [diseases]. [It is] produced in mountain valleys and river valleys.

[Textual Research]

[In the book entitled] *Ming Yi Bie Lu*（《名医别录》，*Special Record of Great Doctors*），[it] says [that Weipi（猬皮，hedgehog hide，Corium Erinacei seu Hemiechini) is] produced in the fields in Chushan（楚山）and [can be] collected at any time.

[In] case [analysis in the book entitled] *Shuo Wen*（《说文》，*On Culture*），[it] says [that there is a kind of animal that looks] like Haozhu（豪猪，hedgehog），or may be called Wei（猬，hedgehog）. [In the book entitled] *Guang Ya*（《广雅》，*The First Chinese Encyclopedic Dictionary*），[it] says [that the so-called] Huwang（虎王）refers to Wei（猬，hedgehog）.

能治疗五种痔疮,阴部侵淫,腐烂下血,赤白带下,血流不止,阴部肿痛,牵引腰背。用酒煮后服用,可以消除各种病患。该物生长在山川河谷之中。

Notes

1. Weipi （猬皮，hedgehog hide，Corium Erinacei seu Hemiechini），also called Ciweipi（刺猬皮），is an animal medicinal，entering the stomach meridian，the large intestine meridian and the kidney meridian，effective in resolving stasis and ceasing pain，restraining and ceasing bleeding，and fixing essence. Clinically it is used to treat pain in the gastric region，hematochezia，uterine bleeding，prolapse of anus，hemorrhoids，seminal emission and enuresis.

本书为国家社科基金项目"中医名词术语英译国际标准化研究"（No.08BYY009）、国家社科基金项目"中医英语翻译理论与方法研究"（No.12BYY024）、国家中医药管理局项目"中国参与世界卫生组织ICTM方案研究"(No.YYS20090010-2)、上海市教委科研创新重点项目"中医英语翻译原则、标准与方法研究"（B-7037-12-000001）、国家外文局重点项目"中医典籍翻译的历史、现状与国际传播调研报告"、上海市教委重点课程建设项目"国学典籍英译"、上海师范大学重点科研项目"国学典籍多译本平行语料库建设"（A-7031-12-002001）的阶段性成果。

Shēn Nóng Běn Cǎo Jīng

神农本草经

Agriculture God's Canon of Materia Medica

孙星衍◎考据 Textually Researched by Sun Xingyan

刘希茹◎今译 Translated in Modern Chinese by Liu Xiru

李照国◎英译 Translated in English by Li Zhaoguo

上海三联书店

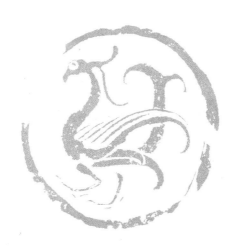

90. 露蜂房

【原文】

味苦,平。

主惊痫瘈疭,寒热邪气,癫疾,鬼精,蛊毒肠痔。火熬之,良。一名蜂肠。生山谷。

【考据】

1.《名医》曰:一名百穿,一名蜂䗖。生牂柯,七月七日采,阴干。

2. 案《淮南子》氾论训云:蜂房不容卵。高诱云:房巢也。

【今译】

味苦,性平。

主治惊风,癫痫,抽搐,寒热邪气,鬼怪性癫痫,虫毒病,肠痔。用火熬后效果更好。又称为蜂肠。该物生长在山谷之中。

90. Lufengfang（Lufengfang（露蜂房，honeycomb of paper wasps，Nidus Polistis Mandarini）[1]

［Original Text］

［Lufengfang（Lufengfang（露蜂房，honeycomb of paper wasps，Nidus Polistis Mandarini），bitter in taste and mild ［in property］，［is mainly used］ to treat epilepsy，convulsion，cold-heat ［disease caused by］ evil-Qi，epilepsy，［disease caused by strange pathogenic factors like］ ghost，［disease caused by］ worm toxin and intestinal hemorrhoids. To be broiled by fire is more effective. ［It is also］ called Fengchang（蜂肠），existing in mountains and valleys.

［Textual Research］

835

［In the book entitled］ *Ming Yi Bie Lu*（《名医别录》，*Special Record of Great Doctors*），［it］ says ［that Lufengfang（Lufengfang（露蜂房，honeycomb of paper wasps，Nidus Polistis Mandarini）is also］ called Baichuan（百穿）and Feng（蜂），existing in Zangke（牂柯）. ［It can be］ collected on July 7th ［in the Chinese lunar calender］ and dried in the shade.

Notes

1. Lufengfang（Lufengfang（露蜂房，honeycomb of paper wasps，Nidus Polistis Mandarini）is an insect medicinal，sweet in taste，mild and toxic in property，entering the liver meridian and the stomach meridian，effective in expelling wind，removing toxin and killing worms. Clinically it is used to treat wind impediment，headache caused by wind attack，whooping cough，epilepsy，urticaria and itching.

91. 鳖甲

【原文】

味咸,平。

主心腹症瘕坚积,寒热,去痞息肉,阴蚀,痔恶肉。生池泽。

【考据】

1.《名医》曰:生丹阳,取无时。

2. 案《说文》云:鳖,甲虫也。

【今译】

味咸,性平。

主治心腹部症瘕,坚硬性聚积,寒热病,能祛除痞证,能治疗息肉,阴部溃疡,痔疮及溃烂恶肉。该物生长在池泽中。

91. Biejia（鳖甲，turtle carapace，Carapax Trionycis）[1]

[Original Text]

[Biejia（鳖甲，turtle carapace，Carapax Trionycis），] salty in taste and mild [in property], [is mainly used] to treat conglomeration and intractable accumulation in the abdomen and cold-heat [disease], and to eliminate lump, plypus, genital ulcer, hemorrhois and necrotic muscles. [It] exists in lakes and swamps.

[Textual Research]

[In the book entitled] *Ming Yi Bie Lu*（《名医别录》，*Special Record of Great Doctors*），[it] says [that Biejia（鳖甲，turtle carapace，Carapax Trionycis）] exists in Danyang（丹阳）and [can be] collected at any time.

Notes

1. Biejia（鳖甲，turtle carapace，Carapax Trionycis）is a turtle medicinal, salty in taste and mild in property, entering the liver meridian, the spleen meridian and the kidney meridian, effective in enriching Yin and subduing Yang, softening hardness and dispersing binding. Clinically it is used to treat tidal fever due to Yin deficiency, night sweating due to bone steaming, hypertension, malaria, amenorrhea and abdominal mass.

92. 蟹

【原文】

味咸,寒。

主脑中邪气,热结痛,喎僻,面肿败漆。烧之致鼠。生池泽。

【考据】

1. 《名医》曰:生伊洛诸水中,取无时。

2. 案《说文》云:蟹有二敖八足旁行,非蛇鳝之穴无所庇,或作鳜,蜅蟹也。

3. 《荀子》勤学扁云:蟹六跪而二螯,非蛇蟺之穴无所寄托。《广雅》云:蜅蟹,蜅也。

4. 《尔雅》云:螖蜢,小者蟧。郭璞云:或曰即蟚蟝也,似蟹而小。

【今译】

味咸,性寒。

主治脑中邪气,热结疼痛,嘴巴喎斜,败漆所致面肿。火烧后可招致老鼠。该物生长在池泽中。

92. Xie（蟹，meat of mitten crab，Caro Eriocheiris）[1]

[Original Text]

[Xie（蟹，meat of mitten crab，Caro Eriocheiris），] salty in taste and cold [in property]，[is mainly used] to treat [headache caused by] evil-Qi in the brain，pain [caused by] heat binding，crooked mouth and swollen face caused by lacquer. [When] broiled by fire，[it can] attract mouse. [It] exists in lakes and swamps.

[Textual Research]

[In the book entitled] *Ming Yi Bie Lu*（《名医别录》，*Special Record of Great Doctors*），[it] says [that Xie（蟹，meat of mitten crab，Caro Eriocheiris）] exists in waters in Yiluo（伊洛）and [can be] collected at any time.

[In] case [analysis in the book entitled] *Shuo Wen*（《说文》，*On Culture*），[it] says [that] Xie（蟹，meat of mitten crab，Caro Eriocheiris）has two touching appendages and eight moving appendages. It only stays in the cave of echidna nocturna. [It is] also called Guixie（蛫蟹）.

Notes

1. Xie（蟹，meat of mitten crab，Caro Eriocheiris）is a crab medicinal，salty in taste and cold in property，entering the liver meridian and the stomach meridian，effective in clearing heat，dispersing blood stasis and curing severe injury. Clinically it is used to treat traumatic injury，fracture，scabies and scald.

93. 柞蝉

【原文】

味咸,寒。

主小儿惊痫,夜啼,癫病,寒热,生杨柳上。

【考据】

1.《名医》曰:五月采,蒸干之。

2. 案《说文》云:蝉以旁鸣者,蜩蝉也。《广雅》云:蜻蚑,蝉也,复育,蜕也,旧作蚱蝉。别录云:蚱者,鸣蝉也,壳一名楛蝉,又名伏蜟,案蚱即柞字。《周礼》考工记云:侈则柞。郑元云:柞读为咋咋然之咋,声大外也。《说文》云:诸、大声也,音同柞,今据作柞。柞蝉即五月鸣蜩之蜩,《夏小正》云:五月良蜩鸣,传良蜩也,五采具。《尔雅》云:蜩、蜋、蜩。《毛诗》云:如蜩。《传》云:蜩、蝉也。方言云:楚谓之蜩,宋卫之间,谓之螗蜩,陈郑之间,谓之螂蜩,秦晋之间,谓之蝉,海岱之间,谓之蜻。论衡云:蝉生于复育,开背而出。而玉扁云:蚱蝉,七月生。陶宏景音蚱作笮云:痤蝉,是为月令之寒蝉,《尔雅》所云蜕矣,《唐本》注非之也。

93. Zhachan（柞蝉，cicada，
Cryptotympana atrata）[1]

［**Original Text**］

［Zhachan（柞蝉，cicada，Cryptotympana atrata），］salty in taste and cold［in property］，［is mainly used］to treat infantile convulsive epilepsy，night crying［of baby］，epilepsy and cold-heat［disease］. ［It］exists on the poplar and willow.

［**Textual Research**］

［In the book entitled］*Ming Yi Bie Lu*（《名医别录》，*Special Record of Great Doctors*），［it］says［that Zhachan（柞蝉，cicada，Cryptotympana atrata）can be］collected in May and dried by steaming.

［In the book entitled］*Fang Yan*（《方言》，*On Dialects*），［it］says［that Zhachan（柞蝉，cicada，Cryptotympana atrata）is］called Tiao（蜩）in the Chu（楚）［State］，Tangtiao（蜣蜩）in the Song（宋）and Wei（卫）［States］，Langtiao（螂蜩）in the Chen（陈）and Zheng（郑）［States］，Chan（蝉）in the Qin（秦）and Jin（晋）［States］，Qi（蜛）in the region between Hai（海）[2] and Dai（岱）[3].

Notes

1. Zhachan（柞蝉，cicada，Cryptotympana atrata）is an insect

【今译】

味咸,性寒。

主治小儿惊风,癫痫,夜哭,癫病,寒热证。该物生长在杨柳树上。

medicinal, salty and sweet in taste, cold in property, entering the liver meridian and the lung meridian, effective in clearing heat, expelling wind and relieving fright. Clinically it is used to treat infantile fever, infantile convulsion, hyperspasmia, epilepsy, night crying and migraine.

2. Hai（海）refers to Bohai（渤海）in the Shandong Province （山东省）.

3. Dai（岱）refers to Taishan（泰山）mountain which is also called Daishan（岱山）mountain.

神农本草经

94. 蛴螬

【原文】

味咸,微温。

主恶血,血淤,(《御览》作血瘤)痹气,破折血在胁下坚满痛,月闭,目中淫肤,青翳,白膜。一名蟦蛴。生平泽。

【考据】

1.《名医》曰:一名蟦齐,一名勃齐,生河内人家积粪草中,取无时,反行者,良。

2. 案《说文》云:蝤、蝤也,蛴,蝤蛴也,蝎、蛴蚍蝎也。《广雅》云:蛭蝏,蚍蝎,地蚕,蠹蟦,蛴螬。《尔雅》云:蟦、蛴螬。郭璞云:在粪土中,又蝤蛴,蝎。

3. 郭璞云:在木中,今虽通名蝎,所在异,又蝎,蛣𧕙。郭璞云:木中蠹虫,蝎、桑蠹。郭璞云:即拮掘。《毛诗》云:领如蝤蛴。《传》云:蝤蛴,蝎虫也。方言云:蛴螬,谓之蟦,自关而东,谓之蝤蛴,或谓之蚕蝎,或谓之蚕蠋,梁益之间,谓之蛒,或谓之蝎或谓之蛭蛒,秦晋之间,谓之蠹,或谓之天蝼。

94. Qicao（蛴螬，dried larva of grub，Larva Holotrichiae）[1]

［Original Text］

［Qicao（蛴螬，dried larva of grub，Larva Holotrichiae），］salty in taste and slightly warm［in property］，［is mainly used］to treat blood stasis and impediment of Qi［due to］blood stasis，to resolve lump，fullness and pain below the rib-side［due to］blood stasis，and to treat amenorrhea，pterygium，blue nebula and albuginea.［It is also］called Feiqi（蟦蛴），existing in plains and swamps.

［Textual Research］

［In the book entitled］*Ming Yi Bie Lu*（《名医别录》，*Special Record of Great Doctors*），［it］says［that Qicao（蛴螬，dried larva of grub，Larva Holotrichiae）is also］called Feiqi（蟹齐）and Pengqi（勃齐），existing in manure and straw in Henei（河内）.［It can be］collected at any time.［Those that］move reversely are better.

Notes

1. Qicao（蛴螬，dried larva of grub，Larva Holotrichiae）is salty in taste，warm and toxic in property，entering the liver meridian，effective in activating the blood，expelling stasis and removing toxin. Clinically it

4.《列子·天瑞篇》云：乌足根为蛴螬。《博物志》云：蛴螬以背行，快于足用，《说文》无蟦字，当借蜰为之，声相近，字之误也。

【今译】

味咸，性微温。

主治因瘀滞所致死血，瘀血闭阻，能破解坚硬瘀血在胁下引起的疼痛，能治疗闭经，目中胬肉、青翳和白膜。又称为蟦蛴。该物生长在平川水泽之中。

846

is used to treat abdominal mass, conglomeration, pain and damage caused by blood stasis, amenorrhea, tetanus, throat impediment and arthralgia.

95. 乌贼鱼骨

【原文】

味咸,微温。

主女子漏下,赤白经汁,血闭,阴蚀,肿痛,寒热,症瘕,无子。生池泽。

【考据】

1.《名医》曰:生东海,取无时。

2. 案《说文》云:鲗、乌鲗,鱼名,或作鲫,左思赋,有乌贼。刘逵注云:乌贼鱼,腹中有墨。陶宏景云:此是鹢乌所化作,今其口脚具存,犹相似尔。

【今译】

味咸,性微温。

主治女子阴道出血淋漓不断,赤白带下,经闭,阴部溃疡,肿痛,寒热病,症瘕,能治疗不孕之症。该物生长在池泽中。

95. Wuzei Yugu（乌贼鱼骨,Os Sepiae；cuttlefish bone）[1]

[Original Text]

[Wuzei Yugu（乌贼鱼骨,Os Sepiae；cuttlefish bone），] salty in taste and slightly warm [in property], [is mainly used] to treat vaginal discharge of red and white liquid，amenorrhea，genital swelling and pain，cold-heat [disease]，abdominal conglomeration and infertility. [It] exists in lakes and swamps.

[Textual Research]

[In the book entitled] *Ming Yi Bie Lu*（《名医别录》,*Special Record of Great Doctors*），[it] says [that Wuzei Yugu（乌贼鱼骨,Os Sepiae；cuttlefish bone）] exists in Donghai（东海,East Sea）and [can be] collected at any time.

Notes

1. Wuzei Yugu（乌贼鱼骨,Os Sepiae；cuttlefish bone）is a fish medicinal，salty in taste，astringent and slightly warm in property，entering the liver meridian and the kidney meridian，effective in restraining activities of certain organs，ceasing bleeding，controlling essence and resolving sourness. Clinically it is used to treat flooding and spotting（metrostaxis and metrorrhagia），hematemesis，nosebleed，hematochezia，seminal emission，premature ejaculation，spontaneous spermatorrhea and leucorrhea.

96. 白僵蚕

【原文】

味咸,平。

主小儿惊痫夜啼,去三虫,减黑皯,令人面色好,男子阴疡病。生平泽。

【考据】

1.《名医》曰:生颍川,四月取自死者。

2. 案《说文》云:蚕任丝也。《淮南子》说林训云:蚕食而不饮,二十二日而化。

3.《博物志》云:蚕三化,先孕而后交,不交者亦生子,子后为鏊,皆无眉目,易伤,收采亦薄,玉篇作僵蚕,正当为僵,旧作殭,非。

【今译】

味咸,性平。

主治小儿惊风,癫痫,夜哭,能祛除三种虫子,能消除面部黑斑,能使人面部美好,能治疗男子阴部溃疡。该物生长在平川水泽之中。

96. Baijiangcan（白僵蚕，silkworm larva，Larva Bombycis） [1]

[Original Text]

[Baijiangcan（白僵蚕，silkworm larva，Larva Bombycis），] salty in taste and mild [in property], [is mainly used] to treat infantile convulsion，epilepsy and night crying，to eliminate three worms，to reduce black spots，to luster facial expression and to treat genital ulcer in men. [It] exists in lakes and pools.

[Textual Research]

[In the book entitled] *Ming Yi Bie Lu*（《名医别录》，*Special Record of Great Doctors*），[it] says [that Baijiangcan（白僵蚕，silkworm larva，Larva Bombycis），] exists in Yingchuan（颍川）and [can be] collected in April [when it] has died naturally.

Notes

1. Baijiangcan（白僵蚕，silkworm larva，Larva Bombycis）is an insect medicinal，salty and pungent in taste，mild in property，entering the liver meridian and the lung meridian，effective in expelling wind and relieving spasm，resolving phlegm and dispersing bind. Clinically it is used to treat wind stroke，convulsion，epilepsy，facial paralysis，headache，vertigo，redness of the eyes，swelling and pain of the throat，skin itching and scrofula.

97. 蛇鱼甲

【原文】

味辛,微温。

主心腹症瘕,伏坚,积聚,寒热,女子崩中,下血五色,小腹阴中相引痛,疮疥,死肌。生池泽。

【考据】

1.《名医》曰:生南海,取无时。

2. 案《说文》云:鳝、鱼名,皮可为鼓鼍,鼍、水虫似蜥,易长大。陶宏景云:蛇即鼍甲也。

【今译】

味辛,性微温。

97. Sheyujia（蛇鱼甲，eel carapace，Carapax Anguilla）[1]

[Original Text]

[Sheyujia（蛇鱼甲，eel carapace，Carapax Anguilla），] pungent in taste and slightly warm [in property]，[is mainly used] to relieve abdominal conglomeration，hardness and accumulation [of pathogenic factors]，and to treat cold-heat [disease]，fulminant vaginal hemorrhea，bleeding with five colors，lower abdominal and genital convulsion and pain，scabies and necrotic mulses. [It] exists in lakes and swamps.

[Textual Research]

[In the book entitled] *Ming Yi Bie Lu* （《名医别录》，*Special Record of Great Doctors* ），[it] says [that Sheyujia（蛇鱼甲，eel carapace，Carapax Anguilla）is also] exists in Nanhai（南海，South Sea）and [can be] collected at any time.

[In] case [analysis in the book entitled] *Shuo Wen* （《说文》，*On Culture* ），[it] says [that] eel is a sort of fish. [Its] carapace is similar to that of alligator. [It is] an insect in waters like lizard，very long and big. "

Notes

1. Sheyujia（蛇鱼甲，eel carapace，Carapax Anguilla）is a fish

主治心腹部癥瘕,伏坚积聚,寒热病,女子阴道突然大量出血,血色混杂,小腹部和阴中相互牵引疼痛,疮疥,肌肉坏死。该物生长在池泽中。

medicinal, salty and sweet in taste, mild and toxic in property, effective in nourishing and strengthening the body, expelling wind and killing worms. Clinically it is used to eliminate worms inside the body, vomiting with clear liquid, bone steaming, flaccidity, emaciation and hematochezia.

98. 樗鸡

【原文】

味苦,平。

主心腹邪气,阴痿,益精,强志,生子好色,补中轻身。生川谷。

【考据】

1.《名医》曰:生河内樗树上,七月采,暴干。

2. 案《广雅》云:樗鸠,樗鸡也。《尔雅》云:鞁、天鸡。李巡云:一名酸鸡。郭璞云:小虫,黑身赤头,一名莎鸡,又曰樗鸡。《毛诗》云:六月莎鸡振羽。陆玑云:莎鸡,如蝗而班色,毛翅数重,某翅正赤,或谓之天鸡,六月中,飞而振羽,索索作声,幽州人谓之蒲错,是也。

【今译】

味苦,性平。

98. Chuji（樗鸡, red lady-bug, Huecchys Sanguinea）[1]

[Original Text]

[Chuji（樗鸡, red lady-bug, Huecchys Sanguinea）,] bitter in taste and mild [in property], [is mainly used] to treat [disease in] the heart and abdomen [caused by] evil-Qi and impotence, to replenish essence, to strengthen memory, [to enable people] to conceive baby, to increase sexuality, to tonify the middle（the internal organs）and to relax the body. [It] exists in mountain valleys and river valleys.

[Textual Research]

[In the book entitled] *Ming Yi Bie Lu*（《名医别录》, *Special Record of Great Doctors*）, [it] says [that Chuji（樗鸡, red lady-bug, Huecchys Sanguinea）] exists in Chushu（樗树, Ailanthus altissima）in Henei（河内）. [It can be] collected in July and dried in the sun.

[In the book entitled] *Guang Ya*（《广雅》, *The First Chinese Encyclopedic Dictionary*）, [it] says [that the so-called] Chujiu（樗鸠）refers to Chuji（樗鸡, red lady-bug, Huecchys Sanguinea）. Li Xun（李巡）said, "[It is also] called Suanji（酸鸡）."Guo Pu（郭璞）said, "[It is] a small insect with black body and red head, also called Shaji（莎鸡）and Chuji（樗鸡）."

857

　　主治心腹中邪气所致之症，阳痿，能补益精气，能增强记忆力，能使人生育子女，能提高性欲，能充实人体内脏，能使人身体轻盈。该物生长在山川河谷之中。

Notes

1. Chuji (樗鸡, red lady-bug, Huecchys Sanguinea) is an insect medicinal, bitter and pungent in taste, mild and toxic in property, entering the liver meridian, effective in activating the blood and breaking stasis, removing toxin and dispersing binding. In ancient times it was used to tonify kidney-Yang and to treat impotence, sterility and infertility. Now it is used to treat scrofula, scabies and amenorrhea due to blood stasis.

99. 蛞蝓

【原文】

味咸,寒。

主贼风,㖞僻,轶筋,及脱肛,惊痫挛缩。一名陵蠡。生池泽。

【考据】

1.《名医》曰:一名土蜗,一名附蜗,生大山及阴地沙石垣下,八月取。

2. 案《说文》云:蝓,虎蝓也,蠃,一石虎蝓。《广雅》云:蠡蠃、蜗牛,蠡蝓也。《中山经》云:青要之山是多仆累。郭璞云:仆累,蜗牛也,《周礼》鳖人,祭祀供蠃。郑云:蠃蠡蝓。《尔雅》云:蚹蠃蠡蝓。郭璞云:即蜗牛也。《名医》曰:别出蜗牛条,非。旧作蛞,《说文》所无。据玉篇云:蛞蛞东,知即活东异文,然则当为活。

【今译】

味咸,性寒。

主治虚贼之风,口角歪斜,筋脉突出,脱肛,惊风,癫痫,四肢挛缩。又称为陵蠡。该物生长在池泽中。

99. Kuoyu（蛞蝓，slug，Limax）[1]

[Original Text]

[Kuoyu（蛞蝓，slug，Limax），] salty in taste and cold [in property], [is mainly used] to treat [disease caused by] thief-like wind，distorted mouth，protrusion of sinews，prolapse of anus，convulsion，epilepsy and spasm. [It is also] called Lingli（陵蠡），existing in lakes and swamps.

[Textual Research]

[In the book entitled] *Ming Yi Bie Lu*（《名医别录》，*Special Record of Great Doctors*），[it] says [that Kuoyu（蛞蝓，slug，Limax）is also] called Tuwo（土蜗）and Fuwo（附蜗），existing in large mountains，shady fields and inside sand. [It can be] collected in August.

Notes

1. Kuoyu（蛞蝓，slug，Limax）is an insect medicinal，salty in taste and cold in property，effective in clearing heat，expelling wind，breaking stasis，unobstructing collaterals，removing toxin and resolving swelling. Clinically it is used to treat distorted mouth due to wind stroke，spasm of sinews and vessels，convulsion，epilepsy，panting，throat impediment，amenorrhea，abdominal conglomeration，hemorrhoids，prolapse of anus and abscess.

100. 石龙子

【原文】

味咸,寒。

主五癃,邪结气,破石淋下血,利小便水道。一名蜥易。生川谷。

【考据】

1.《吴普》曰:石龙子,一名守宫,一名石蜴,一名石龙子,(《御览》)。

2.《名医》曰:一名山龙子,一名守宫,一石石蜴,生平阳及荆山石间,五月取着石上令干。

3. 案《说文》云:蜥、虫之蜥易也,易,蜥易,蝘蜓,守宫也,象形,蝘在壁曰蝘蜓,在草曰蜥易,或作蝘,虭、荣虭蛇,医以注鸣者。《广雅》云:蛤蚧,卢蝘,蚵蚘,蜥蝎也。《尔雅》云:蝾螈,蜥蝎,蝘蜓,守宫也。

4.《毛诗》云:胡为虺蜴,《传》云蜴,螈也。陆玑云:虺蜴,一名蝾螈,蜴也,或谓之蛇医,如蜥蜴,青绿色,大如指,形状可恶。方言云:守宫,秦晋西夏谓之守宫,或谓之卢蜥蜓,或谓之蜥易,其在泽中者,谓之易锡,南楚谓之蛇医,或谓之蝾螈,东齐,海岱谓之蝾螈,北燕谓之祝蜓,

100. Shilongzi（石龙子，skink，Eumeces seu Lygosoma）[1]

[Original Text]

[Shilongzi（石龙子，skink，Eumeces seu Lygosoma），] salty in taste and cold [in property]，[is mainly used] to treat five [kinds of] stranguria[2] and stagnation of evil-Qi，to resolve stony stranguria with bleeding，to promote urination and [to unobstruct] waterway [in the body]. [It] exists in mountain valleys and river valleys.

[Textual Research]

[In the book entitled] *Wu Pu Ben Cao*（《吴普本草》，*Wu Pu's Studies of Materia Medica*），[it] says [that] Shilongzi（石龙子，skink，Eumeces seu Lygosoma）[is also] called Shougong（守宫）and Shixi（石蜴）[according to the book entitled] *Tai Ping Yu Lan*（《太平御览》，*Imperial Studies in Taiping Times*）.

[In the book entitled] *Ming Yi Bie Lu*（《名医别录》，*Special Record of Great Doctors*），[it] says [that] Shilongzi（石龙子，skink，Eumeces seu Lygosoma）[is also] called Shougong（守宫）and Shixi（石蜴），existing in the area between Pingyang（平阳）and Jingshan（荆山）. [It can be] collected in May and dried on stones.

Notes

1. Shilongzi（石龙子，skink，Eumeces seu Lygosoma）is an

桂林之中，守宫大者而能鸣，谓之蛤蚧。

【今译】

味咸，性寒。

主治五种癃闭症，邪气结滞，能破除石淋病症下血，能使小便通畅，能通利水道。又称为蜥易。该物生长在山川河谷之中。

insect medicinal, salty in taste and cold in property, entering the kidney meridian, effective in relieving convulsion, breaking stagnation and promoting urination. Clinically it is used to treat epilepsy, scrofula, stony stranguria and mammary cancer.

2. The five kinds of stranguria include heat stranguria, bloody stranguria, stony stranguria, Qi stranguria and paste stranguria.

101. 木虻

【原文】

味苦,平。

主目赤痛,眦伤,泪出,瘀血,血闭,寒热酸惭无子。一名魂常。生川泽。

【考据】

1.《名医》曰:生汉中,五月取。

2. 案《说文》云:虻齧人飞虫。《广雅》云:𧓤𧓤,虻也此省文。《淮南子》齐俗训云:水蚚为蟙蝱。高诱云:青蛉也。又说山训云:虻、散积血。

【今译】

味苦,性平。

主治眼睛红肿疼痛,眼角受伤,泪流不止,瘀血,经闭,寒热酸痛,能治疗不孕之症。又称为魂常。该物生长在山川和平泽之中。

101. Mumang（木虻, gadfly, Diptera） [1]

[Original Text]

[Mumang（木虻, gadfly, Diptera），] bitter in taste and mild [in property], [is mainly used] to treat redness and pain of eyes, injury of canthus with tearing, amenorrhea [due to] blood stasis, cold-heat [disease], severe pain and infertility. [It is also] called Hunchang（魂常）, existing in valleys and swamps.

[Textual Research]

[In the book entitled] *Ming Yi Bie Lu*（《名医别录》, *Special Record of Great Doctors*）, [it] says [that Mumang（木虻, gadfly, Diptera）] exists in Hanzhong（汉中）and [can be] collected in May.

[In] case [analysis in the book entitled] *Shuo Wen*（《说文》, *On Culture*）, [it] says [that Mumang（木虻, gadfly, Diptera) is] a winged insect [that] stings men.

Notes

1. Mumang（木虻, gadfly, Diptera）is an insect medicinal, bitter in taste and slightly cold in property, entering the liver meiridan, effective in expelling blood stasis and resolving abdominal conglomeration. Clinically it is used to treat amenorrhea due to blood stasis, cold-heat disease and traumatic injury.

102. 蜚虻

【原文】

味苦,微寒。

主逐瘀血,破下血积坚痞症瘕,寒热,通利血脉及九窍。生川谷。

【考据】

1.《名医》曰:生江夏,五月取,腹有血者良。

【今译】

味苦,性微寒。

能消除瘀血,能攻破瘀血积滞,坚硬痞块,症瘕及寒热病。能通利血脉及九窍。该物生长在山川河谷之中。

102. Feimang（蜚虻，dun fly，Tabanus） [1]

[Original Text]

[Feimang（蜚虻，dun fly，Tabanus），] bitter in taste and slightly cold [in property], [is mainly used] to expel blood stasis, to break stagnation of blood, hard lump and conglomeration, to treat cold-heat [disease], to unobstruct blood vessels and nine orifices. [It] exists in mountain valleys and river valleys.

[Textual Research]

[In the book entitled] *Ming Yi Bie Lu* （《名医别录》，*Special Record of Great Doctors*）, [it] says [that Feimang（蜚虻，dun fly，Tabanus）] exists in Jiangxia（江夏）and [can be] collected in May. [The one with] blood in the abdomen is better.

Notes

1. Feimang（蜚虻，dun fly，Tabanus）is an insect medicinal, similar to Mumang（木虻，gadfly，Diptera）.

103. 蜚廉

【原文】

味咸,寒。

主血淤,(《御览》引云逐下血),症坚,寒热,破积聚,喉咽痹,内寒,无子。生川泽。

【考据】

1.《吴普》曰:蜚廉虫。神农黄帝云:治妇人寒热(《御览》)。

2.《名医》曰:生晋阳及人家屋间,立秋采。

3. 案《说文》云:蜚,卢蜚也,蜚、臭虫,负蠜也,蠜、目蠜也。《广雅》云:飞蜚,飞蠊也。《尔雅》云:蜚蜱,蠦.郭璞云:即负盘臭虫。《唐本》注云:汉中人食之下气,名曰石美,一名卢蜚,一石负盘,旧作蠊,据刑禼疏引此作廉。

103. Feilian (蜚廉，cockroach，Blatta seu Periplaneta) [1]

[Original Text]

[Feilian（蜚廉，cockroach，Blatta seu Periplaneta），] salty in taste and cold [in property], [is mainly used] to treat blood stasis, hard conglomeration, cold-head [disease], accumulation [of pathogenic factors], internal cold and infertility. [It] exists in valleys and swamps.

[Textual Research]

[In the book entitled] *Wu Pu Ben Cao*（《吴普本草》，*Wu Pu's Studies of Materia Medica*），[it] says [that] Feilian（蜚廉，cockroach，Blatta seu Periplaneta）is a sort of insect. [According to] Agriculture God（神农）and Yellow Emperor（黄帝），[it can be used] to treat cold-heat [disease] in women [as mentioned in the book entitled] *Tai Ping Yu Lan*（《太平御览》，*Imperial Studies in Taiping Times*）.

[In the book entitled] *Ming Yi Bie Lu*（《名医别录》，*Special Record of Great Doctors*），[it] says [that Feilian（蜚廉，cockroach，Blatta seu Periplaneta）] exists in Jinyang（晋阳）and the houses of those who lived there. [It can be] collected in autumn.

871

Notes

1. Feilian（蜚廉，cockroach，Blatta seu Periplaneta）is an insect

【今译】

味咸,性寒。

主治瘀血,症瘕,寒热病,能破解积聚,喉咽痹,能治疗内寒症和不孕之症。该物生长在山川和平泽之中。

medicinal, salty in taste and cold in property, effective in unobstructing vessels and expelling blood stasis. Clinically it is used to treat cold-heat disease, sore-throat, blood stagnation and abdominal lumps.

104. 蟅虫

【原文】

味咸,寒。

主心腹寒热洗洗,血积症瘕,破坚下血闭,生子,尤良。一名地鳖。生川泽。

【考据】

1.《吴普》曰:(蟅虫)虫,一名土鳖(《御览》)。

2.《名医》曰:一名土鳖,生河东及沙中,人家墙壁下,土中湿处,十月暴干。

3. 案《说文》云:蟅虫属鳖,目鳖也。《广雅》云:负鳖,蟅也。《尔雅》云:草虫,负鳖。郭璞云:常羊也。《毛诗》云:喓喓草虫。《传》云:草虫,常羊也。陆玑云:小大长短如蝗也,奇音,青色,好在茅草中。

【今译】

味咸,性寒。

104. Zhechong（蟅虫，ground beetle，Corydiidae）[1]

[Original Text]

［Zhechong（蟅虫，ground beetle，Corydiidae），］salty in taste and cold［in property］，［is mainly used］to treat cold-heat disease in the heart and abdomen with chilliness and shivering［as well as］conglomeration［due to］blood stagnation，and to break obstinate amenorrhea.［It is］more effective［in promoting］conception of baby.［It is also］called Dibie（地鳖），existing in valleys and swamps.

[Textual Research]

［In the book entitled］*Wu Pu Ben Cao*（《吴普本草》，*Wu Pu's Studies of Materia Medica*），［it］says［that］Zhechong（蟅虫，ground beetle，Corydiidae）［is also］called Tubie（土鳖）［according to the book entitled］*Tai Ping Yu Lan*（《太平御览》，*Imperial Studies in Taiping Times*）.

［In the book entitled］*Ming Yi Bie Lu*（《名医别录》，*Special Record of Great Doctors*），［it］says［that Zhechong（蟅虫，ground beetle，Corydiidae）is also］called Tubie（土鳖），existing in the wet soil below the walls of houses in Hedong（河东）and sand.［It can be］collected in October and dried in the sun.

Notes

　　主治心腹部发冷发热,瑟瑟颤栗,血液停滞,症瘕,能破解顽固性经闭,能使人生育子女,疗效甚佳。又称为地鳖。该物生长在山川和平泽之中。

1. Zhechong（蟅虫, ground beetle, Corydiidae）is an insect medicinal, salty in taste and cold and toxic in property, entering the liver meridian, the heart meridian and the spleen meridian, effective in activating the blood and expelling stasis, unobstructing vessels and ceasing pain. Clinically it is used to treat abdominal conglomeration and accumulation, amenorrhea, dysmenorrhea, abdominal pain due to blood stasis after delivery of baby and traumatic injury.

105. 伏翼

【原文】

味咸,平。

主目瞑,明目,夜视有精光。久服,令人喜乐,媚好无忧。一名蝙蝠。生川谷,(旧作禽部,今移)。

【考据】

1.《吴普》曰:伏翼,或生人家屋间,立夏后,阴干。治目冥,令人夜视有光。(艺文类聚)。

2.《名医》曰:生太山,及人家屋间,立夏后采,阴干。

3. 案《说文》云:蝙、蝙蝠也,蝠、蝙蝠,服翼也。《广雅》云,伏翼,飞鼠,仙鼠,吠蠜也。《尔雅》云:蝙蝠服翼。方言云:蝙蝠,自关而东,谓之伏翼,或谓之飞鼠,或谓之老鼠,或谓之仙鼠,自关而西,秦陇之间,谓之蝙蝠,北燕谓之蚊蟙,李当之云:即天鼠。

上虫、鱼,中品一十七种。旧十六种,考禽部伏翼宜入此。

105. Fuyi（伏翼，bat，Vespertilio）[1]

[Original Text]

[Fuyi（伏翼，bat，Vespertilio），] salty in taste and mild [in property], [is mainly used] to treat blurred vision, and to improve vision to see clearly at night. Long-term taking [of it will] enable people to be happy, beautiful and not anxious. [It is also] called Bianfu（蝙蝠），existing in mountain valleys and river valleys.

[Textual Research]

[In the book entitled] *Wu Pu Ben Cao*（《吴普本草》, Wu Pu's Studies of Materia Medica），[it] says [that] Fuyi（伏翼，bat，Vespertilio) may exist in the houses of people's families. [It can be] collected after summer and dried in the shade to treat blurred vision and enable people to see clearly at night.

[In the book entitled] *Ming Yi Bie Lu*（《名医别录》, *Special Record of Great Doctors*），[it] says [that Fuyi（伏翼，bat，Vespertilio)] exists in Taishan（太山）and the houses of people's families. [It can be] collected after the Summer Solstice and dried in the shade.

Notes

1. Fuyi（伏翼，bat，Vespertilio) is a bird medicinal, salty in taste, mild and non-toxic in property, effective in activating the

【今译】

味咸,性平。

主治目光昏暗,能使眼睛明亮,夜视有精光。长期服用,能令人心情愉悦,形象美好,无忧无愁。又称为蝙蝠。该物生长在山川河谷之中。

blood and tonifying the body. Clinically it is used to treat ocular itching and pain, five kinds of stranguria, leucorrhea, chronic cough with upward counterflow of Qi, chronic malaria, scrofula and injury caused by metal.

106. 梅实

【原文】

味酸,平。

主下气,除热,烦满,安心,肢体痛,偏枯不仁,死肌,去青黑志,恶疾。生川谷。

【考据】

1.《吴普》曰:梅实(《大观本草》作核)。明目,益气,(《御览》)不饥(《大观本草》,引吴氏本草)。

2.《名医》曰:生汉中,五月采,火干。

3. 案《说文》云:蔣,干梅之属,或作蔣,某、酸果也,以梅为楠。《尔雅》云:梅楠。郭璞云:似杏实酢,是以某注梅也,《周礼》笾人,馈食,笾、其实干蔣。郑云:干蔣,干梅也,有桃诸梅诸,是其干者。《毛诗》疏云:梅暴为腊,羹臛齑中,人含之以香口(《大观本草》)。

上果,中品一种,旧同。

106. Meishi（梅实，fruit of Japanese apricot，Fructus Mume）[1]

［Original Text］

［Meishi（梅实，fruit of Japanese apricot，Fructus Mume），］sour in taste and mild［in property］，［is mainly used］to descend Qi，to eliminate heat，vexation and fullness，to tranquilize the heart，to treat pain of limbs，hemiplegia，numbness，necrotic muscles，bluish black spots and severe disease.［It］grows in mountain valleys and river valleys.

［Textual Research］

［In the book entitled］*Wu Pu Ben Cao*（《吴普本草》，*Wu Pu's Studies of Materia Medica*），［it］says［that］Meishi（梅实，fruit of Japanese apricot，Fructus Mume）can improve vision，replenish Qi and［enable people to feel］no hunger［according to the book entitled］*Tai Ping Yu Lan*（《太平御览》，*Imperial Studies in Taiping Times*）.

883

［In the book entitled］*Ming Yi Bie Lu*（《名医别录》，*Special Record of Great Doctors*），［it］says［that Meishi（梅实，fruit of Japanese apricot，Fructus Mume）］grows in Hanzhong（汉中）.［It can be］collected in May and dried through fire.

Notes

1. Meishi（梅实，fruit of Japanese apricot，Fructus Mume）is a

【今译】

味酸,性平。

主治能使气下行降逆,能消除热邪,烦躁和郁闷,能安静心情,能治疗肢体疼痛,偏枯不仁,肌肉坏死,能祛除青黑斑痕,能治疗恶疾。该物生长在山川河谷之中。

herbal medicinal, sour in taste, astringent and warm in property, entering the liver meridian, the spleen meridian, the lung meridian and the large intestine meridian, effective in restraining the lung, astringing the intestines, producing fluid and ceasing bleeding. Clinically it is used to treat chronic cough due to lung deficiency, chronic diarrhea, chronic dysentery, vexation and thirst due to deficiency-heat, abdominal pain due to roundworms, retention of roundworms in the biliary tract, hematochezia, hematuria, flooding and spotting (metrostaxis and metrorrhagia).

107. 大豆黄卷

【原文】

味甘,平。

主湿痹,筋挛,膝痛。生大豆,涂痈肿。煮汁,饮,杀鬼毒,止痛,赤小豆。主下水,排痈肿脓血。生平泽。

【考据】

1.《吴普》曰:大豆黄卷,神农黄帝雷公无毒,采无时,去面䵴,得前胡,乌啄,杏子,牡蛎,天雄,鼠屎,共蜜和佳,不欲海藻龙胆,此法,大豆初出黄土芽是也。生大豆,神农岐伯生熟寒,九月采,杀乌豆毒,并不用元参。赤小豆,神农黄帝咸,雷公甘,九月采(《御览》)。

2.《名医》曰:生大山,九月采。

3. 案《说文》云:椒豆也,象豆生之形也。荅,小椒也,藿椒之少也。《广雅》云:大豆,椒也,小豆,荅也,豆角谓之荚,其叶谓之藿。《尔雅》云,戎叔,谓之荏叔,孙炎云大豆也。

107. Dadou Huangjuan（大豆黄卷，soybean sprout，Semen Glycines Siccus）[1]

［**Original Text**］

［Dadou Huangjuan（大豆黄卷，soybean sprout，Semen Glycines Siccus），］sweet in taste ［and］ mild ［in property］；［is mainly used］ to treat dampness impediment，spasm of sinews and pain of the knees. ［Pound］ raw soybean ［can be used］ to treat abscess. To take the decoction ［of soybean can］ eliminate ［pathogenic factors like］ ghost toxin and relieve pain.

Chixiaodu（赤小豆，rice bean，Semen Phaseoli）［can be used to expel dampness by］ discharging water ［through urination］，to eliminate abscess and to purulent blood.

［It］ grows in plains and swamps.

887

［**Textual Research**］

［In the book entitled］ *Wu Pu Ben Cao*（《吴普本草》，*Wu Pu's Studies of Materia Medica*），［it］ says ［that］ Dadou Huangjuan（大豆黄卷，soybean sprout，Semen Glycines Siccus），［according to］ Agriculture God（神农），Yellow Emperor（黄帝）and Leigong（雷公），［is］ non-toxic ［in property］ and ［can be］ collected at any time. ［It can be used］ to eliminate facial black spots together with Xingzi（杏子，apricot fruit；ansu apricot fruit，Fructus Pruni Armeniacae），Muli（牡蛎，oyster shell，Concha Ostreae），Tianxiong

【今译】

味甘,性平。

主治湿邪所致痹证,筋脉挛急,膝部疼痛。

生大豆,捣烂外敷,能消除痈肿。

煮的豆汁,饮用后能杀除鬼怪似的致病毒物,能消除疼痛。

赤小豆,能去除水湿,排除痈肿脓血。该物生长在平川水泽之中。

（天雄，tianxiong conite，Aconiti Radix Lateralis Tianxiong）and Shushi（鼠屎，bat dung，Faeces Vespertilionis）.［According to］Agriculture God（神农）and Qibo（岐伯），ripe raw soybean［can be］collected in September to eliminate toxin in black beans；［according to］Agriculture God（神农）and Yellow Emperor（黄帝），［it is］salty［in tastc］；［according to］Leigong（雷公），［it is］sweet［in taste］and［can be collected in September［as mentioned in the book entitled］*Tai Ping Yu Lan*（《太平御览》，*Imperial Studies in Taiping Times*）.

　　［In the book entitled］*Ming Yi Bie Lu*（《名医别录》，*Special Record of Great Doctors*），［it］says［that Dadou Huangjuan（大豆黄卷，soybean sprout，Semen Glycines Siccus）］grows in large mountains and［can be］collected in September.

Notes

　　1. Dadou Huangjuan（大豆黄卷，soybean sprout，Semen Glycines Siccus）is a herbal medicinal，sweet in taste and mild in property，entering the spleen meridian and the stomach meridian，effective in reliving pathogenic factors in the superficies and expelling dampness-heat. Clinically it is used to treat common cold due to summer-heat dampness，lumps and oppression in the chest，dysuria，edema and dampness impediment.

108. 粟米

【原文】

味咸,微寒。

主养肾气,去胃脾中热,益气。

陈者,味苦,主胃热,消渴,利小便(《大观本草》,作黑字,据《吴普》增)。

【考据】

1.《吴普》曰:陈粟,神农黄帝苦无毒,治脾热,渴,粟养肾气(《御览》)。

2. 案《说文》云:粟、嘉谷实也。孙炎注《尔雅》粢稷云:粟也,今关中人呼小米为粟米,是。

108. Sumi（粟米，foxtail millet seed, Semen Setariae Italicae）[1]

[Original Text]

[Sumi（粟米，foxtail millet seed，Semen Setariae Italicae），] salty in taste and slightly cold [in property], [is mainly used] to nourish kidney-Qi，to eliminate heat in the stomach and spleen，and to replenish Qi.

Old Sumi（粟米，foxtail millet seed，Semen Setariae Italicae）is bitter in taste [and can be used] to relieve heat in the stomach，[to treat] wasting-thirst and to promote urination.

[Textual Research]

[In the book entitled] *Wu Pu Ben Cao*（《吴普本草》，*Wu Pu's Studies of Materia Medica*），[it] says [that] Sumi（粟米，foxtail millet seed，Semen Setariae Italicae），[according to] Agriculture God（神农）and Yellow Emperor（黄帝），[is] bitter in taste and non-toxic [in property]，and [can be used] to relieve heat in the spleen and thirst，and to nourish kidney-Qi [as mentioned in the book entitled] *Tai Ping Yu Lan*（《太平御览》，*Imperial Studies in Taiping Times*）.

Notes

1. Sumi（粟米，foxtail millet seed，Semen Setariae Italicae）is a

【今译】

味咸,性微寒。

能滋养肾气,能祛除胃脾中的热气,能补益精气。

陈旧的,味苦,主治胃热,消渴,能使小便通畅。

herbal medicinal, effective in harmonizing the middle (internal organs), replenishing the kidney, eliminating heat and removing toxin. Clinically it is used to treat deficiency of the spleen and stomach, regurgitation, vomiting, wasting-thirst, diarrhea, dysentery, vexation and depression.

109. 黍米

【原文】

味甘,温。

主益气补中,多热,令人烦(《大观本》,作黑字,据《吴普》增)。

【考据】

1.《吴普》曰:黍,神农甘无毒,七月取,阴干,益中补气。(《御览》)

2.案《说文》云:黍、禾属而粘者,以大暑而种,故谓之黍。孔子曰:黍可为酒,禾入水也。《广雅》云:粢黍稻,其采谓之禾。齐氏要术引记胜之书曰:黍,忌丑,又曰黍,长于巳,壮于酉,生于戌,老于亥,死于丑,恶于丙午,忌于丑寅卯,按黍,即糜之种也。

上米谷,中品三种,旧二种,大小豆为二,无粟米黍米,今增。

【今译】

味甘,性温。

能补益精气,能充实人体内脏,能消除令人烦躁的发热。

109. Shumi（黍米，fruit of broomcorn millet，Fructus Panici Miliacei）[1]

[Original Text]

[Shumi（黍米，fruit of broomcorn millet，Fructus Panici Miliacei），] sweet in taste and warm [in property], [is mainly used to] replenish Qi, to tonify the middle (the internal organs) and [to relieve] excessive heat [that causes] vexation.

[Textual Research]

[In the book entitled] *Wu Pu Ben Cao*（《吴普本草》，*Wu Pu's Studies of Materia Medica*），[it] says [that] Shumi（黍米，fruit of broomcorn millet，Fructus Panici Miliacei），[according to] Agriculture God（神农），[is] sweet [in taste] and non-toxic [in property]. [It can be] collected in July and dried in the shade [for the purpose of] replenishing the middle (the internal organs) and tonifying Qi [as mentioned in the book entitled] *Tai Ping Yu Lan*（《太平御览》，*Imperial Studies in Taiping Times*）.

Notes

1. Shumi（黍米，fruit of broomcorn millet，Fructus Panici Miliacei） is a herbal medicinal, entering the spleen meridian and the stomach meridian, effective in replenishing Qi, tonifying the spleen, harmonizing the stomach and enabling people to sleep peacefully. Clinically it is used to treat regurgitation, vomiting, diarrhea, insomnia, coronary disease, hypertension, dysuria and dysentery.

110. 蓼实

【原文】

味辛,温。

主明目温中,耐风寒,下水气,面目浮肿,痈疡。

马蓼,去肠中蛭虫,轻身。生川泽。

【考据】

1.《吴普》曰,蓼实一名天蓼,一名野蓼,一名泽蓼。(艺文类聚)。

2.《名医》曰:生雷泽。

3. 案《说文》云:蓼、辛菜蔷虞也,蔷,蔷虞,蓼。《广雅》云:荭、茏、蘜、马蓼也。《尔雅》云:蔷虞,蓼。郭璞云:虞蓼,泽蓼,又荭,茏古,其大者,归。

4. 郭璞云:俗呼荭草为茏鼓,语转耳。《毛诗》云:隰有游龙,《传》云:龙,红草也。

5. 陆玑云:一名马蓼,叶大而赤色生水中,高丈余,又以薅杀蓼。《传》云:蓼,水草也。

110. Liaoshi（蓼实，red-knees fruit，Fructus Polygoni Hydropiperis）[1]

[Original Text]

[Liaoshi （蓼实，red-knees fruit，Fructus Polygoni Hydropiperis），] pungent in taste and warm [in property]，[is mainly used] to improve vision，to warm the middle（the internal organs），to resist wind-cold，to purge retention of water，and to relieve facial dropsy and abscess.

Maliao（马蓼，Polygonum Blumei）[can be used] to eliminate Zhichong（蛭虫，Amphibdellatidae）in the intestines and relax the body.

[It] grows in valleys and swamps.

[Textual Research]

[In the book entitled] *Wu Pu Ben Cao* （《吴普本草》，*Wu Pu's Studies of Materia Medica*），[it] says [that] Liaoshi （蓼实，red-knees fruit，Fructus Polygoni Hydropiperis）[is also] called Tianliao（天蓼），Yeliao（野蓼）and Zeliao（泽蓼）.

[In the book entitled] *Ming Yi Bie Lu* （《名医别录》，*Special Record of Great Doctors*），[it] says [that Liaoshi（蓼实，red-knees fruit，Fructus Polygoni Hydropiperis）] grows in Leize（雷泽）.

Lu Ji（陆玑）said，"[It is also] called Maliao（马蓼）. [Its] leaves are large and red，about one *Zhang*（丈）in length，growing

【今译】

味辛,性温。

能使眼睛明亮,能温煦人体脏器,能使人耐受风寒,能祛除水湿,能消解面目浮肿,能治疗痈疡。

马蓼,能去除肠中蛭虫,能使人身体轻盈。该物生长在山川和平泽之中。

in water."

Notes

1. Liaoshi （蓼实, red-knees fruit, Fructus Polygoni Hydropiperis) is a herbal medicinal, pungent in taste and warm in property, entering the spleen meridian and the liver meridian, effective in warming the middle (the internal organs) and promoting urination, breaking stasis and resolving accumulation. Clinically it is used to treat vomiting, diarrhea, abdominal pain, dysentery, dropsy due to retention of water, conglomeration and distension.

111. 葱实

【原文】

味辛,温。

主明目补中不足,其茎可作汤,主伤寒寒热,出汗,中风面目肿。

【考据】

1.《品汇精要》:"味辛,性温,无毒。"

2.《中药志》:"治肾虚阳痿,目眩。"

【今译】

味辛,性温。

能使眼睛明亮,能充实人体内脏,能补益不足。

葱茎可煎煮成汤剂,主治伤寒,寒热病,能使人出汗,能治疗风邪所致疾病及面目浮肿。

111. Congshi（葱实，seed of fistular onion，Semen Allii Fistulosi）[1]

[Original Text]

[Congshi（葱实，seed of fistular onion，Semen Allii Fistulosi），] pungent in taste and warm [in property]，[is mainly used] to improve vision，tonify insufficiency of the middle (the internal organs).

Its stalks can be boiled into decoction for treating cold damage，cold-heat [disease]，inducing sweating and [curing] facial dropsy.

[Textual Research]

[In the book entitled] *Ping Hui Jing Yao*（《品汇精要》，*Collection of the Essentials*），[it] says [that Congshi（葱实，seed of fistular onion，Semen Allii Fistulosi) is] pungent [in taste]，warm and non-toxic [in property]，[can be used] to improve vision and vertigo.

[In the book entitled] *Zhong Yao Zhi*（《中药志》，*History about Materia Medica*），[it] says [that Congshi（葱实，seed of fistular onion，Semen Allii Fistulosi) can] treat kidney deficiency，impotence and blurred vision.

Notes

1. Congshi（葱实，seed of fistular onion，Semen Allii Fistulosi) is a herbal medicinal，entering the liver meridian，the lung meridian and the kidney meridian，effective in harmonizing the five Zang-organs，dispersing heat，relieving stagnation and invigorating Qi. Clinically it is used to treat abscess，ulcer，wasting-thirst，conglomeration，abdominal distension and scrofula.

112. 薤

【原文】

味辛,温。

主金疮,疮败,轻身不饥耐老。生平泽。

【考据】

1.《名医》曰:生鲁山。

2. 案《说文》云薤菜也,叶似韭。《广雅》云:韭、薤、荞,其华谓之菁。《尔雅》云:薤、鸿荟。郭璞云:即薤菜也,又劲山贲。陶宏景云:葱薤异物,而今共条,本经既无韭,以其同类,故也。

【今译】

味辛,性温。

主治因金属创伤所致的痈疮,败疮,能使人身体轻盈,能减少饥饿感,能使人不易衰老。该物生长在平川水泽之中。

112. Xie（薤，bulb of longstamen onion， Bulbus Allii Macrostemi） [1]

［Original Text］

［Xie（薤，bulb of longstamen onion， Bulbus Allii Macrostemi），］ pungent in taste and warm ［in property］，［is mainly used］ to treat injury ［caused by］ metal and severe sore， to relax the body，［to make people feel］ no hunger and to prevent aging. ［It］ grows in plains and swamps.

［Textual Research］

［In the book entitled］ *Ming Yi Bie Lu* (《名医别录》，*Special Record of Great Doctors*)，［it］ says ［that Xie（薤，bulb of longstamen onion， Bulbus Allii Macrostemi)］ grows in Lushan（鲁山）.

［In］ case ［analysis in the book entitled］ *Shuo Wen* (《说文》，*On Culture*)，［it］ says ［that］ Xie（薤，bulb of longstamen onion， Bulbus Allii Macrostemi) is vegetable with the leaves like chives.

Notes

1. Xie（薤，bulb of longstamen onion， Bulbus Allii Macrostemi) is a herbal medicinal， pungent and bitter in taste， warm in property， entering the lung meridian， the stomach meridian and the large intestine meridian， effective in regulating Qi， soothing the chest， invigorating Yang and dispersing stagnation. Clinically it is used to treat chest impediment， angina， discomfort of the chest， dry nausea， chronic dysentery， cold diarrhea， gastritis， cough with phlegm and retention of fluid， and pain of the rib-side.

113. 水苏

【原文】

味辛,微温。

主下气,辟口臭,去毒,辟恶。久服,通神明,轻身,耐老。生池泽。

【考据】

1.《吴普》曰:荮蒩一名水苏,一名劳祖(《御览》)。

2.《名医》曰:一名鸡苏,一名劳祖,一名芥蒩,一名芥苴,生九真,七月采。

3. 案《说文》云:苏,桂荏也。《广雅》云:芥蒩,水苏也。《尔雅》云:苏、桂、荏。

郭璞云:苏荏类,故名桂荏。方言云:苏、亦荏也,关之东西或谓之苏或谓之荏,周郑之间,谓之公蒉,沅湘之南,谓之蘸,其小者谓之蘸葇,按蘸葇,即香薷也,亦名香菜,《名医》别出香薷条,非,今紫苏薄荷等,皆苏类也,《名医》俱别出之。

上菜,中品三种,旧四种,考葱实宜与薤同条,今并假苏,宜入草部。

113. Shuisu（水苏，Baikal betony herb，Herba Stachydis Baicalensis）[1]

［Original Text］

［Shuisu（水苏，Baikal betony herb，Herba Stachydis Baicalensis），］pungent in taste and slightly warm［in property］，［is mainly used］to promote Qi to flow downwards，to resolve halitosis，and to remove toxin and filthy［factors］. Long-term taking［of it will］invigorate spirit and mentality，relax the body and prevent aging.［It］grows in lakes and swamps.

［Textual Research］

［In the book entitled］*Wu Pu Ben Cao*（《吴普本草》，*Wu Pu's Studies of Materia Medica*），［it］says［that the so-called Qiaozu（荞苴）refers to Shuisu（水苏，Baikal betony herb，Herba Stachydis Baicalensis），also called Laozu（劳祖）［according to the book entitled］*Tai Ping Yu Lan*（《太平御览》，*Imperial Studies in Taiping Times*）.

［In the book entitled］*Ming Yi Bie Lu*（《名医别录》，*Special Record of Great Doctors*），［it］says［that Shuisu（水苏，Baikal betony herb，Herba Stachydis Baicalensis）is also］called Jisu（鸡苏），Laozu（劳祖），Jiezu（芥苴）and Jieju（芥苴）.［It］grows in Jiuzhen（九真）and［can be］collected in July.

【今译】

味辛,性微温。

能使气下行降逆,能清除口臭,能祛除毒邪,能消除污秽恶臭。长期服用,能使神志清晰,精神旺盛,身体轻盈,不易衰老。该物生长在池泽中。

Notes

1. Shuisu （水 苏，Baikal betony herb，Herba Stachydis Baicalensis）is a herbal medicinal pungent in taste，slightly warm and non-toxic in property，effective in descending Qi and removing toxin. Clinically it is used to treat hematemesis，nosebleed，flooding and spotting （metrostaxis and metrorrhagia），flaccidity of the lung，bloody dysentery，leucorrhea，headache due to wind attack，blurred vision，wind stroke and vaginal bleeding after delivery of baby.

下卷 下品

1. 石灰

【原文】

味辛,温。

主疽疡疥搔,热气恶疮,癞疾,死肌,堕眉,杀痔虫,去黑子息肉。一名恶灰.生山谷。

【考据】

1.《名医》曰:一名希灰,生中山。

2. 按恶灰,疑当为垩灰,希、石、声之缓急。

【今译】

味辛,性温。

主治疽疡,疥疮,瘙痒,热邪所致恶疮,麻风所致肌肉坏死,须眉脱落,能祛除痔疮,能杀除蛲虫,能去除黑痣和息肉。又称为恶灰.该物生于山谷之中。

Volume 3   The Third Grade

1. Shihui（石灰，lime，Limestonum seu Calx）[1]

[Original Text]

[Shihui（石灰，lime，Limestonum seu Calx），] pungent in taste and warm [in property], [is mainly used] to treat scabies，ulcer，itching，severe sore [caused by] heat-Qi，leprosy，necrotic muscles and loss of eyebrow，to eliminate hemorrhoids，to kill worms，and to remove black spots and polypus. [It is also] called E'chen（恶疢），existing in mountains and valleys.

[Textual Research]

[In the book entitled] *Ming Yi Bie Lu*（《名医别录》，*Special Record of Great Doctors*），[it] says [that Shihui（石灰，lime，Limestonum seu Calx）is also] called Xichen（希疢），existing in Zhongshan（中山）.

Notes

1. Shihui（石灰，lime，Limestonum seu Calx）is a mineral medicinal，pungent in taste，warm and toxic in property，effective in removing toxin，ceasing bleeding and restraining activities of certain organs. Clinically it is used to treat scald，bleeding caused by traumatic injury，ulcer in the lower limbs and verruca.

2. 礜石

【考据】

味辛,大热。

主寒热,鼠瘘,蚀疮,死肌,风痹,腹中坚,一名青分石,一名立制石,一名固羊石(《御览》引云:除热,杀百兽,《大观本》,作黑字),出山谷。

【今译】

1.《吴普》曰:白巩石,一名鼠乡,神农岐伯辛有毒,桐君有毒,黄帝甘有毒。

2. 李氏云:或生魏兴,或生少室,十二月采(《御览》引云,一名太白,一名泽乳,一名食盐,又云李氏大寒,主温热)

3.《名医》曰:一名白巩石,一名太白石,一名泽乳,一名食盐,生汉中及少室,采无时。

4. 案《说文》云:巩,毒石也,出汉中。《西山经》云:皋涂之山,有白石焉。其名曰巩,可以毒鼠。《范子计然》云:巩石出汉中,色白者善。《淮南子·地形训》云:白天九百岁生白巩,高诱云:白巩,巩石也。又说林训云:人食巩石而死,蚕食之而肥。高诱云:巩石,出阴山,一曰能杀

2. Yushi（礜石，poisonous ore Arsenopyrite） [1]

［Original Text］

［Yushi（礜石，poisonous ore，Arsenopyrite），］pungent in taste and severe heat［in property］，［is mainly used］to treat cold-heat ［disease］，ulcerated scrofula，ulcerated sore，necrotic muscles，wind impediment and abdominal hardness.［It is also］called Qingfenshi（青分石），Lizhishi（立制石）and Guyangshi（固羊石），existing in mountains and valleys.

［Textual Research］

［In the book entitled］*Wu Pu Ben Cao*（《吴普本草》，*Wu Pu's Studies of Materia Medica*），［it］says［that Yushi（礜石，poisonous ore Arsenopyrite）is also］called Baigongshi（白巩石）and Shuxiang （鼠乡）．［According to］Agriculture God（神农）and Qibo（岐伯），［it is］pungent［in taste］and toxic［in property］；［according to］Tongjun（桐均），［it is］toxic［in property］；［according to］Yellow Emperor（黄帝），［it is］sweet［in taste］and toxic［in property］．

Li's（李氏）said，"［Yushi（礜石，poisonous ore Arsenopyrite）］may be found in Weixing（魏兴）or Shaoshi（少室），and［can be］collected in December."［According to the book entitled］*Tai Ping Yu Lan*（《太平御览》，*Imperial Studies in Taiping Times*），［it is also］called Taibai（太白），Zeru（泽乳）and Shiyan（食盐）．［It］has also mentioned Li's（李氏）［explanation that it is］severe cold

鼠。案《西山经》云：毒鼠，即治鼠瘘也。

【原文】

味辛，性大热。

主治寒热病，瘰疬，蚀疮，肌肉坏死，风痹证，腹中坚硬。又称为青分石，又称为立制石，又称为固羊石，存在于山谷之中。

[in property] and can treat warm-heat [disease].

[In the book entitled] *Ming Yi Bie Lu* (《名医别录》, *Special Record of Great Doctors*), [it] says [that Yushi (礜石, poisonous ore Arsenopyrite) is also] called Baigongshi (白巩石), Taibaishi (太白石), Zeru (泽乳) and Shiyan (食盐), existing in Hanzhong (汉中) and Shaoshi (少室). [It can be] collected at any time.

[In] case [analysis in the book entitled] *Shuo Wen* (《说文》, *On Culture*), [it] says [that] Yushi (礜石, poisonous ore Arsenopyrite) is a poisonous ore and exists in Hanzhong (汉中). [In the book entitled] *Xi Shan Jing* (《西山经》 *Canon about the West Mountain*), [it] says [that] in the mountain in Gaotu (皋涂), there exists Yushi (礜石, poisonous ore Arsenopyrite) [which is] called Gong (巩) and [can be used] to treat ulcerated scrofula. [In the book entitled] *Fan Zi Ji Ran* (《范子计然》, *Studies About Fan Li's Teacher*), [it] says [that] Yushi (礜石, poisonous ore Arsenopyrite) exists in Hanzhong (汉中) and the white one is better.

913

Notes

1. Yushi (礜石, poisonous ore Arsenopyrite) is a mineral medicinal, pungent and sweet in taste, heat and toxic in property, entering the lung meridian and the spleen meridian, effective in resolving accumulation, expelling cold and dampness and killing worms. Clinically it is used to treat wind-dampness impediment and pain, abdominal pain due to hard lumps and coldness, malaria, scrofula, beriberi due to cold-dampness and severe sore and scabies.

3. 铅丹

【原文】

味辛,微寒。

主吐逆胃反,惊痫瘨疾,除热下气,炼化还成九光。久服通神明(《御览》引作吐下,云久服成仙)。生平泽。

【考据】

1.《名医》曰:一名铅华,生蜀郡。

2. 案《说文》云:铅,青金也。陶宏景云:即今熬铅所作黄丹也。

【今译】

味辛,性微寒。

主治呕吐反胃,惊风,癫痫,能消除热邪所致之症,能使气下行降逆。烧炼能使其恢复多种色彩。长期服用能使神志清晰,精神旺盛。该物生存在平川水泽之中。

3. Qiandan（铅丹，red lead，Plumbum Preparatium）[1]

[Original Text]

[Qiandan（铅丹，red lead，Plumbum Preparatium），] pungent in taste and slightly cold [in property], [is mainly used] to treat vomiting, regurgitation, convulsion and epilepsy, to eliminate heat and to descend Qi. [When] burnt and refined, [it will] restore nine [kinds of] brightness. Long-term taking [of it will] invigorate spirit and mentality. [It] exists in plains and swamps.

[Textual Research]

[In the book entitled] *Ming Yi Bie Lu*（《名医别录》, *Special Record of Great Doctors*）, [it] says [that Qiandan（铅丹，red lead，Plumbum Preparatium) is also] called Qianhua（铅华）, existing in Shujun（蜀郡）.

[In] case [analysis in the book entitled] *Shuo Wen*（《说文》, *On Culture*）, [it] says [that] Qiandan（铅丹，red lead，Plumbum Preparatium) is a blue metal. Tao Hongjing（陶宏景）said, "Now Qiandan（铅丹，red lead，Plumbum Preparatium) can be boiled into yellow bolus."

Notes

1. Qiandan（铅丹，red lead，Plumbum Preparatium）is a mineral medicinal, pungent in taste, slightly cold and toxic in property, entering the heart meridian and the liver meridian, effective in removing toxin, promoting the growth of muscles, restraining sores, eliminating dampness, killing worms, stopping itching and ceasing pain. Clinically it is used to treat severe sore, ulcer and abscess, bleeding caused by traumatic injury and scald.

4. 粉锡

【原文】

味辛,寒。

主伏尸毒螫,杀三虫。一名解锡,锡镜鼻。主女子血闭,症瘕,伏肠,绝孕。生山谷(旧作二种,今并)。

【考据】

1.《名医》曰:生桂阳。

2. 案《说文》云:锡银铅之间也。

【今译】

味辛,性寒。

主治形若死尸的病患,毒虫螫伤,能杀死三种寄生虫。又称为解锡,锡镜鼻。主治女子经闭,肠中症瘕,不能怀孕。该物生长在山谷之中。

4. Fenxi（粉锡，white lead，Plumbum Pulveratum）[1]

[Original Text]

[Fenxi（粉锡，white lead，Plumbum Pulveratum），] pungent in taste and cold ［in property］, ［is mainly used］ to treat ［unconsciousness like］ corpse ［caused by］ sting of poisonous insect, and to kill three worms. ［It is also］ called Jiexi（解锡）.

Xijingbi（锡镜鼻，a broken mirror made of copper）［can be used as a medicinal for］ treating amenorrhea, conglomeration in the intestines and infertility.

［It］ exists in mountains and valleys.

[Textual Research]

［In the book entitled］ *Ming Yi Bie Lu*（《名医别录》, *Special Record of Great Doctors*）, ［it］ says ［that Fenxi（粉锡，white lead，Plumbum Pulveratum）］ exists in Guiyang（桂阳）.

［In］ case ［analysis in the book entitled］ *Shuo Wen*（《说文》, *On Culture*）, ［it］ says ［that Fenxi（粉锡，white lead，Plumbum Pulveratum）is made of］ tin, silver and lead.

917

Notes

1. Fenxi（粉锡，white lead，Plumbum Pulveratum）is a mineral medicinal, pungent in taste, cold and toxic in property, entering the kidney meridian, effective in resolving accumulation of pathogenic factors, killing worms, removing toxin, promoting growth of muscles and restoring health. Clinically it is used to treat infantile malnutrition and diarrhea, dysentery, abdominal pain due to retention of worms, conglomeration, malaria, scabies, abscess, ulcer, oral sore, erysipelas and scald.

5. 代赭

【原文】

味苦,寒。

主鬼注,贼风,蛊毒,杀精物恶鬼,腹中毒,邪气,女子赤沃漏下。一名须丸。生山谷。

【考据】

1.《名医》曰:一名血师,生齐国,赤红青色如鸡冠,有泽,染爪甲,不渝者良,采无时。

2. 案《说文》云:赭,赤土也。《北山经》云:少阳之山,其中多美赭。《管子·地数篇》云:山上有赭者,其下有铁。《范子计然》云:石赭出齐郡,赤色者善,蜀赭,出蜀郡。据元和郡县志云:少阳山在交城县,其地近代也。

【今译】

味苦,性寒。

5. Daizhe（代赭，hematite，Haematitum）[1]

[Original Text]

[Daizhe（代赭，hematite，Haematitum），] bitter in taste and cold [in property], [is mainly used] to treat tuberculosis, [disease caused by] thief-like wind, [disease caused by] worm toxin, [disease caused by strange pathogenic factors like] monster and ghost, [disease caused by] toxin and evil-Qi in the abdomen and constant vaginal bleeding. [It is also] called Xuwan（须丸）, existing in mountains and valleys.

[Textual Research]

[In the book entitled] *Ming Yi Bie Lu*（《名医别录》, *Special Record of Great Doctors*）, [it] says [that Daizhe（代赭，hematite, Haematitum）is also called] Xueshi（血师）, existing in Qiguo（齐国）. [It is] red and blue like cockscomb, and [can be] collected at any time.

Notes

1. Daizhe（代赭，hematite，Haematitum）is a mineral medicinal, bitter in taste and cold in property, entering the heart meridian and the liver meridian, effective in pacifying the liver and subduing Yang, descending counterflow of Qi, cooling the blood and ceasing bleeding. Clinically it is used to treat exuberance of

主治鬼怪邪气所致之症，虚邪贼风，虫毒所致之病，能杀除妖精恶鬼似的邪物，能消除腹中毒邪，能治疗女子阴道出血淋漓不断。又称为须丸。该物生长在山谷之中。

liver-fire due to hyperactivity of Yang, vertigo, blurred vision, headache, constant stranguria during flooding and spotting (metrostaxis and metrorrhagia) in women, irregular menstruation, cough and panting.

6. 戎盐

【原文】

味咸,寒,无毒。

主明目。目痛,益气,坚肌骨,去毒蛊。

大盐,胃肠结热,喘逆,胸中病,令人吐(《御览》引云,主肠胃结热,《大观本》,作黑字)。

卤盐,味苦寒,主大热,消渴狂烦,除邪及下蛊毒,柔肌肤(《御览》引云,一名寒石,明目益气)。生池泽(旧作三种,今并)。

【考据】

1.《名医》曰戎盐,一名胡盐,生胡盐山,及西羌,北地,酒泉,福禄城东南角,北海青,南海赤,十月采,大盐,生邯郸又河东,卤盐,生河东盐池。

2. 案《说文》云:盐咸也,古者宿沙初作煮海盐,卤,西方咸地也,从西省象盐形,安定有卤县,东方谓之斥,西方谓之卤盐,河东盐池,袤五十一里,广七里,周百十六里。北山经云:景山南望盐贩之泽。郭璞云:即解县盐池也,今在河东猗氏县,案在山西安邑运城。

6. Rongyan（戎盐，halite，Halitum）[1]

[Original Text]

[Rongyan（戎盐，halite，Halitum），] salty in taste，cold and non-toxic [in property]，[is mainly used] to improve vision，to relieve ocular pain，to replenish Qi，to strengthen muscles and bones and to eliminate worm toxin.

Large salt[2] [can be used] to treat [disease caused by] heat binding in the stomach and intestines，panting with dyspnea，disease in the chest [that] leads to vomiting.

Halide salt，bitter in taste and cold [in property]，can treat [disease caused by] severe heat，wasting-thirst with manic vexation，eliminate evil，remove worm toxin and soften muscles. It exists in lakes and swamps.

[Textual Research]

[In the book entitled] *Ming Yi Bie Lu*（《名医别录》，*Special Record of Great Doctors*），[it] says [that] Rongyan（戎盐，halite，Halitum）[is also] called Huyan（胡盐），produced in Huyan（胡盐）mountain，Xiqiang（西羌），Beidi（北地），Jiuquan（酒泉）and southeast in Fulu（福禄）City. [It appears] blue in Beihai（北海，Northern Sea）and red in Nanhai（南海，Southern Sea）. [It can be] collected in October. Large salt is produced in Handan（邯郸）and Hedong（河东）. Halide salt is produced in salt pool in Hedong

【今译】

味咸,性寒,无毒。

能使眼睛明亮,能治疗眼睛肿痛,能补益精气,能坚强肌骨,能祛除毒蛊。

大盐,能治疗胃肠热结,喘息上逆,胸中疾病,能引发呕吐。

卤盐,味苦,性寒,主治身体高热,能治疗消渴,狂躁烦恼,能消除邪气,能祛除虫毒所致之病,能柔和肌肤。该物生长在池泽中。

神农本草经

（河东）.

Notes

1. Rongyan（戎盐，halite，Halitum）is salty in taste and cold in property，entering the heart meridian and the kidney meridian，effective in cooling the blood，promoting urination，relieving inflammation，strengthening the heart and improving vision. Clinically it is used to treat hematuria，bleeding from the tongue，redness，swelling and pain of the eyes，hypertension，rheumatic arthritis and goiter.

7.　白垩

【原文】

味苦，温。

主女子寒热症瘕，月闭，积聚。生山谷。

【考据】

1.《吴普》曰：白垩一名白蟮。（一切经音义）

2.《名医》曰：一名白善，生邯郸，采无时。

3. 案《说文》云：垩，白涂也。《中山经》云：葱聋之山，是多白垩。

【今译】

味苦，性温。

主治女子恶寒发热，症瘕，闭经，积聚。该物生长在山谷之中。

7. Bai'e（白垩，chalk，Calx seu Creta）[1]

[Original Text]

[Bai'e（白垩，chalk，Calx seu Creta），] bitter in taste and warm [in property], [is mainly used] to treat cold-heat [disease] and abdominal conglomeration， amenorrhea and accumulation in women. [It] exists in mountains and valleys.

[Textual Research]

[In the book entitled] *Wu Pu Ben Cao*（《吴普本草》，*Wu Pu's Studies of Materia Medica*），[it] says [that] Bai'e（白垩，chalk，Calx seu Creta）[is also] called Baishan（白蟮）.

[In the book entitled] *Ming Yi Bie Lu*（《名医别录》，*Special Record of Great Doctors*），[it] says [that Bai'e（白垩，chalk，Calx seu Creta）is also] called Baishan（白善），existing in Handan（邯郸）and [can be] collected at any time.

[In the book entitled] *Zhong Shan Jing*（《中山经》，*Central Mountain Canon*），[it] says [that] the mountains in Conglong（葱聋）contain much Bai'e（白垩，chalk，Calx seu Creta）.

Notes

1. Bai'e（白垩，chalk，Calx seu Creta）is a mineral medicinal， entering the spleen meridian， the stomach meridian， the lung meridian and the kidney meridian，effective in tonifying the lung， resolving thirst and clearing heat. Clinically it is used to treat amenorrhea， vulva swelling and pain， vaginal bleeding， diarrhea， dysentery， seminal emission， uterine coldness， infertility， hemorrhoids， hematemesis and abdominal pain.

8. 冬灰

【原文】

味辛,微温。

主黑子,去疣息肉,疽蚀,疥搔。一名藜灰。生川泽。

【考据】

1.《名医》曰:生方谷。

【今译】

味辛,性微温。

主治黑痣,祛除疣子,息肉,能破溃疽疖,能治疗疥疮瘙痒。又称为藜灰。该物生长在山川和平泽之中。

8. Donghui（冬灰，lambsquarters juvenile ash，Cinis Chenopodii Albi Juvenilis）[1]

[Original Text]

［Donghui（冬灰，Cinis Chenopodii Albi Juvenilis; lambsquarters juvenile ash），］pungent in taste and slightly warm ［in property］, ［is mainly used］ to resolve black spots, to eliminate wart and polypus, to treat ulcer, scabies and itching. ［It is also］ called Lihui（藜灰），existing in valleys and swamps.

[Textual Research]

［In the book entitled］ *Ming Yi Bie Lu*（《名医别录》，*Special Record of Great Doctors*），［it］ says ［that Donghui（冬灰，Cinis Chenopodii Albi Juvenilis; lambsquarters juvenile ash）］ exists in Fanggu（方谷）.

Notes

1. Donghui （冬 灰，Cinis Chenopodii Albi Juvenilis; lambsquarters juvenile ash） is a mineral medicinal, effective in ceasing bleeding and removing toxin. Clinically it is used to treat sore, ulcer and necrotic muscles.

9. 青琅玕

【原文】

味辛,平。

主身痒,火疮,痈伤,疥搔,死肌。一名石珠。生平泽。

【考据】

1.《名医》曰:一名青珠,生蜀郡,采无时。

2. 案《说文》云:琅玕似珠者,古文作。禹贡云:雍州贡璆琳琅玕.郑云:琅玕珠也。

上玉石,下品九种,旧十二种,粉锡,锡镜鼻为二,戎盐,大盐,卤盐为非,三考当各为一。

【今译】

味辛,性平。

主治身痒,火烧所致疮疡,感染痈疮,疥疮,瘙痒,肌肉坏死。又称为石珠。该物生长在平川水泽之中。

9. Qinglanggan（青琅玕，rongkol，Acropora pulchra）[1]

〔Original Text〕

〔Qinglanggan（青琅玕，rongkol，Acropora pulchra），〕pungent in taste and mild〔in property〕，〔is mainly used〕to treat itching of the body，scald，abscess，scabies and necrotic muscles.〔It is also〕called Shizhu（石珠），existing in plains and swamps.

〔Textual Research〕

〔In the book entitled〕*Ming Yi Bie Lu*（《名医别录》，*Special Record of Great Doctors*），〔it〕says〔that Qinglanggan（青琅玕，rongkol，Acropora pulchra）is also〕called Qingzhu（青珠）.〔It〕exists in Shujun（蜀郡）and〔can be〕collected at any time.

Notes

1. Qinglanggan（青琅玕，rongkol，Acropora pulchra）is a mineral medicinal，pungent in taste and mild in property，effective in expelling wind and relieving itching，removing toxin and resolving stasis. Clinically it is used to treat tinea tonsure，scabies，abscess，retention of blood stasis and stony stranguria.

10. 附子

【原文】

味辛,温。

主风寒咳逆邪气,温中,金属创伤,破症坚积聚,血瘕,寒湿踒(《御览》作痿)。蹙拘挛,脚痛,不能行步(《御览》引云:为百药之长,《大观本》,作黑字)。生山谷。

【考据】

1.《吴普》曰:附子一名茛,神农辛,岐伯雷公甘有毒,李氏苦有毒,大温,或生广汉,八月采,皮黑肥白(《御览》)。

2.《名医》曰:生楗为及广汉东,月采为附子,春采为乌头(《御览》)。

3. 案《范子计然》云:附子出蜀武都中,白色者善。

【今译】

味辛,性温。

10. Fuzi（附子，aconite，
Radix Aconiti Praeparata）[1]

［Original Text］

［Fuzi（附子，aconite，Radix Aconiti Praeparata），］pungent in taste and warm ［in property］，［is mainly used］ to relieve wind-cold ［syndrome/pattern］ and cough with dyspnea ［caused by］ evil-Qi，to warm the middle，［to heal］ sore ［caused by］ metal，to eliminate obstinate conglomeration，accumulation and scabies，［to treat］ abdominal mass with blood，limp and spasm of legs ［due to］ cold-dampness，inability to walk ［due to］ pain of the feet. ［It］ grows in mountains and valleys.

［Textual Research］

［In the book entitled］ *Wu Pu Ben Cao*（《吴普本草》，*Wu Pu's Studies of Materia Medica*），［it］ says ［that］ Fuzi（附子，aconite，Radix Aconiti Praeparata）［is also］ called Liang（茛）. ［According to］ Agriculture God（神农），［it is］ pungent ［in taste；［according to］ Qibo（岐伯）and Leigong（雷公），［it is］ sweet ［in taste］ and toxic ［in property］；［according to］ Li's（李氏），［it is］ bitter ［in taste］，toxic and quite warm ［in property］. ［It］ may grow in Guanghan（广汉）and ［can be］ collected in August ［according to the book entitled］ *Tai Ping Yu Lan*（《太平御览》，*Imperial Studies in Taiping Times*）.

主治风寒咳嗽气逆,能祛除邪气,能温煦人体脏器,能消除金属创伤,能消散坚硬癌块和体内积聚,能治疗血瘕,寒湿所致腿瘸拘挛,腿脚疼痛,不能行步。该物生长在山谷之中。

[In the book entitled] *Ming Yi Bie Lu* (《名医别录》, *Special Record of Great Doctors*), [it] says [that Fuzi (附子, aconite, Radix Aconiti Praeparata)] grows in Jianwei (犍为) and the east of Guanghan (广汉). [When] collected every month, [it] is Fuzi (附子, aconite, Radix Aconiti Praeparata); [when] collected in spring, [it] is Wutou (乌头, root of Szechwan aconita, Radix Aconiti) [according to the book entitled] *Tai Ping Yu Lan* (《太平御览》, *Imperial Studies in Taiping Times*).

[In the book entitled] *Fan Zi Ji Ran* (《范子计然》, *Studies About Fan Li's Teacher*), [it] says [that] Fuzi (附子, aconite, Radix Aconiti Praeparata) grows in the middle region of Wudu (武都) in Shu (蜀) [State]. The white one is better.

Notes

1. Fuzi (附子, aconite, Radix Aconiti Praeparata) is a herbal medicinal, pungent in taste, heat and toxic in property, entering the heart meridian, the spleen meridian and the kidney meridian, effective in replenishing Yang and tonifying fire, warming the middle (the internal organs) and dispersing cold. Clinically it is used to treat impotence, frequent urination, edema, wind-cold and dampness impediment.

935

11. 乌头

【原文】

味辛,温。

主中风,恶风洗洗,出汗,除寒湿痹,咳逆上气,破积聚,寒热。其汁煎之,名射罔,杀禽兽。一名奚毒,一名即子,一名乌喙。生山谷。

【考据】

1.《吴普》曰:乌头,一名茛,一名千狄,一名毒公,一名卑负(《御览》作果负),一名耿子,神农雷公桐君黄帝甘有毒,正月始生。叶厚、茎方、中空,叶四四相当,与蒿相似。

2. 又云:乌喙,神农雷公桐君黄帝有毒,李氏小寒,十月采,形如乌头,有两岐相合,如乌之喙,名曰乌喙也,所畏恶使,尽与乌头同,一名萴子,一名茛,神农岐伯有大毒,李氏大寒,八月采,阴干。是附子角之大者,畏恶与附子同。(《御览》,《大观本》节文)

3.《名医》曰:生朗陵,正月二月采,阴干,长三寸,已上为天雄。

4. 按《说文》云:萴,乌喙也。《尔雅》云:芨,堇草。郭璞云:即乌头也,江东呼为堇。《范子计然》云:乌头出三辅中,白者善。国语云:骊姬

11. Wutou（乌头，root of Szechwan aconita，Radix Aconiti）[1]

[Original Text]

[Wutou（乌头，root of Szechwan aconita，Radix Aconiti），] pungent in taste and warm [in property], [is mainly used] to treat wind stroke [marked by] aversion to cold with chilliness，shivering and sweating，to eliminate cold-dampness impediment and cough with dyspnea and upward counterflow of Qi，to break accumulation and conglomeration，and [to treat] cold-heat [disease]. Before being decocted，[it is] called Shewang（射罔）and [can be used] to kill birds and beasts. [It is also] called Xidu（奚毒），Jizi（即子）and Wuhui（乌喙），growing in mountains and valleys.

[Textual Research]

[In the book entitled] *Wu Pu Ben Cao*（《吴普本草》，*Wu Pu's Studies of Materia Medica*），[it] says [that] Wutou（乌头，root of Szechwan aconita，Radix Aconiti）[is also] called Lang（莨），Qiandi（千狄），Dugong（毒公），Bifu（卑负）and Gengzi（耿子）. [In the book entitled] *Tai Ping Yu Lan*（《太平御览》，*Imperial Studies in Taiping Times*），[it is also] called Goufu（果负）. [According to] Agriculture God（神农），Leigong（雷公），Tongjun（桐均）and Yellow Emperor（黄帝），[it is] sweet [in taste] and toxic [in property]. [It] begins to sprout in January. [Its] leaves are thick，[its] stalks are square and [its] internal is hallow. [In its structure，] four leaves correspond to each other，similar to artemisia.

置堇于肉。韦昭云：堇，乌头也。《淮南子》主术训云：莫凶于鸡毒。高诱云：鸡毒，乌头也，按鸡毒即奚毒，即子，即荝子侧子也，《名医》别出侧子条，非。

【今译】

味辛，性温。

主治因感受风邪所致病患，恶风颤栗，出汗，能解除寒湿邪气所致痹证，咳嗽，呼吸困难，能破解积聚，能治疗寒热病。乌头的煎汁，名为射罔，可杀死禽兽。又称为奚毒，又称为即子，又称为乌喙。该物生长在山谷之中。

神农本草经

[It] also says, "[According to] Agriculture God（神农），Leigong（雷公），Tongjun（桐均）and Yellow Emperor（黄帝），Wuhui（乌喙）is toxic [in property]; [according to] Li's（李氏），[it is] slightly cold [in property] and [can be] collected in October. [In terms of] structure, [it is] similar to Wutou（乌头，root of Szechwan aconita，Radix Aconiti）. Two stalks are the same, like the beak of a crow. That is why it is called Wuhui（乌喙），[which means the beak of a crow]. Thus [it is] quite the same as Wutou（乌头，root of Szechwan aconita，Radix Aconiti）. [It is also] called Cezi（茡子）and Lang（茛）. [According to] Agriculture God（神农）and Qibo（岐伯），[it is] severely toxic [in property]; [according to] Li's（李氏），[it is] severely cold [in property], and [it can be] collected in August and dried in the shade."

[In the book entitled] *Ming Yi Bie Lu*（《名医别录》，*Special Record of Great Doctors*），[it] says [that Wutou（乌头，root of Szechwan aconita，Radix Aconiti）] grows in Langling（朗陵）. [It can be] collected in January and February, and dried in the shade, about three *Cun*（寸）in length. Above [it] is Tianxiong（天雄，tianxiong conite，Aconiti Radix Lateralis Tianxiong）.

Notes

1. Wutou（乌头，root of Szechwan aconita，Radix Aconiti）is a herbal medicinal，pungent in taste，heat and severely toxic in property，entering the heart meridian and the spleen meridian，effective in expelling wind and dampness，dispersing pathogenic cold and relieving pain. Clinically it is used to treat wind-cold and dampness impediment，paralysis，cold headache，pain of the limbs，coldness and pain in the heart and abdomen，and genital swelling with pus.

12. 天雄

【原文】

味辛,温。

主大风,寒湿痹,沥节痛,拘挛,缓急,破积聚,邪气,金创,强筋骨,轻身健行。一名白幕。(《御览》引云,长阴气,强志,令人武勇,力作不倦,《大观本》,作黑字)生山谷。

【考据】

1.《名医》曰:生少室,二月采根,阴干。

2. 案《广雅》云:蒛,奚毒,附子也,一岁为荝子,二岁为乌喙,三岁为附子,四岁为乌头,五岁为天雄。《淮南子》缪称训云:天雄,乌喙,药之凶毒也,良医以活人。

【今译】

味辛,性温。

主治因重风所致之症,寒湿邪所致痹证,能消解关节游走性疼痛和

12. Tianxiong（天雄，tianxiong conite，Aconiti Radix Lateralis Tianxiong）[1]

[Original Text]

[Tianxiong（天雄，tianxiong conite，Aconiti Radix Lateralis Tianxiong），] pungent in taste and warm [in property]，[is mainly used] to treat great wind[2]，cold-dampness impediment，acute arthralgia and spasm or flaccidity of joints，to break accumulation and conglomeration，[to eliminate] evil-Qi，[to cure] sore [caused by injury of] metal，to strengthen sinews and bones，to relax the body and [to enable people] to walk sturdily. [It is also] called Baimu（白幕），growing in mountains and valleys.

[Textual Research]

[In the book entitled] *Ming Yi Bie Lu*（《名医别录》，*Special Record of Great Doctors*），[it] says [that Tianxiong（天雄，tianxiong conite，Aconiti Radix Lateralis Tianxiong）] grows in Shaoshi（少室）. [Its] root [can be] collected in February and dried in the shade.

[In the book entitled] *Guang Ya*（《广雅》，*The First Chinese Encyclopedic Dictionary*），[it] says [that the so-called] Xidu（奚毒） refers to Fuzi（附子，aconite，Radix Aconiti Praeparata）. [When it has grown for] one year，[it is] Cezi（萴子）；[when it has grown for] two years，[it is] Wuhui（乌喙）；[when it has grown for] three

拘挛,能使挛拘的筋脉舒畅正常,能破解积聚和邪气,能治疗金属创伤,能强健筋骨,能使人身体轻盈,行走有力。又称为白幕。该物生长在山谷之中。

years, [it is] Fuzi (附子, aconite, Radix Aconiti Praeparata); [when it has grown for] four years, [it is] Wutou (乌头, root of Szechwan aconita, Radix Aconiti); [when it has grown for] five years, [it is] Tianxiong (天雄, tianxiong conite, Aconiti Radix Lateralis Tianxiong).

Notes

1. Tianxiong (天雄, tianxiong conite, Aconiti Radix Lateralis Tianxiong) is a herbal medicinal, pungent in taste, warm and severely toxic in property, effective in dispersing pathogenic cold, expelling wind and dampness, regulating vessels, replenishing essence, improving vision, unobstructing the nine orifices and relieving pain. Clinically it is used to treat leprosy, wind-dampness impediment, spasm and pain of joints, flaccidity of limbs, abdominal mass and conglomeration, sweating and sores.

2. Great wind means disease caused by pathogenic wind or leprosy.

13. 半夏

【原文】

味辛,平。

主伤寒,寒热,心下坚,下气,喉咽肿痛,头眩胸张,咳逆肠鸣,止汗。一名地文,一名水玉(已上八字,元本黑字)。生川谷。

【考据】

1.《吴普》曰:半夏一名和姑,生微邱,或生野中,叶三三相偶,二月始生,白华员上(《御览》)。

2.《名医》曰:一名示姑,生槐里,五月、八月,采根暴干。

3. 案月令云:二月半夏生。《范子计然》云:半夏出三辅,色白者善。《列仙传》云:赤松子服水玉以教神农,疑即半夏别名。

【今译】

味辛,性平。

13. Banxia（半夏，pinellia，Rhizoma Pinelliae）[1]

［Original Text］

［Banxia（半夏，pinellia，Rhizoma Pinelliae），］pungent in taste and mild［in property］，［is mainly used］to treat cold damage，cold-heat［disease］and lumps below the heart，［to promote］Qi to flow downwards，［to treat］swelling and pain of the throat，vertigo，chest distension，cough with dyspnea and borborygmus，and to stop sweating.［It is also］called Diwen（地文）and Shuiyu（水玉），growing in mountain valleys and river valleys.

［Textual Research］

［In the book entitled］*Wu Pu Ben Cao*（《吴普本草》，*Wu Pu's Studies of Materia Medica*），［it］says［that］Banxia（半夏，pinellia，Rhizoma Pinelliae）［is also］called Hegu（和姑），growing in Weiqiu（微邱）or in the wild lands.［In terms of its］leaves，three correspond to three.［It］begins to sprout in February with white flowers on the top［according to the book entitled］*Tai Ping Yu Lan*（《太平御览》，*Imperial Studies in Taiping Times*）.

［In the book entitled］*Ming Yi Bie Lu*（《名医别录》，*Special Record of Great Doctors*），［it］says［that Banxia（半夏，pinellia，Rhizoma Pinelliae）is also］called Shigu（示姑），growing in Kuili（槐里）.［Its］root［can be］collected in May and August，and dried in the sun.

　　主治伤寒病，寒热病，心下坚硬，能使气下行降逆，能治疗喉咽肿痛，头目眩晕，胸部胀满，咳嗽气逆，肠鸣，能止汗。又称为地文，又称为水玉。该物生长在山川河谷之中。

Yue Ling （月令） said, "Banxia （半夏, pinellia, Rhizoma Pinelliae) begins to grow in February." [In the book entitled] *Fan Zi Ji Ran* （《范子计然》, *Studies About Fan Li's Teacher*), [it] says [that] Banxia （半夏, pinellia, Rhizoma Pinelliae) grows in the three places and the white one is better.

Notes

1. Banxia （半夏, pinellia, Rhizoma Pinelliae） is a herbal medicinal, pungent in taste, warm and toxic in property, entering the spleen meridian and the stomach meridian, effective in drying dampness and resolving phlegm, reducing counterflow and stopping vomiting, relieving mass and dispersing bind. Clinically it is used to treat retention of phlegm, cough and panting, stagnation of phlegm and headache, vertigo and insomnia, vomiting and nausea, regurgitation and mass in the chest, depression, scabies and abscess.

14. 虎掌

【原文】

味苦,温。

主心痛,寒热,结气,积聚,伏梁,伤筋,痿,拘缓,利水道。生山谷。

【考据】

1.《吴普》曰:虎掌,神农雷公苦无毒,岐伯桐君辛有毒,立秋九月采之(《御览》引云,或生太山,或宛朐)。

2.《名医》曰:生汉中及宛句,二月、八月采,阴干。

3. 案《广雅》云:虎掌,瓜属也。

14. Huzhang（虎掌，root or herb of brooklet anemone，Radix seu Herba Anemones Rivularis）[1]

[Original Text]

[Huzhang（虎掌，root or herb of brooklet anemone，Radix seu Herba Anemones Rivularis），] bitter in taste and warm [in property]，[is mainly used] to treat heartache，cold-heat [disease]，binding of Qi，accumulation and conglomeration，visceral lump，damage of sinews，flaccidity and spasm，and to disinhibit waterway [in the body]. [It] grows in mountains and valleys.

[Textual Research]

[In the book entitled] *Wu Pu Ben Cao*（《吴普本草》，*Wu Pu's Studies of Materia Medica*），[it] says [that] Huzhang（虎掌，root or herb of brooklet anemone，Radix seu Herba Anemones Rivularis），[according to] Agriculture God（神农）and Leigong（雷公），[is] bitter [in taste] and non-toxic [in property]；[according to] Qibo（岐伯）and Tongjun（桐均），[it is] pungent [in taste] and toxic [in property]，and [can be] collected in September. [According to the book entitled] *Tai Ping Yu Lan*（《太平御览》，*Imperial Studies in Taiping Times*），[it] may grow in Taishan（太山）or Wanqu（宛朐）.

[In the book entitled] *Ming Yi Bie Lu*（《名医别录》，*Special Record of Great Doctors*），[it] says [that Huzhang（虎掌，root or

949

【今译】

味苦,性温。

主治心痛,寒热病,气机结滞,病邪积聚,腹部硬块,筋脉受伤,瘰痹证,能使拘急和缓,能通利水道。该物生长在山谷之中。

herb of brooklet anemone，Radix seu Herba Anemones Rivularis)〕 grows in Hanzhong（汉中）and Yuanju（冤句）.〔It can be〕collected in February and August，and dried in the shade.

〔In the book entitled〕*Guang Ya*（《广雅》，*The First Chinese Encyclopedic Dictionary*），〔it〕says〔that〕Huzhang（虎掌，root or herb of brooklet anemone，Radix seu Herba Anemones Rivularis) belongs to melon.

Notes

1. Huzhang（虎掌，root or herb of brooklet anemone，Radix seu Herba Anemones Rivularis) is a herbal medicinal，bitter and pungent in taste，warm and toxic in property，entering the liver meridian，the lung meridian and the spleen meridian，effective in drying dampness and resolving phlegm，expelling wind and relieving fright，resolving swelling and dispersing binding. Clinically it is used to treat wind stroke with stagnation of phlegm，distorted face and eyes，paralysis，vertigo，epilepsy，convulsion，tetanus and cough and panting due to phlegm and dampness.

15. 鸢尾

【原文】

味苦,平。

主蛊毒邪气,鬼注,诸毒,破症瘕积聚,去水,下三虫。生山谷。

【考据】

1.《吴普》曰:鸢尾,治蛊毒(《御览》)。

2.《名医》曰:一名乌园,生九疑山,五月采。

3. 案《广雅》云:鸢尾,乌蓬,射干也(疑当作鸢尾乌园也,乌蓬射干也,是二物)。《唐本》注云:与射干全别。

952

15. Yuanwei (鸢尾, rhizome of roof iris, Rhizoma Iridis Tectori) [1]

[Original Text]

[Yuanwei （鸢尾, rhizome of roof iris, Rhizoma Iridis Tectori）,] bitter in taste and mild [in property], [is mainly used] to treat [disease caused by] worm toxin and evil-Qi and tuberculosis [caused by] various toxin like ghost, to break abdominal lumps, accumulation and conglomeration, to eliminate dampness and to remove three worms. [It] grows in mountains and valleys.

[Textual Research]

[In the book entitled] *Wu Pu Ben Cao* （《吴普本草》, *Wu Pu's Studies of Materia Medica*）, [it] says [that] Yuanwei （鸢尾, rhizome of roof iris, Rhizoma Iridis Tectori） can treat [disease caused by] worm toxin [according to the book entitled] *Tai Ping Yu Lan* （《太平御览》, *Imperial Studies in Taiping Times*）.

[In the book entitled] *Ming Yi Bie Lu* （《名医别录》, *Special Record of Great Doctors*）, [it] says [that Yuanwei （鸢尾, rhizome of roof iris, Rhizoma Iridis Tectori） is also] called Wuyuan （乌园）, growing in Jiuyishan （九疑山）. [It can be] collected in May.

【今译】

味苦,性平。

主治虫毒所致之病,鬼怪之邪所致之症,能消解各种毒邪,能破除症瘕积聚,能消除水湿,能祛除三种虫子。该物生长在山谷之中。

Notes

1. Yuanwei （鸢尾, rhizome of roof iris, Rhizoma Iridis Tectori) is a herbal medicinal, bitter and pungent in taste, cold and slightly toxic in property, effective in activating the blood and reducing stasis, relieving dampness and resolving accumulation, removing toxin and expelling wind. Clinically it is used to treat traumatic injury, wind-dampness impediment and pain, abdominal mass and conglomeration, abdominal pain due to indigestion and difficulty in urination and defecation.

16. 大黄

【原文】

味苦，寒。

主下瘀血，血闭，寒热，破症瘕积聚，留饮，宿食，荡涤肠胃，推陈致新，通利水谷（《御览》，此下有道字），调中化食，安和五脏。生山谷。

【考据】

1.《吴普》曰：大黄一名黄良，一名火参，一名肤如，神农雷公苦有毒，扁鹊苦无毒，李氏小寒，为中将军，或生蜀郡，北部，或陇西，二月花生，生黄赤叶，四四相当，黄茎高三尺许，三月华黄，五月实黑，三月采根，根有黄汁，切，阴干。（《御览》）

2.《名医》曰：一名黄良，生河西及陇西，二月八月采根，火干。

3. 案《广雅》云：黄良大黄也。

【今译】

味苦，性寒。

能排出瘀血，能治疗闭经，寒热病，能破解症瘕积聚，水饮停滞，

16. Dahuang（大黄，rhubarb，
Radix et Rhizoma Rhei） [1]

[Original Text]

［Dahuang（大黄，rhubarb，Radix et Rhizoma Rhei），］ bitter in taste and cold ［in property］，［is mainly used］ to treat blood stasis，amenorrhea and cold-head ［disease］，to purge abdominal mass，conglomeration and accumulation，retention of fluid and indigestion，to activate the intestines and stomach，to bring forth the new by reducing the old，to unobstruct and disinhibit water and food，to regulate the middle（the internal organs），to digest food，and to harmonize the five Zang-organs. ［It］ grows in mountains and valleys.

957

[Textual Research]

［In the book entitled］ *Wu Pu Ben Cao* （《吴普本草》，*Wu Pu's Studies of Materia Medica* ），［it］ says ［that］ Dahuang （大黄，rhubarb，Radix et Rhizoma Rhei）［is also］ called Huangliang（黄良），Huoshen（火参）and Furu（肤如）. ［According to］ Agriculture God（神农）and Leigong（雷公），［it is］ bitter ［in taste］ and toxic ［in property］；［according to］ Bianque（扁鹊），［it is］ bitter ［in taste］ and non-toxic ［in property］；［according to］ Li's（李氏），［it is］ slightly cold ［in property］. ［It］ may grow in the north of Shujun （蜀郡）or Longxi（陇西）. ［In］ February，［it begins］ to blossom

饮食不化,能荡涤肠胃,能清除人体中的糟粕,能纳入新的营养之物,能通利水谷,能调理内脏以消化饮食,能安和五脏。该物生长在山谷之中。

with yellow and red leaves, four corresponding to four; [its] yellow stalks are about three *Chi*（尺）in length; [in] March, [its] flowers become yellow; [in] May, [its] fruits become black; [in] March, [its] root with yellow juice [can be] collected, cut and dried in the shade [according to the book entitled] *Tai Ping Yu Lan*（《太平御览》, *Imperial Studies in Taiping Times*).

[In the book entitled] *Ming Yi Bie Lu*（《名医别录》, *Special Record of Great Doctors*）, [it] says [that Dahuang（大黄, rhubarb, Radix et Rhizoma Rhei) is also] called Huangliang（黄良）, growing in Hexi（河西）and Longxi（陇西）. [Its] root [can be] collected in February and August, and dried through fire.

[In the book entitled] *Guang Ya*（《广雅》, *The First Chinese Encyclopedic Dictionary*）, [it] says [that] Huangliang（黄良）refers to Dahuang（大黄, rhubarb, Radix et Rhizoma Rhei）.

Notes

1. Dahuang（大黄, rhubarb, Radix et Rhizoma Rhei）is a herbal medicinal, bitter in taste and cold in property, entering the stomach meridian, the large intestine meridian and the liver meridian, effective in purging heat toxin, removing stagnation and accumulation and reducing blood stasis. Clinically it is used to treat constipation, delirium, indigestion, diarrhea, dysentery, jaundice, stranguria, redness and pain of the eyes, hematemesis, nosebleed and hematochezia.

17. 亭历（旧作葶苈,《御览》作亭历）

【原文】

味辛,寒。

主症瘕积聚,结气,饮食寒热,破坚逐邪,通利水道。一名大室,一名大适。生平泽,及田野。

【考据】

1.《名医》曰:一名下历,一名蒿,生藁城,立夏后,采实阴干,得酒良。

2. 案《说文》云:草亭历也。《广雅》云:狗荠,大室,亭苈也。《尔雅》云:草,亭历。郭璞云:实叶皆似芥。《淮南子》缪称训云:亭历愈张。西京杂记云:亭历死于盛夏。

【今译】

味辛,性寒。

17. Tingli（亭历，pepperweed seed，fixweed transymustard seed，Semen Lepidii seu Descurainiae）[1]

[Original Text]

[Tingli（亭历，pepperweed seed，fixweed transymustard seed，Semen Lepidii seu Descurainiae），] pungent in taste and cold [in property]， [is mainly used] to treat abdominal mass，conglomeration and accumulation with Qi stagnation and [disease caused by poor] diet and [invasion of] cold-heat，to break hardness，to expel [pathogenic factors] and to unobstruct waterway [in the body]. [It is also] called Dashi（大室）and Dashi（大适）. [It] grows in plains，swamps and fields.

[Textual Research]

[In the book entitled] *Ming Yi Bie Lu*（《名医别录》，*Special Record of Great Doctors*），[it] says [that Tingli（亭历，pepperweed seed，fixweed transymustard seed，Semen Lepidii seu Descurainiae）is also] called Xiali（下历）and Hao（蒿），growing in Gaocheng（藁城）. After the Summer Solstice，[it can be] collected，dried in the shade and used together with wine.

[In the book entitled] *Guang Ya*（《广雅》，*The First Chinese Encyclopedic Dictionary*），[it] says [that Tingli（亭历，Semen Lepidii seu Descurainiae；pepperweed seed；fixweed transymustard seed）is also] called Gouqi（狗荠），Dashi（大室）and Tingli（亭苈）.

　　主治症瘕积聚，气结，因饮食不当而造成的发冷发热，能破除坚固邪气，能通利水道。又称为大室，又称为大适。该物生长在平川水泽之中及田野里。

Guo Pu (郭璞) said, "[Its] leaves look like [that of] mustard." [In the book entitled] *Huai Nan Zi* (《淮南子》, *A Philosophy Book Compiled by Liu An, King in Huainan*), [it] says [that according to the book entitled] *Xi Jing Zha Ji* (《西京杂记》, *Miscellanea about Xijing*), Tingli (亭历, pepperweed seed, fixweed transymustard seed, Semen Lepidii seu Descurainiae) dies in the height of summer.

Notes

1. Tingli (亭历, pepperweed seed, fixweed transymustard seed, Semen Lepidii seu Descurainiae), also called Tinglizi (葶苈子), is a herbal medicinal, pungent and bitter in taste, cold in property, entering the lung meridian, the heart meridian, the liver meridian, the stomach meridian and the bladder meridian, effective in clearing heat, digesting food, purging the lung, descending Qi, expelling phlegm, resolving swelling and promoting urination. Clinically it is used to treat abdominal distension, mass, conglomeration and accumulation, retention of fluid in the chest and abdomen, edema, lung abscess, dysuria, panting due to exhaustion of the heart, tuberculosis and scrofula.

18. 桔梗

【原文】

味辛,微温。

主胸胁痛如刀刺,腹满,肠鸣,幽幽惊恐悸气(《御览》引云:一名利如,《大观本》,作黑字)。生山谷。

【考据】

1.《吴普》曰:桔梗,一名符扈,一名白药,一名利如,一名梗草,一名卢如,神农医和苦无毒,扁鹊黄帝咸,岐伯雷公甘无毒,李氏大寒,叶如荠苨,茎如笔管,紫赤,二月生(《御览》)。

2.《名医》曰:一名利如,一名房图,一名白药,一名梗草,一名荠苨,生蒿高及冤句,二八月采根,暴干。

3. 案《说文》云:桔,桔梗,药名。《广雅》云:犁如。桔梗也。战国策云:今求柴胡,及之睾黍梁父之阴,则郤车而载耳。桔梗于沮泽,则累世不得一焉。

4.《尔雅》云:苨,菧苨。郭璞云:荠苨。据《名医》云是此别名,下又出荠苨条,非,然陶宏景亦别为二矣。

18. Jiegeng（桔梗，platycodon grandiflorum, Radix Platycodi）[1]

［Original Text］

［Jiegeng（桔梗，platycodon grandiflorum，Radix Platycodi），］pungent in taste and slightly warm ［in property］，［is mainly used］to treat pain of the chest and rib-side like being stabbed by knife，abdominal fullness，borborygum like deer crying，terror and palpitation. ［It］grows in mountains and valleys.

［Textual Research］

［In the book entitled］ *Wu Pu Ben Cao*（《吴普本草》，*Wu Pu's Studies of Materia Medica*），［it］says ［that］Jiegeng（桔梗，platycodon grandiflorum，Radix Platycodi）［is also］called Fuhu（符扈），Baiyao（白药），Liru（利如），Gengcao（梗草）and Luru（卢如）. ［According to］Agriculture God（神农）and Yihe（医和），［it is］bitter ［in taste］and non-toxic ［in property］；［according to］Bianque（扁鹊）and Yellow Emperor（黄帝），［it is］salty ［in taste］；［according to］Qibo（岐伯）and Leigong（雷公），［it is］sweet ［in taste］and non-toxic ［in property］；［according to］Li's（李氏），［it is］severely cold ［in property］. ［Its］leaves are like Jini（荠苨，Adenophora trachelioides），［its］stalks are like the brush tube，purple and red. ［It can be］collected in February ［according to the book entitled］ *Tai Ping Yu Lan*（《太平御览》，*Imperial*

【今译】

味辛，性微温。

主治胸胁痛如刀刺，腹部胀满，肠鸣幽幽，惊恐心慌。该物生长在山谷之中。

Studies in Taiping Times).

[In the book entitled] *Ming Yi Bie Lu* (《名医别录》, *Special Record of Great Doctors*), [it] says [that Jiegeng (桔梗, platycodon grandiflorum, Radix Platycodi) is also] called Liru (利如), Fangtu (房图), Baiyao (白药), Gengcao (梗草) and Jini (荠苨), growing in Haogao (蒿高) and Yuanju (冤句). [Its] root [can be] collected in February and August, and dried in the sun.

[In] case [analysis in the book entitled] *Shuo Wen* (《说文》, *On Culture*), [it] says [that the so-called] Jie (桔) is the medicinal name of Jiegeng (桔梗, platycodon grandiflorum, Radix Platycodi). [In the book entitled] *Guang Ya* (《广雅》, *The First Chinese Encyclopedic Dictionary*), [it] says [that the so-called] Liru (犁如) refers to Jiegeng (桔梗, platycodon grandiflorum, Radix Platycodi).

Notes

1. Jiegeng (桔梗, platycodon grandiflorum, Radix Platycodi) is a herbal medicinal, bitter and pungent in taste, mild in property, entering the lung meridian, effective in diffusing the lung, expelling phlegm, disinhibiting the throat and eliminating pus. Clinically it is used to treat cough, excessive phlegm, sore-throat, chest fullness with lump and oppression, lung abscess and vomiting with pus and blood.

19. 莨荡子

【原文】

味苦,寒。

主齿痛出虫,肉痹,拘急,使人健行,见鬼,多食令人狂走。久服轻身,走及奔马,强志益力通神。一名横唐。生川谷。

【考据】

1.《名医》曰:一名行唐,生海滨,及雍州,五月采子。

2. 案《广雅》云:蒁萍,荡蕳也。陶宏景云:今方家多作狼蓎,旧作蓎。案《说文》无蓎蕳字。《史记·淳于意传》云:灾川王美人怀子而不乳,引以莨荡药一撮,本草图经引,作浪荡,是。

【今译】

味苦,性寒。

主治牙齿疼痛并有虫子出现,肌肉麻木不仁且拘急,多服用则使人

19. Langdangzi（莨荡子，seed of black henbane，Semen Hyoscyami Nigri）[1]

[Original Text]

[Langdangzi（莨荡子，seed of black henbane，Semen Hyoscyami Nigri），] bitter in taste and cold [in property], [is mainly used] to treat toothache with worms and muscle impediment with spasm，and to enable people to walk sturdily with visual hallucination. Excessive taking [of it will] make people run about wildly. Long-term taking [of it will] relax the body，run like gallant horse，strengthen memory，replenish Qi and invigorate spirit. [It is] also called Hengtang（横唐）. [It] grows in mountain valleys and river valleys.

969

[Textual Research]

[In the book entitled] *Ming Yi Bie Lu*（《名医别录》，*Special Record of Great Doctors*），[it] says [that Langdangzi（莨荡子，seed of black henbane，Semen Hyoscyami Nigri）is also] called Xingtang（行唐），growing in Haibin（海滨）and Yongzhou（雍州）. [Its] seeds [can be] collected in May.

Notes

1. Langdangzi（莨荡子，seed of black henbane，Semen Hyoscyami Nigri）is a herbal medicinal，bitter in taste，warm and

如见鬼怪一样疯狂,用量过大则使人狂奔乱跑。长期服用,能使人身体轻盈,奔跑时像奔驰的骏马一样,能增强记忆力,能补益气力,能通畅神气。又称为横唐。该物生长在山川河谷之中。

severely toxic in property, entering the lung meridian and the liver meridian, effective in relieving convulsion, ceasing pain, resolving epilepsy and panting, and stopping diarrhea. Clinically it is used to treat epilepsy, mania, pain in the gastric region, asthma and chronic diarrhea.

20. 草蒿

神农本草经

【原文】

味苦,寒。

主疥搔,痂痒,恶疮,杀虫,留热在骨节间。明目。一名青蒿,一名方溃。生川泽。

【考据】

1.《名医》曰:生华阴。

2. 案《说文》云:蒿,菣也,菣,香蒿也,或作莖。《尔雅》云:蒿菣。郭璞云:今人呼青蒿香中炙啖者为菣,《史记·司马相如传》,菴䕲。注《汉书音义》曰:菴䕲,蒿也。陶宏景云:即今青蒿。

【今译】

味苦,性寒。

主治疥疮瘑痒,恶性疮,能杀虱子,能消除在骨节间的体内郁热,能使眼睛明亮。又称为青蒿,又称为方溃。该物生长在山川和平泽之中。

20. Caohao（草蒿，sweet wormwood herb，Herba Artemisiae Annuae）[1]

［Original Text］

［Caohao（草蒿，sweet wormwood herb，Herba Artemisiae Annuae），］ bitter in taste and cold ［in property］，［is mainly used］ to treat scabies，itching，crust and severe sore，to kill worms and to relieve bone steaming with heat in the joints. ［It is also］ called Qinghao（青蒿）and Fangkui（方溃），growing in valleys and swamps.

［Textual Research］

［In the book entitled］ *Ming Yi Bie Lu*（《名医别录》，*Special Record of Great Doctors*），［it］ says ［that Caohao（草蒿，sweet wormwood herb，Herba Artemisiae Annuae）］ grows in Huayin（华阴）.

Notes

1. Caohao（草蒿，sweet wormwood herb，Herba Artemisiae Annuae）is a herbal medicinal，bitter in taste and cold in property，entering the liver meridian and the gallbladder meridian，effective in clearing summer-heat，expelling malaria and killing worms. Clinically it is used to treat common cold，summer-heat attack，low fever in the late period of warm disease，tidal fever in tuberculosis and low fever without clear causes.

21. 旋复花

【原文】

味咸,温。

主结气,胁下满,惊悸,除水,去五脏间寒热,补中下气。一名金沸草,一名盛椹。生川谷。

【考据】

1.《名医》曰:一名戴椹,生平泽,五月采花,日干,二十日成。

2. 案《说文》云:蕧,盗庚也。《尔雅》云:蕧盗庚:郭璞云:旋复似菊。

【今译】

味咸,性温。

21. Xuanfuhua（旋复花，Inula flower，Flos Inula Japonica）[1]

[Original Text]

[Xuanfuhua（旋复花，Inula flower，Flos Inula Japonica），] salty in taste and warm [in property]，[is mainly used] to treat stagnation of Qi，fullness below rib-side，convulsion and palpitation，to expel water and to eliminate cold-heat in the five Zang-organs，to tonify the middle（the internal organs）and to descend Qi. [It is also] called Jinfeicao（金沸草）and Shengzhen（盛椹），growing in mountain valleys and river valleys.

[Textual Research]

[In the book entitled] *Ming Yi Bie Lu*（《名医别录》，*Special Record of Great Doctors*），[it] says [that Xuanfuhua（旋复花，Inula flower，Flos Inula Japonica）is also] called Daizhen（戴椹），growing in lakes and pools. [Its] flowers [can be] collected in May and dried in the sun for twenty days.

[In] case [analysis in the book entitled] *Shuo Wen*（《说文》，*On Culture*），[it] says [that] Xuanfuhua（旋复花，Inula flower，Flos Inula Japonica）[is also] called Daogeng（盗庚）. Guo Pu（郭璞）said，"Xuanfuhua（旋复花，Inula flower，Flos Inula Japonica）looks like chrysanthemums."

主治气结，胁下胀满，惊风，心悸，能消除体内水湿，能祛除五脏间寒热，能充实人体内脏，能使气下行降逆。又称为金沸草，又称为盛椹。

该物生长在山川河谷之中。

Notes

1. Xuanfuhua（旋复花，Inula flower，Flos Inula Japonica）is a herbal medicinal，bitter，salty and pungent in taste，slightly warm in property，entering the lung meridian，the liver meridian and the stomach meridian，effective in resolving phlegm，relieving panting，tonifying the middle（the internal organs），disinhibiting the intestines and descending counterflow of Qi. Clinically it is used to treat cough and panting with excessive phlegm，hiccup，vomiting，edema，distension and fullness below the rib-side，palpation，convulsion，headache due to wind attack，nebula，dysuria and toothache.

22. 藜芦（《御览》作梨芦）

【原文】

味辛,寒。

主蛊毒,咳逆,泄利,肠澼,头疡,疥搔,恶疮,杀诸蛊毒,去死肌。一名葱苒。生山谷。

【考据】

1.《吴普》曰:藜芦,一名葱葵,一名丰芦,一名蕙葵(《御览》引云,一名山葱,一名公苒),神农雷公辛有毒(《御览》引云:玄黄帝有毒),岐伯咸有毒,李氏太寒,大毒,扁鹊苦有毒,大寒,叶根小相连(《御览》引云:二月采根)。

2.《名医》曰:一名葱葵,一名山葱,生太山,三月采根,阴干。

3. 案《广雅》云:藜芦,葱苒也。《范子计然》云:藜芦出河东,黄白者善。《尔雅》云:茖,山葱,疑非此。

22. Lilu（藜芦，root and rhizome of black falsehellebore，Radix et Rhizoma Veratri）[1]

［Original Text］

［Lilu（藜芦，root and rhizome of black falsehellebore，Radix et Rhizoma Veratri），］ pungent in taste and cold ［in property］，［is mainly used］ to treat ［disease caused by］ worm toxin，cough with dyspnea，dysentery，diarrhea，head ulcer，scabies and severe sore，and to eliminate various worm toxin and necrotic muscles. ［It is also］ called Congran（葱苒），growing in mountains and valleys.

［Textual Research］

［In the book entitled］ *Wu Pu Ben Cao*（《吴普本草》，*Wu Pu's Studies of Materia Medica*），［it］ says ［that］ Lilu（藜芦，root and rhizome of black falsehellebore，Radix et Rhizoma Veratri）［is also］ called Congkui（葱葵），Fenglu（丰芦）and Huikui（蕙葵）. ［In the book entitled］ *Tai Ping Yu Lan*（《太平御览》，*Imperial Studies in Taiping Times*），［it］ says ［that Lilu（藜芦，root and rhizome of black falsehellebore，Radix et Rhizoma Veratri）is also］ called Shancong（山葱）and Gongran（公苒）. ［According to］ Agriculture God（神农）and Leigong（雷公），［Lilu（藜芦，root and rhizome of black falsehellebore，Radix et Rhizoma Veratri）is］ pungent ［in taste］ and toxic ［in property］；［according to］ Qibo（岐伯），［it is］ salty ［in taste］ and toxic ［in property］；［according to］ Li's（李氏），

【今译】

味辛,性寒。

主治虫毒所致之病,咳嗽气逆,痢疾,泄泻,头部溃疡,疥疮瘑痒,恶性疮,能杀除各种虫毒,能祛除坏死的肌肉。又称为葱苒。该物生长在山谷之中。

神农本草经

［it is］severely cold and toxic［in property］; ［according to］Bianque
（扁鹊），［it is］ bitter［in taste］, toxic and severely cold［in
property］, the leaves and roots［of which］are connected with each
other. ［According to the book entitled］ *Tai Ping Yu Lan* （《太平御
览》, *Imperial Studies in Taiping Times*）［its］ root［can be］
collected in February.

［In the book entitled］ *Ming Yi Bie Lu* （《名医别录》, *Special
Record of Great Doctors*），［it］says［that Lilu （藜芦, root and
rhizome of black falsehellebore, Radix et Rhizoma Veratri) is also］
called Congtan （葱菼）and Shancong （山葱），growing in Taishan
（太山）. ［Its］root［can be］collected in March and dried in the
shade.

［In the book entitled］ *Fan Zi Ji Ran* （《范子计然》, *Studies
About Fan Li's Teacher*），［it］says［that］ Lilu （藜芦, root and
rhizome of black falsehellebore, Radix et Rhizoma Veratri) grows
in Hedong （河东）and the yellow and white one is better.

Notes

1. Lilu （藜芦, root and rhizome of black falsehellebore, Radix
et Rhizoma Veratri) is a herbal medicinal, bitter and pungent in
taste, cold and severely cold in property, entering the lung meridian
and the stomach meridian, effective in relieving wind and phlegm,
killing worms and removing toxin. Clinically it is used to treat wind
stroke with stagnation of phlegm, epilepsy, scabies, ulcer and
throat impediment.

23. 钩吻（《御览》作肠）

【原文】

味辛,温。

主金属创伤乳痉,中恶风,咳逆上气,水肿,杀鬼注（旧作,《御览》作注,是）蛊毒。一名野葛。生山谷。

【考据】

1. 《吴普》曰:秦钩肠一名毒根,一名野葛,神农辛,雷公有毒杀人,生南越山,或益州,叶如葛,赤茎大如箭、方、根、黄,或生会稽东冶,正月采（《御览》）。

2. 《名医》曰:生傅高山,及会稽东野。

3. 案《广雅》云:莨钩吻也。《淮南子》说林训云:蝮蛇螫人,傅以和堇则愈。高诱云:和堇,野葛,毒药。《博物志》云:钩吻毒,桂心葱叶沸解之。陶宏景云:或云钩吻是毛茛。《沈括补笔谈》云:闽中人呼为吻莽,亦谓之野葛,岭南人谓之胡蔓,俗谓之断肠草,此草人间至毒之物,不入药用,恐本草所出别是一物,非此钩吻也。

23. Gouwen（钩吻，graceful jessamine herb，Herba Gelsemii Elegantis）[1]

[Original Text]

[Gouwen（钩吻，graceful jessamine herb，Herba Gelsemii Elegantis），] pungent in taste and warm [in property], [is mainly used] to treat sore [caused by injury of] metal，breast swelling，[unconsciousness caused by] severe wind，cough with dyspnea and upward counterflow of Qi，edema，tuberculosis and [disease caused by] worm toxin. [It is also] called Yeke（野葛），growing in mountains and valleys.

[Textual Research]

[In the book entitled] *Wu Pu Ben Cao*（《吴普本草》，*Wu Pu's Studies of Materia Medica*），[it] says [that] [Gouwen（钩吻，graceful jessamine herb，Herba Gelsemii Elegantis）is also] called Qingouchang（秦钩肠），Dugen（毒根）and Yeke（野葛）. [According to] Agriculture God（神农），[it is] pungent [in taste]；[according to] Leigong（雷公），[it is] toxic and killing people. [It] grows in Nanyue（南越）mountains or Yizhou（益州）with leaves like [that of] Ge（葛，Pueraria lobata）， red stalks as large as arrow and yellow root. [It] may grow in Dongye（东冶）in Huiji（会稽），and [can be] collected in January [according to the book entitled] *Tai Ping Yu Lan*（《太平御览》，*Imperial Studies in Taiping Times*）.

【今译】

味辛,性温。

主治金属创伤,乳痓,中恶,咳嗽,呼吸困难,水肿,能祛除鬼怪邪气和虫毒所致之病。又称为野葛。该物生长在山谷之中。

[In the book entitled] *Ming Yi Bie Lu* (《名医别录》, *Special Record of Great Doctors*), [it] says [that Gouwen (钩吻, graceful jessamine herb, Herba Gelsemii Elegantis)] grows in the mountains in Fugao (傅高) and the east lands in Huiji (会稽).

[In the book entitled] *Guang Ya* (《广雅》, *The First Chinese Encyclopedic Dictionary*), [it] says [that the so-called] Lang (莨) refers to Gouwen (钩吻, graceful jessamine herb, Herba Gelsemii Elegantis). [In the book entitled] *Bo Wu Zhi* (《博物志》, *History of All Plants*), [it] says [that] toxin in Gouwen (钩吻, graceful jessamine herb, Herba Gelsemii Elegantis) [can be] resolved by boiling with Guixin (桂心) [which is one kind of Rougui (肉桂, cassiabarktree bark, Cortex Cinnamomi)] and the leaves of onion.

Notes

1. Gouwen (钩吻, graceful jessamine herb, Herba Gelsemii Elegantis) is a herbal medicinal, bitter and pungent in taste, warm and severely toxic in property, effective in removing toxin and resolving swelling, killing worms and relieving itching. Clinically it is used to treat sore, abscess, leprosy, traumatic injury, ulcer, scabies and eczema.

24. 射干

【原文】

味苦,平。

主咳逆上气,喉痹咽痛不得消息,散急气,腹中邪逆,食饮大热。一名乌扇,一名乌蒲。生川谷。

【考据】

1.《吴普》曰:射干,一名黄远也(《御览》)。

2.《名医》曰:一名乌痉娑,一名乌吹,一名草姜,生南阳田野,三月三日,采根阴干。

3. 案《广雅》云:鸢尾乌蘧,射干也。《荀子》劝学篇云:西方有木焉,名曰射干,茎长四寸。《范子计然》云:射干根如安定。

【今译】

味苦,性平。

24. Shegan（射干，blackberrylily rhizome，Rhizoma Belamcandae）[1]

[Original Text]

［Shegan （射干，blackberrylily rhizome，Rhizoma Belamcandae），］bitter in taste and mild ［in property］，［is mainly used］to treat cough with dyspnea and upward counterflow of Qi，impediment and pain of the throat and inability to breathe，and to disperse stagnation of Qi，retention of evil in the abdomen and severe heat ［caused by inappropriate］ diet.［It is also］called Wushan（乌扇）and Wupu（乌蒲），growing in mountain valleys and river valleys.

[Textual Research]

［In the book entitled］*Wu Pu Ben Cao*（《吴普本草》，*Wu Pu's Studies of Materia Medica*），［it］says ［that］ Shegan（射干，blackberrylily rhizome，Rhizoma Belamcandae）［is also］called Huangyuan（黄远）［according to the book entitled］*Tai Ping Yu Lan*（《太平御览》，*Imperial Studies in Taiping Times*）.

［In the book entitled］*Ming Yi Bie Lu*（《名医别录》，*Special Record of Great Doctors*），［it］says ［that Shegan （射干，blackberrylily rhizome，Rhizoma Belamcandae）is also］called Wuzhisha（乌痓翣），Wuchui（乌吹）and Caojiang（草姜），growing in the lands in Nanyang（南阳）.［Its］root ［can be］collected on

　　主治咳嗽，呼吸困难，治疗喉痹，咽痛，不能呼吸，能消散气结不畅，腹中邪气逆行，能消除因食饮不节而身体高热。又称为乌扇，又称为乌蒲。该物生长在山川河谷之中。

March 3 and dried in the shade.

[In the book entitled] *Guang Ya* (《广雅》, *The First Chinese Encyclopedic Dictionary*), [it] says [that the so-called] Yuanwei (鸢尾) and Wusha (乌蓬) refer to Shegan (射干, blackberrylily rhizome, Rhizoma Belamcandae). [In the book entitled] *Xun Zi* (《荀子》, *Works Written by Xunzi*[2]) about how to learn, [it] says, "[In] the west there is a sort of wood called Shegan (射干, blackberrylily rhizome, Rhizoma Belamcandae) with the stalks about 4 *Cun* (寸) in length. [In the book entitled] *Fan Zi Ji Ran* (《范子计然》, *Studies About Fan Li's Teacher*), [it] says [that] the root of Shegan (射干, blackberrylily rhizome, Rhizoma Belamcandae) is stable.

Notes

1. Shegan (射干, blackberrylily rhizome, Rhizoma Belamcandae) is a herbal medicinal, bitter in taste, cold and slightly toxic in property, entering the lung meridian and the liver meridian, effective in purging fire and removing toxin, disinhibiting the throat and resolving phlegm, dispersing stasis and stagnation. Clinically it is used to treat sore-throat, cough with phlegm, panting with Qi stagnation, swelling of the liver and spleen, scrofula and tuberculosis.

2. Xunzi (荀子, about 313 BC - 238 BC) was a great scholar in the Warring States Period (475 BC - 221 BC).

25. 蛇合（原注云，合是含字）

【原文】

味苦，微寒。

主惊痫寒热邪气，除热，金创，疽痔，鼠瘘，恶疮，头疡。一名蛇衔。生山谷。

【考据】

1.《名医》曰：生益州，八月采，阴干。

2. 按本草图经云：或云是雀瓢，即是萝摩之别名。据陆玑云：芄兰一名萝摩，幽州谓之雀瓢，则即《尔雅》蘽芄兰也，《唐本》草，别出萝摩条，非，又见女青。

【今译】

味苦，性微寒。

主治惊风，癫痫及寒热邪气所致之病，能消除热邪，能治疗金属创伤，疮肿，痔疮，瘰疬，恶疮，头部溃疡。又称为蛇衔。该物生长在山谷之中。

25. Shehe（蛇合，klein cinquefoil herb with root，Herba Potentillae Kleinianae cum Radice）[1]

［Original Text］

［Shehe （蛇合，klein cinquefoil herb with root，Herba Potentillae Kleinianae cum Radice），］bitter ［in taste］ and slightly cold ［in property］，［is mainly used］ to treat convulsion，epilepsy，cold-heat ［disease caused by］ evil-Qi，to eliminate heat，to treat damage ［caused by injury of］ metal，carbuncle，hemorrhoids，tuberculosis，severe sore and head ulcer. ［It is also］ called Shexian （蛇衔），growing in mountains and valleys.

［Textual Research］

［In the book entitled］ *Ming Yi Bie Lu* （《名医别录》，*Special Record of Great Doctors*），［it］ says ［that Shehe （蛇合，klein cinquefoil herb with root，Herba Potentillae Kleinianae cum Radice）］ grows in Yizhou （益州），［can be］ collected in August and dried in the shade.

Notes

1. Shehe （蛇合，klein cinquefoil herb with root，Herba Potentillae Kleinianae cum Radice），also called Shehan （蛇含），is a herbal medicinal，pungent and bitter in taste，cool in property，effective in clearing heat and removing toxin. Clinically it is used to treat high fever，convulsion，cough，swelling and pain of the throat，dysentery，bleeding caused by metal injury and snake bite.

26. 恒山（旧作常山，《御览》作恒山，是）

【原文】

味苦，寒。

主伤寒，寒热，热发温疟，鬼毒，胸中痰结吐逆。一名互草。生川谷。

【考据】

1.《吴普》曰：恒山，一名漆叶，神农岐伯苦，李氏大寒，桐君辛有毒，二月八月采。

2.《名医》曰：生盖州及汉中，八月采根，阴干。

3. 案《后汉书华陀传》云：陀授以漆叶青黏散，漆叶屑一斗，青黏十四两，以是为率，言久服去三虫，利五脏，轻体，使人头不白。

【今译】

味苦，性寒。

主治伤寒，寒热病，因热而发作的温疟，鬼毒病，胸中痰结，咳喘，呕吐。又称为互草。该物生长在山川河谷之中。

26. Changshan（常山，root of antifebrile dichroa，Radix Dichroae）[1]

［Original Text］

［Changshan（常山，root of antifebrile dichroa，Radix Dichroae），］bitter in taste and cold ［in property］，［is mainly used］ to treat cold damage，cold-heat ［disease］，fever ［due to］ warm malaria，severe toxin ［like a］ ghost，retention of phlegm in the chest with vomiting. ［It is also］ called Hucao（互草），growing in mountain valleys and river valleys.

［Textual Research］

［In the book entitled］ *Wu Pu Ben Cao*（《吴普本草》，*Wu Pu's Studies of Materia Medica*），［it］ says ［that］ Changshan（常山，root of antifebrile dichroa，Radix Dichroae）［is also］ called Qiye（漆叶）. ［According to］ Agriculture God（神农）and Qibo（岐伯），［it is］ bitter ［in taste］；［according to］ Li's（李氏），［it is］ severely cold ［in property］；［according to］ Tongjun（桐均），［it is］ pungent ［in taste］ and toxic ［in property］. ［It can be］ collected in February and August.

［In the book entitled］ *Ming Yi Bie Lu*（《名医别录》，*Special Record of Great Doctors*），［it］ says ［that Changshan（常山，root of antifebrile dichroa，Radix Dichroae）］ grows in Gaizhou（盖州）and Hanzhong（汉中）. ［Its］ root ［can be］ collected in August and dried in the shade.

Notes

1. Changshan（常山，root of antifebrile dichroa，Radix Dichroae）is a herbal medicinal，bitter and pungent in taste，cold and toxic in property，entering the lung meridian，the liver meridian and the heart meridian，effective in relieving heat，reducing phlegm and resolving malaria. Clinically it is used to treat vomiting，malaria，retention of phlegm and fluid，lumps in the chest and diaphragm.

27. 蜀漆

【原文】

味辛,平。

主疟及咳逆,寒热,腹中症坚,痞结,积聚邪气,蛊毒,鬼注(旧作疰,《御览》作蛀)。生川谷。

【考据】

1.《吴普》曰:蜀漆叶,一名恒山,神农岐伯雷公辛有毒,黄帝辛,一经酸,如漆叶蓝青相似,五月采(《御览》)。

2.《名医》曰:生江陵山,及蜀汉中常山,苗也,五月采叶,阴干。

3. 案《广雅》云:恒山蜀漆也。《范子计然》云:蜀漆出蜀郡。

【今译】

味辛,性平。

27. Shuqi（蜀漆，dichroa，
Ramulus et Folium Dichroae）[1]

［Original Text］

［Shuqi（蜀漆，dichroa，Ramulus et Folium Dichroae），］pungent in taste and mild ［in property］，［is mainly used］ to treat malaria，cough with dyspnea，cold-heat ［disease］，abdominal lump，conglomeration and accumulation ［due to］ evil-Qi，［disease caused by］ worm toxin ［and strange pathogenic factors like］ ghost. ［It］ grows in mountain valleys and river valleys.

［Textual Research］

［In the book entitled］ *Wu Pu Ben Cao*（《吴普本草》，*Wu Pu's Studies of Materia Medica*），［it］ says ［that］ Shuqi（蜀漆，dichroa，Ramulus et Folium Dichroae）［is also］ called Hengshan（恒山）. ［According to］ Agriculture God（神农），Qibo（岐伯）and Leigong（雷公），［it is］ pungent ［in taste］ and toxic ［in property］；［according to］ Yellow Emperor（黄帝），［it is］ pungent ［in taste］. ［It is］ sometimes sour ［in taste］. ［Its leaves are］ similar to the blue and green leaves of lacquer. ［It can be］ collected in May ［according to the book entitled］ *Tai Ping Yu Lan*（《太平御览》，*Imperial Studies in Taiping Times*）.

［In the book entitled］ *Ming Yi Bie Lu*（《名医别录》，*Special Record of Great Doctors*），［it］ says ［that Shuqi（蜀漆，dichroa，

　　主治疟疾，咳嗽气逆，寒热病，腹中坚硬性癥瘕，结块，邪气积聚，能治疗虫毒所致之病，鬼怪之邪所致之症。该物生长在山川河谷之中。

Ramulus et Folium Dichroae)] grows in Jiangling（江陵）mountain and Hanzhong（汉中）and Changshan（常山）in the Shu（蜀）[State]. [Its] leaves [can be] collected in May and dried in the shade.

[In the book entitled] *Guang Ya*（《广雅》, *The First Chinese Encyclopedic Dictionary*），[it] says [that the so-called] Hengshan（恒山）refers to Shuqi（蜀漆，dichroa，Ramulus et Folium Dichroae）. [In the book entitled] *Fan Zi Ji Ran*（《范子计然》, *Studies About Fan Li's Teacher*），[it] says [that] Shuqi（蜀漆，dichroa，Ramulus et Folium Dichroae）grows in Shujun（蜀郡）.

Notes

1. Shuqi（蜀漆，dichroa，Ramulus et Folium Dichroae）is a herbal medicinal，bitter and pungent in taste，warm and toxic in property，entering the liver meridian，effective in reducing heat and resolving malaria. Clinically it is used to treat various malaria，infantile convulsion，epilepsy and disease caused by severe pathogenic factors.

28. 甘遂

【原文】

味苦,寒。

主大腹疝瘕,腹满,面目浮肿,留饮宿食,破症坚积聚,利水谷道。一名主田。生川谷。

【考据】

1.《吴普》曰:甘遂一名主田,一名曰泽,一名重泽,一名鬼丑,一名陵藁,一名甘槁,一名甘泽,神农桐君苦有毒,岐伯雷公有毒,须二月八月采(《御览》)。

2.《名医》曰:一名甘藁,一名陵藁,一名陵泽,一名重泽,生中山,二月采根,阴干。

3. 案《广雅》云:陵泽,甘遂也。《范子计然》云:甘遂,出三辅。

【今译】

味苦,性寒。

28. Gansui（甘遂，kansui，Radix Kansui）[1]

［Original Text］

［Gansui（甘遂，kansui，Radix Kansui），］bitter in taste and cold ［in property］，［is mainly used］ to treat hernia and conglomeration in the major abdomen，abdominal fullness，dropsy of the face and eyes，retention of fluid and retention of undigested food，to break lump and accumulation，and to promote urination and defecation. ［It is also］ called Zhutian（主田），growing in mountain valleys and river valleys.

［Textual Research］

［In the book entitled］ *Wu Pu Ben Cao*（《吴普本草》，*Wu Pu's Studies of Materia Medica*），［it］ says ［that］ Gansui（甘遂，kansui，Radix Kansui）［is also］ called Zhutian（主田），Ze（泽），Zhongze（重泽），Guichou（鬼丑），Linggao（陵藁），Gangao（甘槀）and Ganze（甘泽）. ［According to］ Agriculture God（神农）and Tongjun（桐均），［it is］ bitter ［in taste］ and toxic ［in property］；［according to］ Qibo（岐伯）and Leigong（雷公），［it is］ toxic ［in property］ and ［can be］ collected in February and August ［as mentioned in the book entitled］ *Tai Ping Yu Lan*（《太平御览》，*Imperial Studies in Taiping Times*）.

［In the book entitled］ *Ming Yi Bie Lu*（《名医别录》，*Special Record of Great Doctors*），［it］ says ［that Gansui（甘遂，kansui，

　　主治腹部疝瘕隆起,腹部胀满,面目浮肿,饮食不化而滞留,能消散坚硬痞块和体内积聚,能通利大小便。又称为主田。该物生长在山川河谷之中。

Radix Kansui）is also⌉ called Gangao（甘藁），Linggao（陵藁），Lingze（陵泽）and Zhongze（重泽），growing in Zhongshan（中山）. ⌈Its⌉ root ⌈can be⌉ collected in February and dried in the shade.

⌈In the book entitled⌉ *Guang Ya* （《广雅》，*The First Chinese Encyclopedic Dictionary*），⌈it⌉ says ⌈that⌉ Lingze（陵泽）refers to Gansui（甘遂，kansui, Radix Kansui）. ⌈In the book entitled⌉ *Fan Zi Ji Ran* （《范子计然》，*Studies About Fan Li's Teacher*），⌈it⌉ says ⌈that⌉ Gansui（甘遂，kansui，Radix Kansui）grows in the three places.

Notes

1. Gansui（甘遂，kansui, Radix Kansui）is a herbal medicinal，bitter in taste，cold and toxic in property，entering the spleen meridian and the lung meridian，effective in purging retention of fluid，breaking accumulation and conglomeration，promoting urination and defecation. Clinically it is used to treat edema，abdominal fullness，dysuria，constipation，accumulation and conglomeration in the chest and abdomen，scabies and epilepsy.

29. 白敛

【原文】

味苦,平。

主痈肿疽疮,散结气,止痛除热,目中赤,小儿惊痫,温疟,女子阴中肿痛。一名免核,一名白草,生山谷。

【考据】

1.《名医》曰:一名白根,一名昆仑,生衡山,二月八月,采根暴干。

2.案《说文》云:莶,白莶也,或作蔹。《毛诗》云:蔹蔓于野。陆玑疏云:蔹似栝楼,叶盛而细,其子正黑,如燕荑,不可食也,幽人谓之乌服,其茎叶鬻以哺牛,除热。《尔雅》云:萰,菟荄。郭璞云:未详。据玉篇云:萰,白蔹也。经云:一名菟核,核与荄声相近,即此矣。

【今译】

味苦,性平。

主治痈肿,疽疮,能消散结聚之气,能消除疼痛,能治疗热邪所致之病,眼睛肿痛,小儿惊风,癫痫,温疟,女子阴部肿痛。又称为免核,又称为白草,该物生长在山谷之中。

29. Bailian（白敛，ampelopsis，Radix Ampelopsis）[1]

[Original Text]

[Bailian（白敛，ampelopsis，Radix Ampelopsis），] bitter in taste and mild [in property], [is mainly used] to treat abscess，sore and ulcer，to disperse stagnation of Qi，to cease pain，to eliminate heat，and to resolve redness in the eyes，infantile convulsion，epilepsy，worm malaria，vulva swelling and pain. [It is]also called Mianhe（免核）and Baicao（白草）. [It] grows in mountains and valleys.

[Textual Research]

[In the book entitled] *Ming Yi Bie Lu*（《名医别录》，*Special Record of Great Doctors*），[it] says [that Bailian（白敛，ampelopsis，Radix Ampelopsis）is also] called Baigen（白根）and Kunlun（昆仑），growing in Hengshan（衡山）. [Its] root [can be] collected in February and August，and dried in the sun.

Notes

1. Bailian（白敛，ampelopsis，Radix Ampelopsis）is a herbal medicinal，bitter and pungent in taste，slightly cold in property，entering the heart meridian and the spleen meridian，effective in purging fire and dispersing stagnation，promoting growth of muscles and ceasing pain. Clinically it is used to treat ulcer，sore，abscess，scabies，epilepsy，traumatic injury，scald，leucorrhea，warm malaria，hemorrhoids and diarrhea.

30. 青葙子

【原文】

味苦,微寒。

主邪气,皮肤中热,风搔,身痒,杀三虫。

子名草决明,疗唇口青。一名青蒿,一名萎蒿。生平谷。

【考据】

1.《名医》曰:生道傍,三月三日采茎叶,阴干,五月六日,采子。

案《魏略》云:初平中有青牛先生,常服青葙子,葙当作箱字。

【今译】

味苦,性微寒。

主治邪气所致之症,皮肤发热,因风侵袭而瘙痒,能杀死三种寄生虫。

其子名为草决明,可治疗唇口黑青。又称为青蒿,又称为萎蒿。该物生长在平谷中。

30. Qingxiangzi（青葙子，seed of feather cockscomb，Semen Celosiae）[1]

〔Original Text〕

〔Qingxiangzi（青葙子，seed of feather cockscomb，Semen Celosiae），bitter in taste and slightly cold〔in property〕，〔is mainly used〕to treat〔disease caused by〕evil-Qi，heat in the skin，wind scratching and body itching，and to kill three worms.

〔Its〕seed，called Caojueming（草决明），〔can be used〕to treat bluishness of the lips and mouth.〔It is also〕called Qinghao（青蒿）and Qihao（萋蒿），growing in plains and valleys.

〔Textual Research〕

〔In the book entitled〕*Ming Yi Bie Lu*（《名医别录》，*Special Record of Great Doctors*），〔it〕says〔that Qingxiangzi（青箱子，seed of feather cockscomb，Semen Celosiae）〕grows in the sides of roads.〔Its〕stalks and leaves〔can be〕collected on March 3 and dried in the shade.〔Its〕seed〔can be〕collected on May 6.

Notes

1. Qingxiangzi（青葙子，seed of feather cockscomb，Semen Celosiae）is a herbal medicinal，bitter in taste and slightly cold in property，entering the heart meridian and the liver meridian，effective in clearing liver fire，killing worms，expelling wind，improving vision and relieving itching. Clinically it is used to treat swelling and pain of the eyes，nebula，albuginea，hypertension，vertigo，nosebleed，sore and scabies.

31. 藋菌

【原文】

味咸,平。

主心痛,温中,去长虫,白疢,蛲虫,蛇螫毒,症瘕,诸虫。一名藋芦。
生池泽。

【考据】

1.《名医》曰:生东海及渤海,章武,八月采,阴干。

2. 案《尔雅》云:滇藋茵芝,文选注,引作菌。声类云:滇藋茵芝也,
疑即此藋菌,或一名滇,一名芝,未敢定之。

【今译】

味咸,性平。

主治心痛,能温煦人体脏器,能祛除蛔虫,白癣,蛲虫,能治疗毒蛇
咬伤,癥瘕和虫毒所致各种病症。又称为藋芦。该物生长在池泽中。

31. Guanjun（藋菌，reeds fungi，Ageratum Houstonianum） [1]

[Original Text]

[Guanjun（藋菌，reeds fungi，Ageratum Houstonianum），] salty in taste and mild [in property], [is mainly used] to treat heartache，to warm the middle（the internal organs），and to eliminate roundworm，tinea alba，pinworm，bite by snake，conglomeration and various worms. [It is also] called Guanlu（藋芦），growing in lakes and swamps.

[Textual Research]

[In the book entitled] *Ming Yi Bie Lu*（《名医别录》，*Special Record of Great Doctors*），[it] says [that Guanjun（藋菌，reeds fungi，Ageratum Houstonianum）] grows in Donghai（东海，East Sea），Baohai（渤海）and Zhangwu（章武）. [It can be] collected in August and dried in the shade.

Notes

1. Guanjun（藋菌，reeds fungi，Ageratum Houstonianum）is a herbal medicinal，salty in taste and mild in property，effective in warming the middle（the internal organs）and killing worms. Clinically it is used to treat heartache，diseases caused by roundworms and pinworms，scabies，tinea tonsure and severe sore.

32. 白芨（《御览》作芨）

【原文】

味苦,平。

主痈肿,恶疮,败疽,伤阴,死肌,胃中邪气,贼风,鬼击,痱缓,不收。一名甘根,一名连及草。生川谷。

【考据】

1.《吴普》曰:神农苦,黄帝辛,李氏大寒,雷公辛无毒,茎叶似生姜,藜芦,十月华,直上,紫赤,根白连,二月八月九月采。

2.《名医》曰:生北山及冤句,及越山。

3. 案隋羊公服黄精法云:黄精一名白及亦为黄精别名,今《名医》别出黄精条。

【今译】

味苦,性平。

32. Baiji（白芨，tuber of common bletilla，Rhizoma Bletillae）[1]

[Original Text]

[Baiji（白芨，tuber of common bletilla，Rhizoma Bletillae），] bitter in taste and mild [in property]，[is mainly used] to treat abscess，severe sore，refractory ulcer，genital injury，necrotic muscles，evil-Qi in the stomach，thief-like wind，[fulminant disease caused by severe pathogenic factors like] ghost attack，and sequelae [after wind stroke] difficult to resolve. [It is also] called Gangen（甘根）and Lianjicao（连及草），growing in mountain valleys and river valleys.

[Textual Research]

[In the book entitled] *Wu Pu Ben Cao*（《吴普本草》，*Wu Pu's Studies of Materia Medica*），[it] says [that Baiji（白芨，tuber of common bletilla，Rhizoma Bletillae）]，[according to] Agriculture God（神农），is bitter [in taste]；[according to] Yellow Emperor（黄帝），[it is] pungent [in taste]；[according to] Li's（李氏），[it is] severely cold [in property]；[according to] Leigong（雷公），[it is] pungent [in taste] and non-toxic [in property]. [Its] stalks and leaves are similar to [that of] Shengjiang（生姜，rhizome of common ginger，Rhizoma Zingiberis Recens）and Lilu（藜芦，root and rhizome of black falsehellebore，Radix et Rhizoma Veratri）. [In]

主治痈肿,恶性疮,溃败疮肿,阴器受伤,肌肉坏死,胃中有邪气,虚邪贼风,鬼怪邪气袭击,中风后遗症,肢体不收。又称为甘根,又称为连及草。该物生长在山川河谷之中。

October，[it begins] to blossom straight upward in purple and red [color]. [Its] root is white and [can be] collected in February，August and September.

[In the book entitled] *Ming Yi Bie Lu* (《名医别录》，*Special Record of Great Doctors*)，[it] says [that Baiji（白芨，tuber of common bletilla，Rhizoma Bletillae）] grows in Beishan（北山），Yuanju（冤句）and Yueshan（越山）.

Notes

1. Baiji（白芨，tuber of common bletilla，Rhizoma Bletillae），also known as Baiji（白及），is a herbal medicinal，bitter and sweet in taste，astringent and slightly cold in property，entering the lung meridian and the stomach meridian，effective in restraining the lung and ceasing bleeding，resolving swelling and promoting growth of muscles. Clinically it is used to treat tuberculosis，hemoptysis，bleeding due to bronchiectasis，bleeding caused by gastric and duodenal ulcer，nosebleed，abscess，scabies，bleeding caused by traumatic injury，scald and rhagadia.

33. 大戟

【原文】

味苦,寒。

主蛊毒,十二水肿,腹满,急痛,积聚,中风,皮肤疼痛,吐逆。一名邛钜(案此无生川泽三字者,古或与泽漆为一条)。

【考据】

1.《名医》曰:生常山,十二月采根,阴干。

2. 案《尔雅》云:荞,邛钜。郭璞云:今药草大戟也。《淮南子》缪称训云:大戟去水。

【今译】

味苦,性寒。

主治虫毒所致之病,多种水肿,腹部胀满,拘急疼痛,邪气积聚,因感受风邪而导致的疾病,皮肤疼痛,呕吐气逆。又称为邛钜。

33. Daji（大戟，root of Peking euphorbia，Radix Euphorbiae Pekinensis）[1]

［Original Text］

［Daji （大戟，root of Peking euphorbia， Radix Euphorbiae Pekinensis)，］ bitter in taste and cold ［in property］， ［is mainly used］ to treat ［disease caused by］ worm toxin， various edema， abdominal fullness and sharp pain， accumulation， aggregation， wind stroke， cutaneous pain and vomiting. ［It is also］ called Qiongju （邛钜）.

［Textual Research］

［In the book entitled］ *Ming Yi Bie Lu* （《名医别录》，*Special Record of Great Doctors*)， ［it］ says ［that Daji （大戟，root of Peking euphorbia， Radix Euphorbiae Pekinensis)］ grows in Changshan （常山）. ［Its］ root ［can be］ collected in December and dried in the shade.

1013

Notes

1. Daji （大戟，root of Peking euphorbia， Radix Euphorbiae Pekinensis) is a herbal medicinal， bitter in taste， cold and toxic in property， entering the lung meridian， the spleen meridian and the kidney meridian， effective in expelling water and promoting defecation， resolving swelling and dispersing stagnation. Clinically it is used to treat edema， panting， retention of fluid in the abdomen， chest pain， scrofula， abscess， scabies and ulcer.

34. 泽漆

【原文】

味苦,性微寒。

主皮肤热,大腹,水气,四肢面目浮肿,丈夫阴气不足。生川泽。

【考据】

1.《名医》曰:一名漆茎,大戟苗也,生太山,三月三日,七月七日,采茎叶,阴干。

2. 案《广雅》云:黍茎,泽漆也。

【今译】

味苦,性微寒。

主治身体发热,腹部积水,四肢面目浮肿,男子阳痿。该物生长在山川和平泽之中。

34. Ziqi（泽漆，sun spurge，
Herba Euphorbiae Helioscopiae） [1]

［Original Text］

［Ziqi（泽漆，sun spurge，Herba Euphorbiae Helioscopiae），］bitter in taste and slightly cold［in property］，［is mainly used］to treat heat in the skin，retention of fluid in the abdomen，dropsy of the limbs，face and eyes and impotence.［It］grows in valleys and swamps.

［Textual Research］

［In the book entitled］*Ming Yi Bie Lu*（《名医别录》，*Special Record of Great Doctors*），［it］says［that Ziqi（泽漆，sun spurge，Herba Euphorbiae Helioscopiae）is also］called Qijing（漆茎），the seedling of Daji（大戟，root of Peking euphorbia，Radix Euphorbiae Pekinensis），growing in Taishan（太山）.［Its］stalks and leaves ［can be］collected on March 3 and July 7，and dried in the shade.

［In the book entitled］*Guang Ya*（《广雅》，*The First Chinese Encyclopedic Dictionary*），［it］says［that the so-called］Shujng（黍茎）refers to Ziqi（泽漆，sun spurge，Herba Euphorbiae Helioscopiae）.

Notes

1. Ziqi（泽漆，sun spurge，Herba Euphorbiae Helioscopiae）is a herbal medicinal，pungent and bitter in taste，cool and toxic in property，entering the spleen meridian，the lung meridian，the small intestine meridian and the large intestine meridian，effective in disinhibiting water，relieving swelling，resolving phlegm，dispersing stagnation and killing worms. Clinically it is used to treat abdominal retention of fluid，dropsy，phlegm retention，panting and cough，scrofula and tuberculosis.

35. 茵芋

【原文】

味苦,温。

主五脏邪气,心腹寒热,羸瘦如疟状,发作有时,诸关节风湿痹痛。生川谷。

【考据】

1.《吴普》曰:茵芋,一名卑共。微温有毒,状如莽草,而细软(《御览》)。

2.《名医》曰:一名莞草,一名卑共。生太山,三月三日,采叶阴干。

35．Yinyu（茵芋，stem and leaf of reeves skimmia，Caulis et Folium Skimmiae Reevesianae） [1]

［Original Text］

［Yinyu（茵芋，stem and leaf of reeves skimmia，Caulis et Folium Skimmiae Reevesianae），］bitter［in taste］and warm［in property］，［is mainly used］to treat［disease in］the five Zang-organs［caused by］evil-Qi，cold and heat in the heart and abdomen，weakness and emaciation like malaria［that］occurs occasionally，wind-dampness impediment and pain of various joint. ［It］grows in mountain valleys and river valleys.

［Textual Research］

［In the book entitled］*Wu Pu Ben Cao*（《吴普本草》，*Wu Pu's Studies of Materia Medica*），［it］says［that］Yinyu（茵芋，stem and leaf of reeves skimmia，Caulis et Folium Skimmiae Reevesianae）［is also］called Beigong（卑共），slightly warm and toxin［in property］like Mangcao（莽草，leaf of lanceleaf anisetree，Folium Illicii Lanceolati），thin and soft，［according to the book entitled］*Tai Ping Yu Lan*（《太平御览》，*Imperial Studies in Taiping Times*）.

［In the book entitled］*Ming Yi Bie Lu*（《名医别录》，*Special Record of Great Doctors*），［it］says［that Yinyu（茵芋，stem and leaf of reeves skimmia，Caulis et Folium Skimmiae Reevesianae）is also］called Guancao（莞草）and Beigong（卑共），growing in Taishan（太

【今译】

味苦,性温。

主治五脏中的邪气,心腹部寒热病,身体消瘦如疟疾,病情随时发作,能治疗关节风湿痹痛。该物生长在山川河谷之中。

山）．[Its] leaves [can be] collected on March 3 and dried in the shade.

Notes

1. Yinyu（茵芋，stem and leaf of reeves skimmia，Caulis et Folium Skimmiae Reevesianae）is a herbal medicinal，bitter in taste，warm and toxic in property，entering the liver meridian and the kidney meridian，effective in removing toxin，relieving heat and wind，invigorating essence and ceasing pain. Clinically it is used to treat abdominal coldness，heat and pain，joint impediment，flaccidity of lower limbs，spasm of limbs，weakness and emaciation.

36. 贯众

【原文】

味苦，性微寒。

主腹中邪，热气，诸毒，杀三虫。一名贯节，一名贯渠，一名百头（《御览》作白），一名虎卷，一名扁符。生山谷。

【考据】

1.《吴普》曰：贯众一名贯来，一名贯中，一名渠母，一名贯钟，一名伯芹，一名药藻，一名扁符，一名黄钟，神农岐伯苦有毒，桐君扁鹊苦，一经甘有毒，黄帝咸酸，一经苦无毒，叶黄，两两相对，茎，黑毛聚生，冬夏不老，四月花，八月实，黑聚相连，卷旁行生，三月八月采根，五月采药（《御览》）。

2.《名医》曰：一名伯萍，一名药藻，此谓草鸱头，生元山及冤句，少室山，二月八月，采根阴干。

3. 案《说文》云：苻草也。《广雅》云：贯节、贯众也。《尔雅》云：泺贯众。郭璞云：叶，圆锐，茎，毛黑，布地，冬夏不死，一名贯渠。又上云：扁符止。郭璞云：未详。据经云：一名篇符，即此也。《尔雅》当云：篇

36．Guanzhong（贯众，rhizome of male fern，Rhizoma Dryopteris Crassirhizomae）[1]

［Original Text］

［Guanzhong（贯众，rhizome of male fern，Rhizoma Dryopteris Crassirhizomae），］bitter in taste and slightly cold［in property］，［is mainly used］to treat［disease in］the abdomen［caused by］evil，heat-Qi and various toxin，and to kill three worms．［It is also］called Guanjie（贯节），Guanqu（贯渠），Baitou（百头），Hujuan（虎卷）and Bianfu（扁符），growing in mountains and valleys．

［Textual Research］

［In the book entitled］*Wu Pu Ben Cao*（《吴普本草》，*Wu Pu's Studies of Materia Medica*），［it］says［that］Guanzhong（贯众，rhizome of male fern，Rhizoma Dryopteris Crassirhizomae）［is also］called Guanlai（贯来），Guanzhong（贯中），Qumu（渠母），Guanzhong（贯钟），Baiqin（伯芹），Yaozao（药藻），Bianfu（扁符）and Huangzhong（黄钟）．［According to］Agriculture God（神农）and Qibo（岐伯），［it is］bitter［in taste］and toxic［in property］；［according to］Tongjun（桐均）and Bianque（扁鹊），［it is］bitter［in taste］and［will be］toxic［if］sweet［in taste］；［according to］Yellow Emperor（黄帝），［it is］salty and sour［in taste］and［will be］non-toxic［if］bitter］．［Its］leaves are yellow，double corresponding to double．［Its］stalks are black with wools and never become old in winter and summer．［In］April，［it begins］to

符,止,泺贯众。

【今译】

味苦,性微寒。

主治腹中热邪所致之病,能消除各种毒邪,能杀死三种寄生虫。又称为贯节,又称为贯渠,又称为百头,又称为虎卷,又称为扁符。该物生长在山谷之中。

blossom；［in］August，［it begins to bear］fruits］，spreading and connected with each other. ［Its］root ［can be］collected in March and August， ［it can be］ collected for medicinal ［purpose］ ［according to the book entitled］ *Tai Ping Yu Lan*（《太平御览》，*Imperial Studies in Taiping Times*）.

［In the book entitled］ *Ming Yi Bie Lu*（《名医别录》，*Special Record of Great Doctors*），［it］says［that Guanzhong（贯众，rhizome of male fern，Rhizoma Dryopteris Crassirhizomae）is also］called Boping（伯萍），Yaozao（药藻）and Caochitou（草鸱头），growing in Yuanshan（元山），Yuanju（冤句）and Shaoshi（少室）mountains.［In］February and August，［its］root［can be］collected and dried in the shade.

［In the book entitled］ *Guang Ya*（《广雅》，*The First Chinese Encyclopedic Dictionary*），［it］says［that the so-called］Guanjie（贯节）refers to Guanzhong（贯众，rhizome of male fern。，Rhizoma Dryopteris Crassirhizomae）. Guo Pu（郭璞）said，"［Its］leaves are round and sharp；［its］stalks are black with wools.［It］spreads all over the land，never dying in winter and summer，also called Guanqu（贯渠）or Bianfuzhi.

Notes

1. Guanzhong （贯众，rhizome of male fern，Rhizoma Dryopteris Crassirhizomae）is a herbal medicinal，bitter in taste，slightly cold and toxic in property，entering the liver meridian and the spleen meridian，effective in clearing heat，removing toxin，killing worms，cooling the blood and ceasing bleeding. Clinically it is used to treat common cold，spots in warm disease，hematemesis，hematochezia， hematuria， vaginal bleeding， and mumps，ringworms，roundworms and pinworms.

37. 莞花

【原文】

味苦,平寒。

主伤寒温疟,下十二水,破积聚,大坚,症瘕,荡涤肠胃中留癖饮食,寒热邪气,利水道。生川谷。

【考据】

1.《名医》曰:生咸阳及河南中牟,六月采花,阴干。

【今译】

味苦,性平寒。

主治伤寒,温疟,各种水肿病症,能破解积聚,坚硬症瘕,能荡涤肠胃中的饮食积聚,寒热邪气,能通利水道。该物生长在山川河谷之中。

37. Raohua（荛花, canescent Flos Wikstroemia Canescens）[1]

［Original Text］

［Raohua（荛花, canescent Flos Wikstroemia Canescens），］bitter in taste，mild and cold［in property］，［is mainly used］to treat cold damage，warm malaria，and various edeam，to break accumulation，aggregation，hard mass and conglomeration，to resolve retention of undigested food，cold-heat and evil-Qi in the intestines and stomach，and to disinhibit waterway［in the body］.［It］grows in mountain valleys and river valleys.

［Textual Research］

［In the book entitled］*Ming Yi Bie Lu*（《名医别录》，*Special Record of Great Doctors*），［it］says［that Raohua（荛花, canescent Flos Wikstroemia Canescens）］grows in Xianyang（咸阳）and Zhongmou（中牟）in Henan（河南）.［Its］flowers［can be］collected in June and dried in the shade.

Notes

1. Raohua（荛花, canescent Flos Wikstroemia Canescens）is a herbal medicinal，pungent and bitter in taste，cold and toxic in property，entering the intestine meridian and the stomach meridian，effective in purging retention of water，breaking accumulation and aggregation. Clinically it is used to treat retention of fluid，edema，cough with dyspnea and upward counterflow of Qi，abdominal mass and conglomeration.

38. 牙子

【原文】

味苦,寒。

主邪气热气,疥瘙,恶疡疮,痔,去白虫。一名狼牙。生川谷。

【考据】

1.《吴普》曰:狼牙一名支兰,一名狼齿,一名犬牙,一名抱子,神农黄帝苦有毒,桐君或咸,岐伯雷公扁鹊苦无毒,生冤句,叶青,根黄赤,六月七月华,八月实,黑,正月八月采根(《御览》)。

2.《名医》曰:一名狼齿,一名狼子,一名犬牙,生淮南及冤句,八月采根,暴干。

3. 案《范子计然》云:狼牙出三辅,色白者善。

【今译】

味苦,性寒。

38. Yazi（牙子，rose root，Radix Indigofera pseudotinctoria） [1]

[Original Text]

[Yazi（牙子，rose root，Radix Indigofera pseudotinctoria），] bitter in taste and cold [in property], [is mainly used] to treat [disease caused by] evil-Qi and heat-Qi, scabies, severe sore and hemorrhoids, and to kill tapeworms. [It is also] called Langya（狼牙）, growing in mountain valleys and river valleys.

[Textual Research]

[In the book entitled] *Wu Pu Ben Cao*（《吴普本草》，*Wu Pu's Studies of Materia Medica*）, [it] says [that] Yazi（牙子，rose root，Radix Indigofera pseudotinctoria） [is also] called Zhilan（支兰）, Langchi（狼齿）, Quanya（犬牙） and Baozi（抱子）. [According to] Agriculture God（神农） and Yellow Emperor（黄帝）, [it is] bitter [in taste] and toxic [in property]; [according to] Tongjun（桐均）, [it is] salty [in taste]; [according to] Qibo（岐伯）, Leigong（雷公） and Bianque（扁鹊）, [it is] bitter [in taste] and toxic [in property], growing in Yuanju（冤句） with green leaves and yellow and red roots. [It begins] to blossom in June and July. [In] August, [it begins] to bear fruits black [in color]. [In] January and August, [its] root [can be] collected [as mentioned in the book entitled] *Tai Ping Yu Lan*（《太平御览》，*Imperial Studies in Taiping Times*）.

主治邪气所致之症以及热邪所致之病,能消除疥疮,瘙痒,恶疮溃疡和痔疮,能祛除绦虫。又称为狼牙。该物生长在山川河谷之中。

[In the book entitled] *Ming Yi Bie Lu* (《名医别录》, *Special Record of Great Doctors*), [it] says [that Yazi (牙子, rose root, Radix Indigofera pseudotinctoria) is also] called Langchi (狼齿), Langzi (狼子) and Quanya (犬牙), growing in Huainan (淮南) and Yuanju (冤句). [Its] root [can be] collected in August and dried in the sun.

[In the book entitled] *Fan Zi Ji Ran* (《范子计然》, *Studies About Fan Li's Teacher*), [it] says [that] Yazi (牙子, rose root, Radix Indigofera pseudotinctoria) grows in the three places. The white one is better.

Notes

1. Yazi (牙子, rose root, Radix Indigofera pseudotinctoria) is a herbal medicinal, bitter in taste, mild in property, entering the lung meridian, the liver meridian and the spleen meridian, effective in restraining certain organs, ceasing bleeding, and removing toxin. Clinically it is used to treat malaria, dysentery, hemoptysis, hematemesis, vaginal bleeding, damage caused by overstrain, abscess, scabies, genital itching and leucorrhea.

39. 羊踯躅

【原文】

味辛,温。

主贼风在皮肤中,淫淫痛,温疟。恶毒,诸痹。生川谷。

【考据】

1.《吴普》曰:羊踯躅花,神农雷公辛有毒,生淮南,治贼风恶毒诸邪气(《御览》)。

2.《名医》曰:一名玉支,生太行山,及淮南山,三月采花,阴干。

3.案《广雅》云:羊踯躅,英光也。古今注云:羊踯躅花,黄羊食之,则死,羊见之则踯躅分散,故名羊踯躅。陶宏景云:花苗似鹿葱。

39. Yangzhizhu（羊踯躅，root of Chinese azalea，Radix Rhododendri Mollis）[1]

〔Original Text〕

〔Yangzhizhu （羊 踯 躅，root of Chinese azalea， Radix Rhododendri Mollis），〕pungent in taste and warm 〔in property〕，〔is mainly used〕to treat wandering pain 〔caused by invasion of〕thief-like wind into the skin，warm malaria，〔disease caused by〕severe toxin and various impediment. 〔It〕grows in mountain valleys and river valleys.

〔Textual Research〕

〔In the book entitled〕*Wu Pu Ben Cao* （《吴普本草》，*Wu Pu's Studies of Materia Medica* ），〔it〕says 〔that〕the flower of Yangzhizhu （羊 踯 躅，Chinese azalea， Rhododendri Mollis ），〔according to〕Agriculture God （神农）and Leigong （雷公），〔is〕pungent 〔in taste〕and toxic 〔in property〕. 〔It〕grows in Huainan （淮南）and 〔can be used〕to treat 〔disease caused by〕thief-like wind，severe toxin and various evil-Qi 〔as mentioned in the book entitled〕*Tai Ping Yu Lan* （《太平御览》，*Imperial Studies in Taiping Times* ）.

〔In the book entitled〕*Ming Yi Bie Lu* （《名医别录》，*Special Record of Great Doctors* ），〔it〕says 〔that Yangzhizhu （羊踯躅，root of Chinese azalea，Radix Rhododendri Mollis) is also〕called Yuzhi

【今译】

味辛,性温。

主治皮肤中的虚邪贼风所致的流窜性疼痛和温疟病,能治疗恶性传染病和各种痹证。该物生长在山川河谷之中。

（玉支），growing in Taihang（太行）mountain and Huainan（淮南）mountain. ［Its］ flower ［can be］ collected in March and dried in the shade.

［In the book entitled］ *Guang Ya* （《广雅》，*The First Chinese Encyclopedic Dictionary*），［it］ says ［that］ Yangzhizhu（羊踯躅，root of Chinese azalea，Radix Rhododendri Mollis） is bright. ［According to］ the explanation made in ancient times and at present，Huangyang（黄羊，yellow sheep，Procapra Przewalskii） will die ［if it has］ eaten the flowers of Yangzhizhu（羊踯躅，Chinese azalea，Rhododendri Mollis）. ［So when］ seeing Yangzhizhu（羊踯躅，Chinese azalea，Rhododendri Mollis），it immediately runs away. That is why Yangzhizhu（羊踯躅，root of Chinese azalea，Radix Rhododendri Mollis） is so named. Tao Hongjing（陶宏景）said，"［Its］ seedling is like Lucong（鹿葱，Lycoris squamigera）."

Notes

1. Yangzhizhu （羊踯躅，root of Chinese azalea，Radix Rhododendri Mollis） is a herbal medicinal，pungent in taste，warm and severely toxic in property，entering the liver meridian，effective in expelling wind，eliminating dampness and ceasing pain. Clinically it is used to treat wind-dampness impediment and pain，traumatic injury，fracture，scabies and bleeding due to worm toxin.

40. 商陆

【原文】

味辛,平。

主水张,疝瘕,痹,熨除痈肿,杀鬼精物,一名荡根,一名夜呼。生川谷。

【考据】

1.《名医》曰:如人行者,有神,生咸阳。

2. 案《说文》:蔏草,枝枝相值,叶叶相当。《广雅》云:常蓼,马尾,商陆也。

3.《尔雅》云:蓫薚马尾。郭璞云:今关西亦呼为薚,江东为当陆。周易夬云:苋陆夬夬。郑元云:苋陆、商陆也,盖蔏即荡俗字,商即荡假音。

【今译】

味辛,性平。

主治水肿,腹部胀满,疝瘕和痹证,能通过外贴消除痈肿,能杀除鬼怪之邪。又称为根,又称为夜呼。该物生长在山川河谷之中。

40. Shanglu（商陆，phytolacca，Radix Phytolaccae）[1]

［Original Text］

［Shanglu（商陆，phytolacca，Radix Phytolaccae），］pungent in taste and mild ［in property］，［is mainly used］ to treat distension ［and fullness due to］ edema，conglomeration and impediment，to eliminate abscess ［through］ external application and ［strange pathogenic factors like］ ghost and monster. ［It is also］ called Tanggen（葛根）and Yehu（夜呼），growing in mountain valleys and river valleys.

［Textual Research］

［In the book entitled］ *Ming Yi Bie Lu*（《名医别录》，*Special Record of Great Doctors*），［it］ says ［that Shanglu（商陆，phytolacca，Radix Phytolaccae）］，looking like a walking man or a spirit，grows in Xianyang（咸阳）.

［In the book entitled］ *Guang Ya*（《广雅》，*The First Chinese Encyclopedic Dictionary*），［it］ says ［that the so-called］ Changliao（常蓼）and Mawei（马尾）refer to Shanglu（商陆，phytolacca，Radix Phytolaccae）.

Notes

1. Shanglu（商陆，phytolacca，Radix Phytolaccae）is a herbal medicinal，bitter in taste，cold and toxic in property，entering the spleen meridian and the bladder meridian，effective in purging water and resolving swelling. Clinically it is used to treat edema，distension and fullness，dysuria，sore and scabies.

41. 羊蹄

【原文】

味苦,寒。

主头秃,疥搔,除热,女子阴蚀(《御览》此四字作无字)。一名东方宿,一名连虫陆,一名鬼目。生川泽。

【考据】

1.《名医》曰:名蓄,生陈留。

2. 案《说文》云:董草也,读若厘,藋,厘草也,芨董草也。《广雅》云:莄,羊蹄也。《毛诗》云:言采其蓫。《笺》云:蓫,牛蘈也。陆德明云:本又作蓄。陆玑云:今人谓之羊蹄。陶宏景云:今人呼秃菜,即是蓄音之讹。诗云:言,采其蓄,案陆英,疑即此草之花,此草一名连虫陆,又陆英,即蒴藋,一名董也,亦苦寒。

41. Yangti（羊蹄，root of Japanese dock，Radix Rumicis）[1]

[Original Text]

[Yangti（羊蹄，root of Japanese dock，Radix Rumicis），] bitter in taste and cold [in property]，[is mainly used] to treat baldhead with ulcer and itching，and to expel heat and valvar ulcer．[It is also] called Dongfangsu（东方宿），Lianchonglu（连虫陆）and Guimu（鬼目），growing in valleys and swamps．

[Textual Research]

[In the book entitled] *Ming Yi Bie Lu*（《名医别录》，*Special Record of Great Doctors*），[it] says [that Yangti（羊蹄，root of Japanese dock，Radix Rumicis）is also] called Xu（蓄）and grows in Chenliu（陈留）．

[In the book entitled] *Guang Ya*（《广雅》，*The First Chinese Encyclopedic Dictionary*），[it] says [that the so-called] Li（蓮）refers to Yangti（羊蹄，root of Japanese dock，Radix Rumicis）．Luying（陆英，flower of Chinese elder，Flos Sambuci Chinensis）perhaps is the flower of Yangti（羊蹄，root of Japanese dock，Radix Rumicis）which is also called Lianchonglu（连虫陆）．Besides，Luying（陆英，flower of Chinese elder，Flos Sambuci Chinensis）is Shuodiao（蒴藋，Chinese elder herb or root，Herba seu Radix Sambuci Chinensis），also called Li（蓮），bitter [in taste] and cold

【今译】

味苦,性寒。

主治头秃,疥疮瘑痒,能清除热气及女子阴部溃疡。又称为东方宿,又称为连虫陆,又称为鬼目。该物生长在山川池泽中。

[in property].

Notes

1. Yangti (羊蹄, root of Japanese dock, Radix Rumicis) is a herbal medicinal, bitter and sour in taste, cold and slightly toxic in property, effective in cooling the blood and ceasing bleeding, clearing heat and removing toxin, promoting defecation and killing worms. Clinically it is used to treat nosebleed, hematemesis, hematochezia, uterine bleeding, stanguria, jaundice, inflammation around the anus and constipation.

42. 萹蓄

【原文】

味辛,平。

主浸淫,疥搔疽痔,杀三虫(《御览》引云:一名篇竹,《大观本》无文)。生山谷。

【考据】

1.《吴普》曰:萹蓄一名蓄辩,一名萹蔓(《御览》)。

2.《名医》曰:生东莱,五月采,阴干。

3. 案《说文》云:萹,萹茿也,茿,萹也,茿水萹,茿,读若督。《尔雅》云:竹萹,蓄。郭璞云:似水蓼,赤茎节,好生道旁,可食,又杀虫。《毛诗》云:绿竹猗猗。《传》云:竹,萹竹也。韩诗茿云:藩,萹茿也,石经同。

42. Bianxu (萹蓄, common knotgrass herb, Herba Polygoni Avicularis) [1]

[Original Text]

[Bianxu (萹蓄, common knotgrass herb, Herba Polygoni Avicularis),] pungent in taste and mild [in property], [is mainly used] to treat spreading [of pathogenic factors in the skin], ulcer, scabies and hemorrhoids, and to kill three worms. [It] grows in mountains and valleys.

[Textual Research]

[In the book entitled] *Wu Pu Ben Cao* (《吴普本草》, *Wu Pu's Studies of Materia Medica*), [it] says [that] Bianxu (萹蓄, common knotgrass herb, Herba Polygoni Avicularis) [is also] called Xubian (蓄辩) and Bianman (萹蔓) [according to the book entitled] *Tai Ping Yu Lan* (《太平御览》, *Imperial Studies in Taiping Times*).

[In the book entitled] *Ming Yi Bie Lu* (《名医别录》, *Special Record of Great Doctors*), [it] says [that Bianxu (萹蓄, common knotgrass herb, Herba Polygoni Avicularis)] grows in Dongcai (东菜). [It can be] collected in May and dried in the shade.

Guo Pu (郭璞) said, "[Bianxu (萹蓄, common knotgrass herb, Herba Polygoni Avicularis) looks] like Shuili (水藜, waternut corm, Cormus Eleocharitis Dulcis) with red stalks and joints, usually growing in roadsides and edible. [It can be used] to kill worms.

【今译】

味辛,性平。

主治浸淫,疥瘙,瘘痒,疮肿,痔疮,能杀死三种寄生虫。该物生长在山谷之中。

Notes

1. Bianxu（萹蓄, common knotgrass herb, Herba Polygoni Avicularis）is a herbal medicinal, bitter in taste and cold in property, entering the bladder meridian, effective in clearing heat, promoting urination and killing worms. Clinically it is used to treat infection of urethra, urethral stones, jaundice, dysentery, ascaridiasis and ancylostomiasis.

43. 狼毒

【原文】

味辛,平。

主咳逆上气,破积聚,饮食寒热,水气恶疮,鼠瘘,疽蚀,鬼精,蛊毒,杀飞鸟走兽。一名续毒。生山谷。

【考据】

1.《名医》曰:生秦亭及奉高,二月八月,采根阴干。

2. 案《广雅》云:狼毒也,疑上脱续毒二字。《中山经》云:大騩之山有草焉,其状如蓍而毛,青华而白实,其名曰蒗,服之不夭,可以不腹病。

【今译】

味辛,性平。

主治咳嗽,呼吸困难,能破解积聚,能消除饮食所致的寒热病,

43. Langdu（狼毒，Chinese stellera root，fischer euphorbia root，Radix Stellerae Chamaejasmis seu Euphorbiae Fischerianae）[1]

［Original Text］

［Langdu（狼毒，Chinese stellera root，fischer euphorbia root，Radix Stellerae Chamaejasmis seu Euphorbiae Fischerianae），］ pungent in taste and mild ［in property］，［is mainly used］ to relieve cough with dyspnea with upward counterflow of Qi ［due to improper］ diet，to break accumulation and aggregation，and to treat cold-heat ［disease］，edema，severe sore，tuberculosis，abscess，scabies，［disease cause by pathogenic factors like］ ghost and worm toxin，and to kill bird and animals. ［It is also］ called Xudu（续毒） and grows in mountains and valleys.

［Textual Research］

［In the book entitled］ *Ming Yi Bie Lu*（《名医别录》，*Special Record of Great Doctors*），［it］ says ［that Langdu（狼毒，Chinese stellera root，fischer euphorbia root，Radix Stellerae Chamaejasmis seu Euphorbiae Fischerianae）］ grows in Qinting（秦亭） and Fenggao（奉高）. ［Its］ root ［can be］ collected in February and August，and dried in the shade.

能治疗水湿所致的恶性痈疮，瘰疬，疮肿溃疡，能祛除鬼怪邪气和虫毒所致之病，能杀除飞鸟走兽。又称为续毒。该物生长在山谷之中。

Notes

1. Langdu（狼毒，Chinese stellera root，fischer euphorbia root，Radix Stellerae Chamaejasmis seu Euphorbiae Fischerianae）is a herbal medicinal，pungent and bitter in taste，mild and severely toxic in property，entering the liver meridian and the spleen meridian，effective in expelling water and phlegm，dispersing stagnation，ceasing pain and killing worms. Clinically it is used to treat edema，abdominal distension，phlegm erosion，retention of undigested food，accumulation of worms，abdominal hernia and pain，retention of fluid and phlegm，cough and panting.

44. 白头翁

【原文】

味苦,温。

主温疟,狂易,寒热,症瘕积聚,瘿气,逐血,止痛,疗金疮。一名野丈人,一名胡王使者。生山谷。

【考据】

1.《吴普》曰:白头翁,一名野丈人,一名奈河草,神农扁鹊苦无毒,生嵩山川谷,破气狂寒热,止痛(《御览》)。

2.《名医》曰:一名奈河草,生高山及田野,四月采。

3. 案陶宏景云:近根处有白茸状似人白头,故以为名。

【今译】

味苦,性温。

44. Baitouweng（白头翁，pulsatilla，Radix Pulsatillae）[1]

［**Original Text**］

［Baitouweng（白头翁，pulsatilla，Radix Pulsatillae），］bitter in taste and warm［in property］，［is mainly used］to treat warm malaria，mania，cold-heat［disease］，abdominal conglomeration，accumulation and aggregation and goiter，to expel blood［stasis］，to relieve pain and to cure sore［caused by injury of］metal．［It is also］called Yezhangren（野丈人）and Huwang Shizhe（胡王使者），growing in mountains and valleys．

［**Textual Research**］

［In the book entitled］*Wu Pu Ben Cao*（《吴普本草》，*Wu Pu's Studies of Materia Medica*），［it］says［that］Baitouweng（白头翁，pulsatilla，Radix Pulsatillae）［is also］called Yezhangren（野丈人）and Naihecao（奈河草）．［According to］Agriculture God（神农）and Bianque（扁鹊），［it is］bitter［in taste］and non-toxic［in property］．［It］grows in mountains and valleys in Songshan（嵩山）and stops pain［according to the book entitled］*Tai Ping Yu Lan*（《太平御览》，*Imperial Studies in Taiping Times*）．

［In the book entitled］*Ming Yi Bie Lu*（《名医别录》，*Special Record of Great Doctors*），［it］says［that Baitouweng（白头翁，pulsatilla，Radix Pulsatillae）is also］called Naihecao（奈河草），

主治温疟,发狂,寒热病,症瘕,积聚,瘿瘤,能祛除瘀血,能消除疼痛,能治疗金属创伤。又称为野丈人,又称为胡王使者。该物生长在山谷之中。

growing in high mountains and lands. [It can be] collected in April.

Tao Hongjing (陶宏景) said, "There are antlers near the root [of Baitouweng (白头翁, pulsatilla, Radix Pulsatillae)], like hoary head. That is why it is so named."

Notes

1. Baitouweng (白头翁, pulsatilla, Radix Pulsatillae) is a herbal medicinal, bitter in taste and cold in property, entering the stomach meridian and the large intestine meridian, effective in clearing heat and removing toxin, cooling the blood and relieving dysentery. Clinically it is used to treat amebic dysentery, bacillary dysentery, malaria and leucorrhea.

45. 鬼臼

神农本草经

【原文】

味辛,温。

主杀蛊毒鬼注,精物,辟恶气不祥,逐邪,解百毒。一名爵犀,一名马目毒公,一名九臼。生山谷。

【考据】

1.《吴普》曰:一名九臼,一名天臼,一名雀犀,一名马目公,一名解毒。生九真山谷及冤句,二月八月采根(《御览》)。

2.《名医》曰:一名天臼,一名解毒,生九真及冤句,二月八月采根。

【今译】

味辛,性温。

45. Guijiu（鬼臼，common dysosma，Rhizoma Dysosmae Versipellis）[1]

[Original Text]

[Guijiu （鬼臼，common dysosma，Rhizoma Dysosmae Versipellis），] pungent in taste and warm [in property]，[is mainly used] to treat [disease caused by] worm toxin and [strange pathogenic factors like] ghost and monster，to expel vicious and non-auspicious Qi，to dispel evils and to resolve various toxin. [It is also] called Juexi（爵犀），Mamu Dugong（马目毒公）and Jiujiu（九臼），growing in mountains and valleys.

[Textual Research]

[In the book entitled] *Wu Pu Ben Cao*（《吴普本草》，*Wu Pu's Studies of Materia Medica*），[it] says [that Guijiu（鬼臼，common dysosma，Rhizoma Dysosmae Versipellis）is also] called Jiujiu（九臼），Tianjiu（天臼），Quexi（雀犀），Mamugong（马目公）and Jiedu（解毒），growing in mountains and valleys in Jiuzhen（九真）and Yuanju（冤句）. [Its] root [can be] collected in February and August [according to the book entitled] *Tai Ping Yu Lan*（《太平御览》，*Imperial Studies in Taiping Times*）.

[In the book entitled] *Ming Yi Bie Lu*（《名医别录》，*Special Record of Great Doctors*），[it] says [that Guijiu（鬼臼，common dysosma，Rhizoma Dysosmae Versipellis）is also] called Tianjiu（天

主治能杀除虫毒鬼怪病邪,能避免遭受精怪不祥恶气的伤害,能祛除邪气,能消解各种毒气。又称为爵犀,又称为马目毒公,又称为九臼。该物生长在山谷之中。

臼) and Jiedu（解毒），growing in Jiuzhen（九真）and Yuanju（冤句）. [Its] root [can be] collected in February and August.

Notes

1. Guijiu （鬼臼，common dysosma，Rhizoma Dysosmae Versipellis) is a herbal medicinal，bitter and pungent in taste，warm and toxic in property，effective in removing toxin，dispersing blood stasis and resolving swelling. Clinically it is used to treat injury caused by snake bite，abscess，scabies，traumatic injury，lymphadenitis，mumps and herpes zoster.

46. 羊桃

【原文】

味苦,寒。

主燔热,身暴赤色,风水积聚,恶疡,除小儿热。一名鬼桃,一名羊肠。生川谷。

【考据】

1.《名医》曰:一名苌楚,一名御弋,一名铫弋,生山林及田野,二月采,阴干。

2. 案《说文》云:苌,苌楚铫弋,一名羊桃。《广雅》云:鬼桃铫戈羊桃也。《中山经》云:丰山多羊桃,状如桃而方,茎可以为皮张。《尔雅》云:长楚姚铫。郭璞云:今羊桃也,或曰鬼桃,叶似桃华,白子如小麦,亦似桃。《毛诗》云:隰有铫楚。《传》云:苌楚,铫弋也。陆玑云:今羊桃是也,叶长而狭,华紫赤色,其枝茎弱过一尺,引蔓于草上,今人以为汲灌,重而善没,不如杨柳也,近下根,刀切其皮,著热灰中,脱之,可韬笔管。

46. Yangtao（羊桃，fruit of yangtao actinidia，Fructus Actinidiae Chinensis）[1]

[Original Text]

[Yangtao（羊桃，fruit of yangtao actinidia，Fructus Actinidiae Chinensis），] bitter in taste and cold [in property], [is mainly used] to treat severe heat [disease marked by] fierce redness of the body, wind-water [disease marked by] accumulation and aggregation, severe sore and infantile heat [disease]. [It is also] called Guitao（鬼桃）and Yangchang（羊肠），growing in mountain valleys and river valleys.

[Textual Research]

[In the book entitled] *Ming Yi Bie Lu*（《名医别录》，*Special Record of Great Doctors*），[it] says [that Yangtao（羊桃，fruit of yangtao actinidia，Fructus Actinidiae Chinensis）is also] called Changcu（苌楚），Yuyi（御弋）and Diaoyi（铫弋），growing in mountains and lands. [It can be] collected in February and dried in the shade.

[In] case [analysis in the book entitled] *Zhong Shan Jing*（《中山经》，*Central Mountain Canon*），[it] says [that] there are many Yangtao（羊桃，fruit of yangtao actinidia，Fructus Actinidiae Chinensis）in Fengshan（丰山），similar to peach. Guo Pu（郭璞）said，"Now Yangtao（羊桃，fruit of yangtao actinidia，Fructus

【今译】

味苦,性寒。

主治发作迅速凶狂的火热病症,身体突然发红,风水证,积聚证,恶疮溃疡,能清除小儿发热。又称为鬼桃,又称为羊肠。该物生长在山川河谷之中。

Actinidiae Chinensis) may be called Guitao (鬼桃). [Its] leaves are similar to the flowers of peach and [its] white seeds are like wheat and also similar to that of peach."

Notes

1. Yangtao (羊桃,fruit of yangtao actinidia, Fructus Actinidiae Chinensis) is a herbal medicinal sweet and sour in taste, cold in property, entering the stomach meridian and the kidney meridian, effective in relieving heat, ceasing thirst and resolving stranguria. Clinically it is used to treat vexing fever, wasting-thirst, poor appetite, indigestion, jaundice, stones in urethra and hemorrhoids.

47. 女青

【原文】

味辛，平。

主蛊毒，逐邪恶气，杀鬼温疟，辟不祥。一名雀瓢（《御览》作翲）。

【考据】

1.《吴普》曰：女青一名霍由祇，神农黄帝辛（《御览》）。

2.《名医》曰：蛇衔根也，生朱崖，八月采，阴干。

3. 案《广雅》云：女青，乌葛也。《尔雅》云：藋芄兰。郭璞云：藋芄蔓生。断之，有白汁可啖。《毛诗》云：芄兰之支。《传》云：芄兰草也。陆玑云：一名萝摩，幽州人，谓之雀瓢。别录云：雀瓢白汁，注虫蛇毒，即女青苗汁也，《唐本》草，别出萝摩条，非。

47. Nǔqing（女青，Japanese metaplexis，Metaplexis Japonica）[1]

[Original Text]

[Nǔqing（女青，Japanese metaplexis，Metaplexis Japonica），] pungent in taste and mild [in property], [is mainly used] to treat [disease caused by] worm toxin, to expel evil and vicious Qi, to dispel warm malaria [like] ghost and to prevent non-auspicious [pathogenic factors]. [It is also] called Quepiao（雀瓢）.

[Textual Research]

[In the book entitled] *Wu Pu Ben Cao*（《吴普本草》, *Wu Pu's Studies of Materia Medica*）, [it] says [that] Nǔqing（女青，Japanese metaplexis，Metaplexis Japonica）[is also] called Huoyouzhi（霍由祇）. [According to] Agriculture God（神农）and Yellow Emperor（黄帝），[it is] pungent [in taste], [as mentioned in the book entitled] *Tai Ping Yu Lan*（《太平御览》, *Imperial Studies in Taiping Times*）.

[In the book entitled] *Ming Yi Bie Lu*（《名医别录》, *Special Record of Great Doctors*）, [it] says [that Nǔqing（女青，Japanese metaplexis，Metaplexis Japonica）is also] called Shexiangen（蛇衔根），growing in Zhuya（朱崖）. [It can be] collected in August and dried in the shade.

【今译】

味辛,性平。

主治虫毒所致之病,能祛除邪恶之气,能杀除鬼怪之病,能治疗温疟,能消除不祥之气。又称为雀瓢。

Notes

1. Nǔqing (女青, Japanese metaplexis, Metaplexis Japonica) is a herbal medicinal, effective in tonifying Qi and replenishing essence, improving deficiency and assisting Yang, strengthening the body and invigorating energy, moving Qi and activating the blood, resolving swelling and removing toxin. Clinically it is used to treat impotence, leucorrhea, insufficiency of milk, sore, cough with phlegm, whooping cough, seminal emission, bleeding due to external injury, scabies and injury caused by snake bite.

48. 连翘

【原文】

味苦,平。

主寒热,鼠瘘,瘰疬,痈肿,恶疮,瘿瘤,结热,蛊毒。一名异翘,一名兰华,一名轵,一名三廉。生山谷。

【考据】

1.《名医》曰:一名折根,生太山,八月采,阴干。

2. 案《尔雅》云:连,异翘。郭璞云:一名连苕,又名连本草云。

【今译】

味苦,性平。

主治寒热病,能治疗鼠瘘,瘰疬,痈肿,恶性痈疮,瘿瘤,结热证以及虫毒所致之病。又称为异翘,又称为兰华,又称为轵,又称为三廉。该物生长在山谷之中。

48. Lianqiao（连翘, fruit of weeping forsythia，Fructus Forsythiae）[1]

[Original Text]

[Lianqiao （连翘, fruit of weeping forsythia， Fructus Forsythiae），] bitter in taste and mild [in property], [is mainly used] to treat cold-heat [disease], tuberculosis, scrofula, abscess, severe sore, goiter, tumor, heat stagnation and worm toxin. [It is also] called Yiqiao（异翘），Lanhua （兰华），Zhi（轵）and Sanlian （三廉），growing in mountains and valleys.

[Textual Research]

[In the book entitled] *Ming Yi Bie Lu* （《名医别录》，*Special Record of Great Doctors*），[it] says [that Lianqiao（连翘, fruit of weeping forsythia，Fructus Forsythiae）is also] called Zhegen（折根），growing in Taishan（太山）. [It can be] collected in August and dried in the shade.

Notes

1. Lianqiao（连翘, fruit of weeping forsythia，Fructus Forsythiae）is a herbal medicinal, bitter in taste, slightly cold in property, entering the lung meridian, the heart meridian and the gallbladder meridian, effective in clearing heat and removing toxin, resolving abscess and dispersing stagnation, expelling wind and dispelling heat. Clinically it is used to treat abscess, scabies, scrofula, subcutaneous nodule, warm disease at the early period, vertigo and delirium.

49. 兰茹(《御览》作问,是)

【原文】

味辛,寒。

主蚀恶肉,败疮,死肌,杀疥虫,排脓恶血,除大风热气,善忘不乐。生川谷。

【考据】

1.《吴普》曰:间茹一名离楼,一名屈居,神农辛,岐伯酸咸有毒,李氏大寒,二月采,叶员黄,高四五尺,叶四四相当,四月华黄,五月实黑,根黄有汁,亦同黄,三月五月采根,黑头者良(《御览》)。

2.《名医》曰:一名屈据,一名离娄,生代郡,五月采,阴干。

3. 案《广雅》云:屈居,芦茹也。《范子计然》云:间茹出武都,黄色者善。

【今译】

味辛,性寒。

49. Lanru（兰茹，Lanru herb，Herba Lanru）^[1]

[Original Text]

[Lanru（兰茹，Lanru herb，Herba Lanru），] pungent in taste and cold [in property], [is mainly used] to erode vicious muscles, to treat putrid sore with necrotic muscles, to kill sarcoptic mite, to expel pus and blood stasis, to dispel severe wind and heat-Qi, and to cure amnesia and depression. [It] grows in mountain valleys and river valleys.

[Textual Research]

[In the book entitled] *Wu Pu Ben Cao*（《吴普本草》，*Wu Pu's Studies of Materia Medica*），[it] says [that] Lanru（兰茹，Lanru herb，Herba Lanru）[is also] called Lilou（离楼）and Quju（屈居）. [According to] Agriculture God（神农），[it is] pungent [in taste]; [according to] Qibo（岐伯，[it is] sour and salty [in taste] and toxic [in property]; [according to] Li's（李氏），[it is] severely cold [in property]. [It can be] collected in February. [Its] leaves are round and yellow, about 4 to 5 *Chi*（尺）in length，four corresponding to four. [In] April [it begins to blossom with] yellow flowers; [in] May [it begins to bear] black fruits; [its] root is yellow with juice; [in] March and May，[its] root [can be collected]; the black one is better [according to the book entitled] *Tai Ping Yu Lan*（《太平御览》，*Imperial Studies in Taiping Times*）.

能消除恶肉,久治不愈之疮和肌肉坏死,能杀除疥虫,能排出脓肿,能治疗脓液瘀血,严重的风热病,虚妄不乐的郁闷病症。该物生长在山川河谷之中。

［In the book entitled］ *Ming Yi Bie Lu*（《名医别录》，*Special Record of Great Doctors*），［it］says［that Lanru（兰茹，Lanru herb，Herba Lanru）is also］called Quju（屈据）and Lilou（离娄），growing in Daijun（代郡）.［It can be］collected in May and dried in the shade.

［In the book entitled］ *Fan Zi Ji Ran*（《范子计然》，*Studies About Fan Li's Teacher*），［it］says［that］Lanru（兰茹，Lanru herb，Herba Lanru）grows in Wudu（武都）and the yellow one is better.

Notes

1. Lanru（兰茹，Lanru herb，Herba Lanru）is a herbal medicinal，pungent in taste，cold and slightly toxic in property，effective in eroding vicious muscles，killing worms，clearing heat，removing toxin and expelling pus and blood stasis. Clinically it is used to treat leprosy，heat impediment，abdominal mass，accumulation，conglomeration and aggregation，and polypus.

50. 乌韭

【原文】

味甘,寒。

主皮肤往来寒热,利小肠膀胱气。生山谷石上。

【考据】

1. 案《广雅》云:昔邪,乌韭也,在屋曰昔邪,在墙曰垣衣。《西山经》云:草荔,状如乌韭。《唐本》注云:即石衣也,亦名石苔,又名石发。按《广雅》又云:石发,石衣也,未知是一否。

【今译】

味甘,性寒。

主治皮肤病和往来寒热病,能通利小肠和膀胱气。该物生长在山谷之中的石上。

50. Wujiu（乌韭，leaf of common wedgelet fern，Folium Stenolomatis）[1]

[Original Text]

[Wujiu（乌韭，leaf of common wedgelet fern，Folium Stenolomatis），] sweet in taste and cold [in property]，[is mainly used] to treat alternate cold and heat in the skin，and to disinhibit Qi in the small intestine and bladder. [It] grows over the stones in mountains and valleys.

[Textual Research]

[In the book entitled] *Guang Ya*（《广雅》，*The First Chinese Encyclopedic Dictionary*），[it] says [that the so-called] Xixie（昔邪） refers to Wujiu（乌韭，leaf of common wedgelet fern，Folium Stenolomatis）. [If growing in] the house，[it is] called Xixie（昔邪）；[if growing] on the wall，[it is] called Yuanyi（垣衣）. [In the book entitled] *Xi Shan Jing*（《西山经》，*Canon About West Mountains*），[it] says [that the so-called] Bili（草荔）looks like Wujiu（乌韭，leaf of common wedgelet fern，Folium Stenolomatis）.

Notes

1. Wujiu（乌韭，leaf of common wedgelet fern，Folium Stenolomatis）is a herbal medicinal，bitter in taste and cold in property，effective in clearing heat，removing toxin，expelling dampness and ceasing bleeding. Clinically it is used to treat common cold，cough，tonsillitis，mumps，enteritis，dysentery，hepatitis，leucorrhea，hematemesis，hematochezia and hematuria.

51. 鹿藿

【原文】

味苦,平。

主蛊毒,女子腰腹痛,不乐肠痈,瘰疬(《御览》作历),疡气。生山谷。

【考据】

1.《名医》曰:生汶山。

2. 案《说文》云:蘆,鹿藿也,读若剽。《广雅》云:蘆,鹿藿也。《尔雅》云:蔨,鹿藿,其实莥。郭璞云:今鹿豆也,叶似大豆,根黄而香,蔓延生。

51. Luhuo（鹿藿，twining rhynchosia herb，Herba Rhynchosiae Volubilis）[1]

[Original Text]

[Luhuo（鹿藿，twining rhynchosia herb，Herba Rhynchosiae Volubilis），] bitter in taste and mild [in property], [is mainly used] to treat [disease caused by] worm toxin，pain of the waist and abdomen in women，depression，acute appendicitis，scrofula and ulcer. [It] grows in mountains and valleys.

[Textual Research]

[In the book entitled] *Ming Yi Bie Lu*（《名医别录》，*Special Record of Great Doctors*），[it] says [that Luhuo（鹿藿，twining rhynchosia herb，Herba Rhynchosiae Volubilis）] grows in Wenshan（汶山）.

[In] case [analysis in the book entitled] *Shuo Wen*（《说文》，*On Culture*）and [in the book entitled] *Guang Ya*（《广雅》，*The First Chinese Encyclopedic Dictionary*），[it] says [that the so-called] Biao（藨）refers to Luhuo（鹿藿，twining rhynchosia herb，Herba Rhynchosiae Volubilis）. [In the book entitled] *Er Ya*（《尔雅》，*On Elegance*），[it] says [that] Juan（菌）refers to Luhuo（鹿藿，twining rhynchosia herb，Herba Rhynchosiae Volubilis）.

Guo Pu（郭璞）said，"Now the leaves of [the so-called] deer bean are similar to [that of] soybean with yellow and fragrant root，

【今译】

味苦,性平。

主治虫毒所致之病,女子腰腹部疼痛,抑郁不乐,肠痛,瘰疬和疮疡。该物生长在山谷之中。

spreading prosperously in growth. "

Notes

1. Luhuo (鹿藿, twining rhynchosia herb, Herba Rhynchosiae Volubilis) is a herbal medicinal, bitter in taste and mild in property, entering the stomach meridian and the kidney meridian, effective in removing toxin, expelling wind-dampness and ceasing pain. Clinically it is used to treat disease caused by worm toxin, scrofula, abscess, suppurative tissue disease, headache, pain of the waist and leg, abdominal pain and postpartum perspiration.

52. 蚤休

【原文】

味苦,微寒。

主惊痫,摇头弄舌,热气在腹中,癫疾,痈疮,阴蚀,下三虫,去蛇毒。一名蚩休。生川谷。

【考据】

1.《名医》曰:生山阳及冤句。

2. 案郑樵云:蚤休,曰螫休,曰重楼金绵,曰重台,曰草,甘遂,今人谓之紫河车,服食家所用,而茎叶亦可爱,多植庭院间。

52. Zaoxiu（蚤休，rhizome of multileaf paris，rhizome of pubescent paris，rhizome of narrowleaf paris，Rhizoma Paridis）[1]

[Original Text]

[Zaoxiu（蚤休，rhizome of multileaf paris，rhizome of pubescent paris，rhizome of narrowleaf paris，Rhizoma Paridis），] bitter in taste and slightly cold [in property]，[is mainly used] to treat convulsion，epilepsy with head shivering and tongue protruding，heat-Qi in the abdomen，epileptic disease，abscess and genital ulcer，to expel three worms and to eliminate snake toxin. [It is also] called Chixiu（蚩休），growing in mountain valleys and river valleys.

[Textual Research]

[In the book entitled] *Ming Yi Bie Lu*（《名医别录》，*Special Record of Great Doctors*），[it] says [that Zaoxiu（蚤休，rhizome of multileaf paris，rhizome of pubescent paris，rhizome of narrowleaf paris，Rhizoma Paridis）] grows in Shanyang（山阳）and Yuanju（冤句）.

Zheng Qiao（郑樵）said，"Zaoxiu（蚤休，rhizome of multileaf paris，rhizome of Chinese paris，rhizome of pubescent paris，rhizome of narrowleaf paris，rhizome of Yunnan manyleaf paris，Rhizoma Paridis）[is also] called Shixiu（螫休），Chonglou Jinmian（重楼金绵），Chongtai（重台），Cao（草）and Gansui（甘遂）. People

【今译】

味苦,性微寒。

主治惊风,癫痫,摇头吐舌,热邪在腹中,癫痫,痈疮,阴部溃疡,能祛除三种虫子和蛇毒。又称为蚩休。该物生长在山川河谷之中。

神农本草经

now call it Ziheche (紫河车) and plant it at home. The leaves and stalks are excellent and usually grow in the courtyard."

Notes

1. Zaoxiu (蚤休, rhizome of multileaf paris, rhizome of pubescent paris, rhizome of narrowleaf paris, Rhizoma Paridis) is a herbal medicinal, bitter in taste, cold and mildly toxic in property, entering the heart meridian and the liver meridian, effective in clearing heat, removing toxin, resolving swelling, relieving convulsion and stopping cough. Clinically it is used to treat injury caused by snake bite, sore, abscess, mumps, infantile convulsion due to high fever, epidemic B encephalitis, tonsillitis, pneumonia and cough.

53. 石长生

【原文】

味咸，微寒。

主寒热，恶疮，火热，辟鬼气不祥(《御览》作辟恶气，不祥，鬼毒)。一名丹草(《御览》引云：丹沙草)。生山谷。

【考据】

1.《吴普》曰：石长生，神农苦，雷公辛，一经甘，生咸阳(《御览》)。

2.《名医》曰：生咸阳。

53. Changshengshi（石长生，maidenhair herb，Herba Adiantum Monochlamys）[1]

[Original Text]

[Changshengshi（石长生，maidenhair herb，Herba Adiantum Monochlamys），] salty in taste and slightly cold [in property]，[is mainly used] to treat cold-heat [disease]，severe sore and [disease caused by] fire-heat，and to eliminate non-auspicious [pathogenic factors like] ghost. [It is also] called Dancao（丹草）. It grows in mountains and valleys.

[Textual Research]

[In the book entitled] *Wu Pu Ben Cao*（《吴普本草》，*Wu Pu's Studies of Materia Medica*），[it] says [that] Changshengshi（石长生，maidenhair herb，Herba Adiantum Monochlamys），[according to] Agriculture God（神农），[is] bitter [in taste]；[according to] Leigong（雷公），[it is] pungent [in taste] and sometimes sweet [in taste]，growing in Xianyang（咸阳）[as mentioned in the book entitled] *Tai Ping Yu Lan*（《太平御览》，*Imperial Studies in Taiping Times*）.

[In the book entitled] *Ming Yi Bie Lu*（《名医别录》，*Special Record of Great Doctors*），[it] says [that Changshengshi（石长生，maidenhair herb，Herba Adiantum Monochlamys）] grows in Xianyang（咸阳）.

【今译】

味咸,性微寒。

主治寒热病,恶性痈疮,火热病,能避免不祥的鬼怪邪气。又称为丹草。该物生长在山谷之中。

Notes

1. Changshengshi（石长生，maidenhair herb，Herba Adiantum Monochlamys）is a herbal medicinal，salty in taste and slightly cold in property，entering the lung meridian，the large intestine meridian and the stomach meridian，effective in clearing heat，resolving phlegm and removing toxin. Clinically it is used to treat ascaridiasis，oxyuriasis，scabies，cough due to lung heat，common cold with fever，ulcer and sore.

54. 陆英

【原文】

味苦,寒。

主骨间诸痹,四肢拘挛,疼酸,膝寒痛,阴痿,短气,不足,脚肿。生川谷。

【考据】

1.《名医》曰:生熊耳及冤句,立秋采,又曰蒴藋,味酸温有毒,一名堇(今本误作堇),一名芨,生四野,春夏采叶,秋冬采茎根。

2.案《说文》云:堇草也,读若厘,芨堇草也,读若急,藋厘草也。《广雅》云:盆,陆英苺也。《尔雅》云:芨堇草。《唐本》注陆英云:此物蒴藋是也,后人不识,浪出蒴藋条。今注云:陆英,味苦寒无毒,蒴藋味酸温有毒,既此不同,难谓一种,盖其类尔。

54. Luying（陆英，flower of Chinese elder herb，Flos Sambuci Chinensis）[1]

[Original Text]

[Luying（陆英，flower of Chinese elder，Flos Sambuci Chinensis），] bitter in taste and cold [in property], [is mainly used] to treat various impediment in the bones，spasm and ache of the four limbs，coldness and pain of the knees，impotence，shortness of breath and swelling of the feet. [It] grows in mountain valleys and river valleys.

[Textual Research]

[In the book entitled] *Ming Yi Bie Lu*（《名医别录》，*Special Record of Great Doctors*），[it] says [that Luying（陆英，flower of Chinese elder，Flos Sambuci Chinensis）] grows in Xiong'er（熊耳）and Yuanju（冤句）. [It can be] collected in the Autumn Solstice，also called Shuodiao（蒴藋）. [It is] sour [in taste]，warm and toxic [in property]，also called Li（堇）and Ji（芨），growing in all places. [Its] leaves [can be] collected in spring and summer，[its] stalks and roots [can be] collected in autumn and winter.

Notes

1. Luying（陆英，flower of Chinese elder，Flos Sambuci Chinensis）is a herbal medicinal，bitter and pungent in taste，cold in

【今译】

味苦,性寒。

主治骨间各种痹证,四肢拘挛疼酸,膝部寒冷疼痛,阳痿,呼吸气短,少气不足,腿脚肿痛。该物生长在山川河谷之中。

property, entering the liver meridian and the kidney meridian, effective in activating the blood and dispersing stasis, soothing the liver and fortifying the spleen, expelling wind and activating the collaterals, inducing sweating and promoting urination. Clinically it is used to treat traumatic injury, hepatitis, rheumatalgia, dislocation, fracture, edema in nephritis, beriberi and urticaria.

55. 荩草

【原文】

味苦,平。

主久咳上气喘逆,久寒,惊悸,痂疥,白秃,疡气,杀皮肤小虫。生川谷。

【考据】

1.《吴普》曰:王刍一名黄草,神农雷公口,生太山山谷,治身热邪气,小儿身热气(《御览》)。

2.《名医》曰:可以染黄,作金色,生青衣,九月十月采。

3. 案《说文》云:荩草也,荩,王刍也。《尔雅》云:荩,王刍。郭璞云:荩,蓐也,今呼鸱脚莎。《毛诗》云:绿竹猗猗。《传》云:荩,王刍也。《唐本》注云:荩草,俗名菉蓐草。《尔雅》所谓王刍。

【今译】

味苦,性平。

55. Jincao（荩草，hispid arthraxon herb，Herba Arthraxonis Hispidi）[1]

[Original Text]

[Jincao（荩草，hispid arthraxon herb，Herba Arthraxonis Hispidi），] bitter in taste and mild [in property]，[is mainly used] to treat chronic cough，dyspnea，panting，chronic cold [disease]，convulsion，palpitation，scabies，tinea tonsure and ulcer，and to kill small worms in the skin. [It] grows in the mountain valleys and river valleys.

[Textual Research]

[In the book entitled] *Wu Pu Ben Cao*（《吴普本草》，*Wu Pu's Studies of Materia Medica*），[it] says [that Jincao（荩草，hispid arthraxon herb，Herba Arthraxonis Hispidi）is also] called Wangchu（王刍）and Huangcao（黄草）. [According to] Agriculture God（神农）and Leigong（雷公），[it] grows in the mountains and valleys in Taishan（太山），treating fever [due to] evil-Qi and infantile fever，[as mentioned in the book entitled] *Tai Ping Yu Lan*（《太平御览》，*Imperial Studies in Taiping Times*）.

[In the book entitled] *Ming Yi Bie Lu*（《名医别录》，*Special Record of Great Doctors*），[it] says [that Jincao（荩草，hispid arthraxon herb，Herba Arthraxonis Hispidi）] can be dyed yellow as golden，growing in Qingyi（青衣）. [It can be] collected in

　　主治长期咳嗽,呼吸困难,喘息气逆,长期有寒冷感,惊恐,心悸,痂疥,白秃和疮疡,能杀除皮肤中的小虫。该物生长在山川河谷之中。

September and October.

Notes

1. Jincao （荩草, hispid arthraxon herb, Herba Arthraxonis Hispidi） is a herbal medicinal, bitter in taste and mild in property, effective in clearing heat, ceasing cough, killing worms, removing toxin and expelling wind and dampness. Clinically it is used to treat hepatitis, chronic cough and panting, pharyngolaryngitis, stomatitis, rhinitis and lymphadenitis.

56. 牛扁

【原文】

味苦,微寒。

主身皮疮,热气,可作浴汤,杀牛虱小虫,又疗牛病。生川谷。

【考据】

1.《名医》曰:生桂阳。

2. 案陶宏景云:太常贮名扁特,或名扁毒。

【今译】

味苦,性微寒。

主治皮肤中因热邪生疮,可煎煮成洗浴用的汤剂。能杀除牛身上的虱子和小虫,能治疗牛病。该物生长在山川河谷之中。

56. Niubian（牛扁，root of stem and leaf of puberulent monkshood，Radix Caulis et Folium Aconitis Puberuli） [1]

〔Original Text〕

〔Niubian（牛扁，root of stem and leaf of puberulent monkshood，Radix Caulis et Folium Aconitis Puberuli），〕 bitter in taste and slightly cold〔in property〕，〔is mainly used〕to treat sore and heat-Qi in the body skin.〔It〕can be boiled for bathing.〔It is also used〕to kill small worms in the skin of cow and treat disease in cow.〔It〕grows in mountain valleys and river valleys.

〔Textual Research〕

〔In the book entitled〕*Ming Yi Bie Lu*（《名医别录》，*Special Record of Great Doctors*），〔it〕says〔that Niubian（牛扁，root of stem and leaf of puberulent monkshood，Radix Caulis et Folium Aconitis Puberuli）〕grows in Guiyang（桂阳）.

Notes

1. Niubian（牛扁，root of stem and leaf of puberulent monkshood，Radix Caulis et Folium Aconitis Puberuli）is a herbal medicinal，bitter in taste，slightly cold and non-toxic in property，entering the liver meridian and the lung meridian，effective in expelling wind，ceasing pain，stopping cough，resolving phlegm，clearing heat，removing toxin and killing worms. Clinically it is used to treat rheumatism with swelling and pain，pain of the waist and legs，panting and cough，scrofula，ulcer and scabies.

57. 夏枯草

【原文】

味苦辛,寒。

主寒热,瘰疬,鼠瘘,头疮,破颓,散瘿,结气,脚肿,湿痹,轻身。一名夕句,一名乃东。生川谷。

【考据】

1.《名医》曰:一名燕面,生蜀郡,四月采。

【今译】

味苦、辛,性寒。

主治寒热病,瘰疬,鼠瘘,头疮,能破解颓疝,能消散瘿瘤和结气,能治疗腿脚肿痛,和湿邪所致痹证,能使人身体轻盈。又称为夕句,又称为乃东。该物生长在山川河谷之中。

57. Xiakucao（夏枯草，common selfheal spike，Spica Prunellae）[1]

[Original Text]

[Xiakucao（夏枯草，common selfheal spike，Spica Prunellae），] bitter and pungent in taste and cold [in property]，[is mainly used] to treat scrofula，tuberculosis and head sore，to break collapsed hernia，to disperse goiter [due to] stagnation of Qi，[to resolve] swelling of feet and dampness impediment，and to relax the body. [It is also] called Xiju（夕句）and Naidong（乃东），growing in mountain valleys and river valleys.

[Textual Research]

[In the book entitled] *Ming Yi Bie Lu*（《名医别录》，*Special Record of Great Doctors*），[it] says [that Xiakucao（夏枯草，common selfheal spike，Spica Prunellae）is also] called Yanmian（燕面），growing in Shujun（蜀郡）. [It can be] collected in April.

Notes

1. Xiakucao（夏枯草，common selfheal spike，Spica Prunellae）is a herbal medicinal，bitter and pungent in taste，cold in property，entering the liver meridian and the gallbladder meridian，effective in clearing heat，purging fire，dispersing stagnation，resolving swelling and improving vision. Clinically it is used to treat redness，swelling and pain of the eyes，hypertension，headache，vertigo，acute hepatitis，pulmonary tuberculosis，scrofula，goiter，tumor，breast cancer，mumps，sore，ulcer and scabies.

58. 芫华

【原文】

味辛,温。

主咳逆上气,喉鸣,喘咽肿,短气,蛊毒,鬼疟,疝瘕,痈肿,杀虫鱼。一名去水。生川谷(旧在木部,非)。

【考据】

1.《吴普》曰:芫华一名去水,一名败华,一名儿草根,一名黄大戟,神农黄帝有毒,扁鹊岐伯苦,李氏大寒,二月生,叶青,加厚则黑,华有紫赤白者,三月实落尽,叶乃生,三月五月采华,芫花根,一名赤芫根,神农雷公苦有毒,生邯郸,九月八月采,阴干,久服令人泄,可用毒鱼(《御览》亦见图经节文)。

2.《名医》曰:一名毒鱼,一名杜芫,其根名蜀桑,可用毒鱼,生淮源,三月三日采花,阴干。

3. 案《说文》云:芫,鱼毒也,《尔雅》云:杬,鱼毒。郭璞云:杬,大木,子似栗,生南方,皮厚,汁赤,中脏卵果。《范子计然》云:芫华出三辅,《史记·仓公传》,临菑女子病蛲瘕,饮以芫花一撮,出蛲可数升,病

58. Yuanhua（芫华，immature flower of lilac daphne，Flos Genkwa）[1]

[Original Text]

[Yuanhua （芫华，immature flower of lilac daphne，Flos Genkwa），] pungent in taste and warm [in property]，[is mainly used] to treat cough with dyspnea and upward counterflow of Qi，laryngeal stridor，gurgling with sputum，swelling of the throat，shortness of breath，[disease caused by] worm toxin，severe malaria，hernia with conglomeration and abscess. [It can be used] to kill worms and fish. [It is also] called Qushui（去水），growing in mountain valleys and river valleys.

[Textual Research]

[In the book entitled] *Wu Pu Ben Cao*（《吴普本草》，*Wu Pu's Studies of Materia Medica*），[it] says [that] Yuanhua （芫华，immature flower of lilac daphne，Flos Genkwa）[is also] called Qushui（去水），Baihua（败华），Caogen（草根）and Huangdaji（黄大戟）. [According to] Agriculture God（神农）and Yellow Emperor（黄帝），[it is] toxic [in property]；[according to] Bianque（扁鹊）and Qibo（岐伯），[it is] bitter [in taste]；[according to] Li's（李氏），[it is] severely cold [in property]. [It begins] to sprout in February. [Its] leaves are green. [If] enriched，[the leaves will] become black. [Its] flowers are purple，red and white. [In]

已颜师古注急就篇云：郭景纯说，误耳，其生南方用脏卵果，自别一杬木，乃左思所云：绵杬枕栌者耳，非毒鱼之杬。

右草，下品四十九种，旧四十八种，考木部芫华宜入此。

【今译】

味辛，性温。

主治咳嗽，呼吸困难，喉中喘鸣，咽喉肿痛，呼吸气短，能治疗虫毒所致之病，鬼怪试的疟疾，疝瘕和痈肿，能杀死虫鱼。又称为去水。该物生长在山川河谷之中。

March，all [the flowers have] faded and the leaves begin to sprout. [Its] flowers [can be] collected in March and May. The root of lilac daphne is called red lilac daphne root. [According to] Agriculture God（神农）and Leigong（雷公），[it is] bitter [in taste] and toxic [in property]，growing in Handan（邯郸）. [It can be] collected in September and August，and dried in the shade. Long-term taking [of it will] lead to diarrhea.

[In the book entitled] *Ming Yi Bie Lu*（《名医别录》，*Special Record of Great Doctors*），[it] says [that Yuanhua（芫华，immature flower of lilac daphne，Flos Genkwa）is also] called Duyu（毒鱼）and Duyuan（杜芫）. Its root is called Shusang（蜀桑），growing in Huaiyuan（淮源）. [Its] flowers [can be] collected on March 3 and dried in the shade.

[In the book entitled] *Fan Zi Ji Ran*（《范子计然》，*Studies About Fan Li's Teacher*），[it] says [that] Yuanhua（芫华，immature flower of lilac daphne，Flos Genkwa）grows in the three places.

Notes

1. Yuanhua（芫华，immature flower of lilac daphne，Flos Genkwa）is a herbal medicinal，pungent and bitter in taste，warm and toxic in property，entering the lung meridian，the spleen meridian and the kidney meridian，effective in purging water，expelling retention of fluid and killing worms. Clinically it is used to treat edema with distension and fullness，cough and panting with retention of phlegm，pain extending to the chest and rib-side and mental disorder.

59. 巴豆

【原文】

味辛,温。

主伤寒,温疟,寒热,破症瘕,结聚坚积,留饮淡癖,大腹水张,荡练五脏六府,开通闭塞,利水谷道,去恶肉,除鬼毒蛊注邪物(《御览》作鬼毒邪注),杀虫鱼,一名巴叔(旧作椒,《御览》作菽),生川谷。

【考据】

1.《吴普》曰:巴豆,一名巴菽,神农岐伯桐君辛有毒,黄帝甘有毒,李氏主温热寒,叶如大豆,八月采(《御览》)。

2.《名医》曰:生巴郡,八月采,阴干,用之,去心皮。

3. 案《广雅》云:巴菽,巴豆也。《列仙传》云:元俗饵巴豆。《淮南子·说林训》云:鱼食巴菽而死,人食之而肥。

【今译】

味辛,性温。

主治伤寒,温疟,寒热病,能破除症瘕,能解除坚硬的聚积和结滞,

59. Badou（巴豆，croton，Fructus Crotonis）[1]

［Original Text］

［Badou（巴豆，croton，Fructus Crotonis），］pungent in taste and warm［in property］，［is mainly used］to treat cold damage，warm malaria and cold-heat［disease］，to break conglomeration，stagnated aggregation and hard accumulation，retention of fluid with hypochondriac lump and enlarged abdomen［due to］retention of water，to scour the five Zang-organs and six Fu-organs，to unobstruct block and closure，to promote urination and defecation，to remove necrotic muscles and to eliminate vicious toxin［like］ghost and accumulation of worms and evil factors.［It can be used］to kill worms and fish.［It is also］called Bajiao（巴椒），growing in mountain valleys and river valleys.

［Textual Research］

［In the book entitled］*Wu Pu Ben Cao*（《吴普本草》，*Wu Pu's Studies of Materia Medica*），［it］says［that］Badou（巴豆，croton，Fructus Crotonis）［is also］called Bashu（巴菽）.［According to］Agriculture God（神农），Qibo（岐伯）and Tongjun（桐均），［it is］pungent［in taste］and toxic［in property］；［according to］Yellow Emperor（黄帝），［it is］sweet［in taste］and toxic［in property］；［according to］Li's（李氏），［it can］treat warm，heat and cold［diseases］.［Its］leaves are like［that of］soybean.［It can be］

能治疗留饮所致癖证,腹部积水肿胀,能荡涤五脏六腑,能开通闭塞,能通利大小便,能去掉恶肉,能祛除鬼毒蛊注等各种邪物,能杀死虫、鱼。又称为巴叔,该物生长在山川河谷之中。

collected in August ⌊according to the book entitled⌋ *Tai Ping Yu Lan*（《太平御览》, *Imperial Studies in Taiping Times*）.

⌈In the book entitled⌉ *Ming Yi Bie Lu*（《名医别录》, *Special Record of Great Doctors*）, ⌈it⌉ says ⌈that Badou（巴豆, croton, Fructus Crotonis)⌉ grows in Bajun（巴郡）. ⌈It can be⌉ collected in August and dried in the shade for medical purpose. The kernel and bark ⌈can be⌉ removed.

⌈In the book entitled⌉ *Guang Ya*（《广雅》, *The First Chinese Encyclopedic Dictionary*）⌈it⌉ says ⌈that the so-called⌉ Bashu（巴菽）is Badou（巴豆, croton, Fructus Crotonis）.

Notes

1. Badou（巴豆, croton, Fructus Crotonis）is a herbal medicinal, pungent in taste, heat and severely toxic in property, entering the stomach meridian and the large intestine meridian, effective in purging cold accumulation, expelling phlegm, moving water and killing worms. Clinically it is used to treat distension, fullness and pain in the chest and abdomen, constipation, retention of phlegm, edema, ascites, epilepsy and mania.

1103

60. 蜀椒

【原文】

味辛,温。

主邪气咳逆,温中,逐骨节,皮肤死肌,寒湿,痹痛,下气,久服之,头不白,轻身增年,生川谷。

【考据】

1.《名医》曰:一名巴椒,一名蓎藙,生武都及巴郡,八月采实,阴干。案《范子计然》云:蜀椒出武都,赤色者善。陆玑云:蜀人作茶,又见秦椒,即《尔雅》菽.陶宏景云:俗呼为樛。

【今译】

味辛,性温。

主治邪气所致的咳嗽气逆,能温煦人体脏器,能祛除骨节病气,能

60. Shujiao（蜀椒，fruit of Sichuan redpepper，Fructus Capsici Frutescentis Sichuan）[1]

[Original Text]

[Shujiao（蜀椒，fruit of Sichuan redpepper，Fructus Capsici Frutescentis Sichuan），] pungent in taste and warm [in property]，[is mainly used] to treat cough with dyspnea [due to] evil-Qi，to warm the middle（internal organs），to resolve [disorder of] joints with necrotic skin and muscles，cold-dampness impediment and pain，and to descend Qi. Long-term taking [of it will] prevent white hair，relax the body and prolong life. [It] grows in mountain valleys and river valleys.

[Textual Research]

[In the book entitled] *Ming Yi Bie Lu*（《名医别录》，*Special Record of Great Doctors*），[it] says [that Shujiao（蜀椒，fruit of Sichuan redpepper，Fructus Capsici Frutescentis Sichuan）is also] called Bajiao（巴椒）and Tangyi（蓎藙），growing in Wudu（武都）and Bajun（巴郡）. [Its] fruit [can be] collected in August and dried in the shade.

[In the book entitled] *Fan Zi Ji Ran*（《范子计然》，*Studies About Fan Li's Teacher*），[it] says [that] Shujiao（蜀椒，fruit of Sichuan redpepper，Fructus Capsici Frutescentis Sichuan）grows in Wudu（武都）. The red one is better.

终止皮肤肌肉坏死,能治疗寒湿病,痹痛,能使气下行降逆。长期服用之,能使人头发不变白,身体轻盈,延长寿命,该物生长在山川河谷之中。

神农本草经

Notes

1. Shujiao (蜀椒, fruit of Sichuan redpepper, Fructus Capsici Frutescentis Sichuan) is a herbal medicinal, pungent in taste, warm and mildly toxic in property, entering the spleen meridian, the stomach meridian and the kidney meridian, effective in warming the middle (the internal organs), dispersing cold, relieving pain, drying dampness and killing worms. Clinically it is used to treat oxyuriasis, heartache, abdominal pain, cold damage, warm malaria, nebula, edema, jaundice, diarrhea and dysentery.

61. 皂荚

【原文】

味辛咸,温。

主风痹,死肌,邪气,风头,泪出,利九窍,杀精物。生川谷。

【考据】

1.《名医》曰:生雍州,及鲁邹县,如猪牙者良,九月十月采,阴干。

2. 案《说文》云:荚草实。《范子计然》云:皂荚出三辅,上价一枚一钱。广志曰:鸡栖子,皂荚也(《御览》),皂即草省文。

61. Zaojia（皂荚，gleditsia，Radix Gleditsiae）[1]

[Original Text]

[Zaojia（皂荚，gleditsia， Radix Gleditsiae），] pungent and salty [in taste] and warm [in property]，[is mainly used] to treat wind impediment，necrotic muscles and [headache due to invasion of pathogenic] wind and evil-Qi into the head with tearing，to disinhibit the nine orifices and to kill [vicious pathogenic factors like] monster. [It] grows in the mountain valleys and river valleys.

[Textual Research]

[In the book entitled] *Ming Yi Bie Lu*（《名医别录》，*Special Record of Great Doctors*），[it] says [that Zaojia（皂荚，gleditsia，Radix Gleditsiae）] grows in Yongzhou（雍州） and Luzou（鲁邹） county. [The one that appears] like pig tooth is better. [It can be] collected in September and October，and dried in the shade.

[In] case [analysis in the book entitled] *Shuo Wen*（《说文》，*On Culture*），[it] says [that Zaojia（皂荚，gleditsia，Radix Gleditsiae）] is the fruit of Jiacao（荚草，Angiospermae）. [In the book entitled] *Fan Zi Ji Ran*（《范子计然》，*Studies About Fan Li's Teacher*），[it] says [that] Zaojia（皂荚，gleditsia，Radix Gleditsiae） grows in the three places.

【今译】

味辛、咸,性温。

主治风邪所致痹证和肌肉坏死,能祛除邪气,能治疗风邪伤头,泪流不止,能使九窍通畅,能杀除鬼怪邪物。该物生长在山川河谷之中。

神农本草经

Notes

1. Zaojia（皂荚, gleditsia, Radix Gleditsiae）is a herbal medicinal, pungent in taste, warm and mildly toxic in property, entering the lung meridian and the large intestine meridian, effective in opening orifices, removing phlegm, promoting defecation, resolving swelling and killing worms. Clinically it is used to treat unconsciousness due to invasion of wind and stagnation of phlegm, lockjaw, headache due to invasion of wind into the head, epilepsy, cough and panting.

62. 柳华

【原文】

味苦,寒。

主风水黄疸,面热黑。一名柳絮。叶主马疥痂疮。实主溃痈,逐脓血。子汁疗渴。生川泽。

【考据】

1.《名医》曰:生琅邪。

2.案《说文》云:柳,小杨也。柽,河柳也,杨木也。《尔雅》柽,河柳。郭璞云:今河旁赤茎小杨,又旄泽柳。郭璞云:生泽中者,又杨,蒲柳。郭璞云:可以为箭,左传所谓董泽之蒲。《毛诗》云:无折我树杞。《传》云:杞木名也。陆玑云:杞,柳属也。

【今译】

味苦,性寒。

主治风水证,黄疸病,面部发热变黑。又称为柳絮。

柳华叶,主治马身上的疥疮痂。

62.　Liuhua（柳华，flower of babylon weeping willow，Flos Salicis Babylonicae）[1]

[Original Text]

[Liuhua（柳华，flower of babylon weeping willow，Flos Salicis Babylonicae），] bitter in taste and cold [in property], [is mainly used] to treat edema，jaundice with black face [as if being] scorched. [It is also] called Liuxu（柳絮）.

[Its] leaves [can be used] to treat horses with scabies and sores.

[Its] fruit [can be used] to treat ulcerated abscess and to expel purulent blood.

Juice [obtained from its] seed [can be used] to treat thirst.

[It] grows in valleys and swamps.

[Textual Research]

[In the book entitled] *Ming Yi Bie Lu*（《名医别录》，*Special Record of Great Doctors*），[it] says [that Liuhua（柳华，flower of babylon weeping willow，Flos Salicis Babylonicae）] grows in Langxie（琅邪）.

[In] case [analysis in the book entitled] *Shuo Wen*（《说文》，*On Culture*），[it] says [that] Liuhua（柳华，flower of babylon weeping willow，Flos Salicis Babylonicae）is a small poplar tree.

柳华果实，主治溃痈，祛除脓血。

柳华子的汁液，能治疗口渴。

该物生长在山川和平泽之中。

Notes

1. Liuhua（柳华，flower of babylon weeping willow，Flos Salicis Babylonicae）is a herbal medicinal, bitter in taste and cold in property, effective in expelling wind and removing dampness, ceasing bleeding and dispersing stasis. Clinically it is used to treat edema, jaundice, hemoptysis, hematemesis, hematochezia and amenorrhea.

63. 楝实

【原文】

味苦,寒。

主温疾伤寒,大热烦狂,杀三虫疥疡,利小便水道。生山谷。

【考据】

1.《名医》曰:生荆山。

2. 案《说文》云:楝木也。《中山经》云:其实如楝。郭璞云:楝,木名,子如指头,白而粘,可以浣衣也。《淮南子·时则训》云:七月其树楝。高诱云:楝实,凤凰所食,今雒城旁有楝树,实,秋熟。

63. Lianshi（楝实，fruit of Szechwan chinaberry，toosendan fruit，Fructus Toosendan）[1]

［Original Text］

［Lianshi（楝实，fruit of Szechwan chinaberry，toosendan fruit，Fructus Toosendan），］bitter in taste and cold ［in property］，［is mainly used］to treat warm disease，cold damage and high fever with vexation and mania，to eliminate three worms，scabies and ulcer，and to promote urination. ［It］grows in mountains and valleys.

［Textual Research］

［In the book entitled］*Ming Yi Bie Lu*（《名医别录》，*Special Record of Great Doctors*），［it］says ［that Lianshi（楝实，fruit of Szechwan chinaberry，toosendan fruit，Fructus Toosendan）］grows in Jingshan（荆山）.

Guo Pu（郭璞）said，"［The so-called］Lian（楝）is the name of a kind of wood，the fruit ［of which is］like a finger，white and sticky，and can be used to wash clothes."

Gao You（高诱）said，"Phoenix likes to eat Lianshi（楝实，fruit of Szechwan chinaberry，toosendan fruit，Fructus Toosendan）. Now there are Lianshu （楝树，chinaberry，Melia azedarach）［growing］around Luocheng（雒城，a city in the Sichuan Province），the fruit ［of which］ripens in autumn."

【今译】

味苦,性寒。

主治温热病,伤寒病,身体高热,烦躁狂妄,能杀死三种寄生虫,能治疗疥疮溃烂,能使小便通畅,水道通利。该物生长在山谷之中。

Notes

1. Lianshi（楝实，Fructus Toosendan; fruit of Szechwan chinaberry; toosendan fruit）is a herbal medicinal, bitter in taste, cold and mildly toxic in property, entering the liver meridian, the stomach meridian and the small intestine meridian, effective in clearing dampness and heat, regulating Qi, relieving pain and killing worms. Clinically it is used to treat pain in the liver, stomach and rib-side, hernia with pain, dysmenorrhea, abdominal pain due to accumulation of worms and mastitis.

64. 郁李仁

【原文】

味酸,平。

主大腹水肿,面目四肢浮肿、利小便水道。根,主齿龈肿,龋齿,生坚。一名爵李。生坚齿川谷。

【考据】

1.《吴普》曰:郁李,一名雀李,一名车下李,一名棣(《御览》)。

2.《名医》曰:一名车下李,一名棣,生高山及邱陵上,五月六月采根。

3. 案《说文》云:棣,白棣也。《广雅》云:山李,雀其霺也。《尔雅》云:常棣,棣。

4. 郭璞云:今关西有棣树,子如樱桃可食。《毛诗》云:六月食郁。《传》云:郁,棣属。刘稹《毛诗义问》云:其树高五六尺,其实大如李,正赤,食之甜。又诗云:常棣之华。《传》云:常棣,棣也。陆玑云:奥李。一名雀李,一曰车下李,所在山中皆有其花,或白或赤,六月中熟大,子如李子可食。《沈括补笔谈》云:晋宫阁铭曰:华林园中有车下李,三百

64. Yuliren（郁李仁，seed of dwarf flowering cherry，seed of longpedicel Chinese buscherry，Semen Pruni）[1]

〔Original Text〕

〔Yuliren（郁李仁，seed of dwarf flowering cherry，seed of longpedicel Chinese buscherry，Semen Pruni），〕 sour in taste and mild〔in property〕，〔is mainly used〕to treat enlarged abdomen with edema，dropsy of the face，eyes and four limbs，and to disinhibit urination.

〔Its〕root〔can be used〕to treat swollen gum and caries，and to strengthen teeth.

〔It is also〕called Jueli（爵李），growing in mountain valleys and river valleys.

〔Textual Research〕

〔In the book entitled〕 Wu Pu Ben Cao（《吴普本草》，Wu Pu's Studies of Materia Medica），〔it says〔that〕Yuliren（郁李仁，seed of dwarf flowering cherry，seed of longpedicel Chinese buscherry，Semen Pruni）〔is also〕called Queli（雀李），Chexiali（车下李）and Di（棣）〔according to the book entitled〕Tai Ping Yu Lan（《太平御览》，Imperial Studies in Taiping Times）.

〔In the book entitled〕 Ming Yi Bie Lu（《名医别录》，Special Record of Great Doctors），〔it〕says〔that Yuliren（郁李仁，seed of dwarf flowering cherry，seed of longpedicel Chinese buscherry，

一十四株,薁李一株。

【今译】

味酸,性平。

主治腹部严重水肿,面部、眼睛和四肢浮肿,能使小便通畅,水道通利。

郁李仁根,主治齿龈肿通和龋齿,能使牙齿坚固。

又称为爵李。该物生长在山川和山谷中。

神农本草经

Semen Pruni) is also] called Chexiali (车下李) and Di (棣), growing in high mountains and hills. [Its] root [can be] collected in May and June.

Notes

1. Yuliren (郁李仁, seed of dwarf flowering cherry, seed of longpedicel Chinese buscherry, Semen Pruni) is a herbal medicinal, pungent, bitter and sweet in taste and mild in property, entering the spleen meridian, the large intestine meridian and the small intestine meridian, effective in moistening the intestines, promoting defecation, disinhibiting urination and resolving swelling. Clinically it is used to treat constipation due to intestinal dryness, edema, abdominal distension and fullness, beriberi, dysuria and edema.

65. 莽草

【原文】

味辛,温。

主风头痈肿,乳痈,疝瘕,除结气疥搔(《御览》有痂疮二字),杀虫鱼。生山谷。

【考据】

1.《吴普》曰:莽草一名春草,神农辛,雷公桐君苦有毒,生上谷山谷中,或冤句,五月采,治风(《御览》)。

2.《名医》曰:一名葞,一名春草,生上谷及冤句,五月采叶,阴干。

3. 案《中山经》云:朝歌之山有草焉,名曰莽草,可以毒鱼,又葂山有木焉,其状如棠而赤,叶可以毒鱼,《尔雅》云:葞,春草。郭璞云:一名芒草。本草云:《周礼》云,翦氏掌除蠹物,以熏草莽之。《范子计然》云:莽草,出三辅者善。

陶宏景云:字亦作两。

65. Mangcao（莽草，leaf of lanceleaf anisetree，Folium Illicii Lanceolati）[1]

[Original Text]

[Mangcao（莽草，leaf of lanceleaf anisetree，Folium Illicii Lanceolati），] pungent in taste and warm [in property], [is mainly used] to treat [headache due to invasion of] wind into the head，abscess，acute mastitis，hernia and conglomeration，to eliminate stagnation of Qi and scabies，and to kill worms and fish. [It] grows in mountains and valleys.

[Textual Research]

[In the book entitled] *Wu Pu Ben Cao*（《吴普本草》，*Wu Pu's Studies of Materia Medica*），[it] says [that] Mangcao（莽草，leaf of lanceleaf anisetree，Folium Illicii Lanceolati）[is also] called Chuncao（春草）. [According to] Agriculture God（神农），[it is] pungent [in taste]；[according to] Leigong（雷公）and Tongjun（桐均），[it is] bitter [in taste] and toxic [in property]，growing in mountains and valleys，or in Yuanju（冤句）. [It can be] collected in May and [can be used] to treat [disease caused by] wind [according to the book entitled] *Tai Ping Yu Lan*（《太平御览》，*Imperial Studies in Taiping Times*）.

[In the book entitled] *Ming Yi Bie Lu*（《名医别录》，*Special Record of Great Doctors*），[it] says [that Mangcao（莽草，leaf of

【今译】

味辛,性温。

主治风邪袭击头部,痈肿,乳痈和疝瘕,能清除气结,疥疮和瘑痒,能杀死虫、鱼。该物生长在山谷之中。

lanceleaf anisetree, Folium Illicii Lanceolati) is also] called Mi (蒳) and Chuncao (春草), growing in the high valleys and Yuanju (冤 句). [Its] leaves [can be] collected in May and dried in the shade.

[In] case [analysis in the book entitled] *Zhong Shan Jing* (《中 山经》, *Central Mountain Canon*), [it] says [that] there is herb in the mountain in Chaoge (朝歌) called Mangcao (莽草, leaf of lanceleaf anisetree, Folium Illicii Lanceolati). [It] can poison fish. There is another tree [which is] as red as birchleaf pear, and [its] leaves can poison fish. [In the book entitled] *Fan Zi Ji Ran* (《范子 计然》, *Studies About Fan Li's Teacher*), [it] says [that] Mangcao (莽草, leaf of lanceleaf anisetree, Folium Illicii Lanceolati) [that] grows in the three places is better.

Notes

1. Mangcao (莽草, leaf of lanceleaf anisetree, Folium Illicii Lanceolati) is a herbal medicinal, pungent in taste, warm and toxic in property, effective in expelling wind and dampness, resolving swelling and distension. Clinically it is used to treat headache caused by wind attack, edema, abscess, skin impediment, scrofula, mastitis, sore-throat, hernia and toothache.

66. 雷丸（《御览》作雷公丸）

【原文】

味苦,寒。

主杀三虫,逐毒气,胃中热,利丈夫,不利女子。作摩膏,除小儿百病(《御览》引云:一名雷矢,《大观本》,作黑字)。生山谷。

【考据】

1.《吴普》曰:雷丸,神农苦,黄帝岐伯桐君甘有毒,扁鹊甘无毒,李氏大寒(《御览》引云:一名雷实,或生汉中,八月采)。

2.《名医》曰:一名雷矢,一名雷实,生石城及汉中土中,八月采根暴干。

3. 案《范子计然》云:雷矢,出汉中,色白者善。

【今译】

味苦,性寒。

66. Leiwan（雷丸，stone-like omphalia，Omphalia Lapidescens）[1]

[Original Text]

[Leiwan（雷丸，stone-like omphalia，Omphalia Lapidescens），] bitter in taste and cold [in property], [is mainly used] to kill three worms, to expel poisonous Qi and [to dispel] heat in the stomach. [It is] effective [in treating] men, but ineffective [in treating] women. [When] made into paste, [it can] treat infantile diseases. [It] grows in mountains and valleys.

[Textual Research]

[In the book entitled] *Wu Pu Ben Cao*（《吴普本草》，*Wu Pu's Studies of Materia Medica*），[it] says [that] Leiwan（雷丸，stone like omphalia，Omphalia），[according to] Agriculture God（神农），[is] bitter [in taste]；[according to] Yellow Emperor（黄帝），Qibo（岐伯）and Tongjun（桐均），[it is] sweet [in taste] and toxic [in property]；[according to] Bianque（扁鹊），[it is] sweet [in taste] and non-toxic [in property]；[according to] Li's（李氏），[it is] severely cold [in property]. [According to the book entitled] *Tai Ping Yu Lan*（《太平御览》，*Imperial Studies in Taiping Times*），[it is also] called Leishi（雷实），growing in Hanzhong（汉中）. [It can be] collected in August.

[In the book entitled] *Ming Yi Bie Lu*（《名医别录》，*Special*

能杀死三种寄生虫，能祛除毒气和胃中热邪。该物所治之病有利男子，不利于女子。摩制成膏，能治疗各种小儿疾病。该物生长在山谷之中。

Record of Great Doctors）, ［it］ says ［that Leiwan（雷丸, stone-like omphalia, Omphalia Lapidescens) is also］ called Leishi（雷矢）and Leishi（雷实）, growing in Shicheng（石城）and Hanzhong（汉中）. ［Its］root ［can be］ collected in August and dried in the sun.

［In the book entitled］ *Fan Zi Ji Ran*（《范子计然》, *Studies About Fan Li's Teacher*）, ［it］ says ［that］ Leishi（雷矢, stone-like omphalia, Omphalia Lapidescens) grows in Hanzhong（汉中）. The white one is better.

Notes

1. Leiwan（雷丸, stone-like omphalia, Omphalia Lapidescens) is a herbal medicinal, bitter in taste, cold and mildly toxic in property, entering the stomach meridian and the large intestine meridian, effective in killing parasites in the intestines. Clinically it is used to treat taeniasis, ancylostomiasis, ascaridiasis and cerebral cysticercosis.

神农本草经

67. 桐叶

【原文】

味苦，寒。

主恶蚀疮，著阴。皮，主五痔，杀三虫。华，主传猪疮，饲猪，肥大三倍。生山谷。

【考据】

1.《名医》曰：生桐柏山。

2. 案《说文》云：桐，荣也，梧，梧桐木，一名榇。《尔雅》云：榇梧。郭璞云：今梧桐，又荣桐木。郭璞云：即梧桐。《毛诗》云：梧桐生矣。《传》云：梧桐柔木也。

【今译】

味苦，性寒。

主治恶性溃烂疮疾，可外敷于阴部。

67. Tongye （桐叶，leaf of fortune paulownia; leaf of royal paulownia，Folium Paulowniae） [1]

［Original Text］

［Tongye （桐叶，leaf of fortune paulownia; leaf of royal paulownia，Folium Paulowniae），］ bitter in taste and cold ［in property］，［is mainly used］ to treat severe sore ［by applying the medicinal to］ the genitals.

［Its］ bark ［can be used］ to treat five ［kinds of］ hemorrhoids and to kill three worms.

［Its］ flower ［can be used］ to treat sore in pigs. To feed a pig ［with its flower will enable it to grow］ three times as big as ［that of others］.

［It］ grows in mountains and valleys.

［Textual Research］

［In the book entitled］ *Ming Yi Bie Lu* （《名医别录》，*Special Record of Great Doctors*），［it］ says ［that Tongye （桐叶，leaf of fortune paulownia; leaf of royal paulownia，Folium Paulowniae）］ grows in Tongbai （桐柏） mountain.

Notes

1. Tongye （桐叶，leaf of fortune paulownia; leaf of royal paulownia，Folium Paulowniae） is a herbal medicinal，bitter in taste

桐叶皮，能治疗五种痔疮，能杀死三种寄生虫。

桐叶花，外敷能治疗猪疮，喂猪能使其比一般的肥大三倍。该物生长在山谷之中。

and cold in property, entering the heart meridian and the liver meridian, effective in clearing heat and removing toxin, resolving blood stasis and stopping bleeding. Clinically it is used to treat furuncle, acute mastitis, intestinal abscess, periappendicular abscess, erysipelas, traumatic injury, blood stasis, Qi stagnation and carbuncle.

68. 梓白皮

【原文】

味苦,寒。

主热,去三虫,叶捣传猪疮,饲猪肥大三倍,生山谷。

【考据】

1.《名医》曰:生河内。

2. 案《说文》云:梓,楸也,或作榟,椅梓也,楸,梓也,櫄,楸也。《尔雅》云:槐小叶曰榎.郭璞云:槐为楸楸,当细叶者为榎,又大而榎,楸。郭璞云:老乃皮粗,皵者为楸,又椅梓。郭璞云:即楸。《毛诗》云椅,桐梓漆,《传》云椅,梓属。陆玑云:梓者楸之,疏,理,白色而生子者,曰梓,梓实,桐皮,曰椅。

【今译】

味苦,性寒。

主治发热,能祛除三种虫子。

梓白皮叶,捣烂外敷能治疗猪疮,喂猪能使其比一般的肥大三倍。该物生长在山谷之中。

68．Zibaipi（梓白皮，root-bark of ovate catalpa，Cortex Catalpae Ovatae Radicis） [1]

[Original Text]

［Zibaipi（梓白皮，root-bark of ovate catalpa，Cortex Catalpae Ovatae Radicis），］ bitter in taste and cold ［in property］，［is mainly used］ to treat fever and eliminate three worms.

［To treat］ sore in pigs，［its］ leaves ［can be］ pounded for external application. To feed a pig ［with the pounded leaves will enable it to grow］ three times as big as ［that of others］.

[Textual Research]

［In the book entitled］ *Ming Yi Bie Lu*（《名医别录》，*Special Record of Great Doctors*），［it］ says ［that Zibaipi（梓白皮，root-bark of ovate catalpa，Cortex Catalpae Ovatae Radicis）］ grows in Henei（河内）.

Notes

1. Zibaipi（梓白皮，root-bark of ovate catalpa，Cortex Catalpae Ovatae Radicis） is a herbal medicinal，bitter in taste and cold in property，entering the gallbladder meridian and the stomach meridian，effective in clearing heat，removing toxin and relieving dampness. Clinically it is used to treat warm disease with fever，jaundice，edema，scabies and ulcer.

69. 石南

【原文】

味辛,平。

主养肾气,内伤,阴衰,利筋骨皮毛。实,杀蛊毒,破积聚,逐风痹。一名鬼目。生山谷。

【考据】

1.《名医》曰:生华阴,二月四月采实,阴干。

【今译】

味辛,性平。

能滋养肾气,能治疗内伤和阴器衰弱,能通利筋骨和皮毛。

石南果实,能杀除虫毒,能破解积聚,能祛除风痹。

又称为鬼目。该物生长在山谷之中。

69. Shinan（石南，fruit of Chinese photinia，Fructus Photiniae Serrulatae）[1]

[Original Text]

[Shinan（石南，fruit of Chinese photinia，Fructus Photiniae Serrulatae），] pungent in taste and mild [in property]，[is mainly used] to nourish kidney-Qi，to treat internal injury and decline of Yin，and to fortify sinews，bones，skin and hair.

[Its] fruit can eliminate worm toxin，break accumulation and aggregation，and expel wind impediment.

[It is also] called Guimu（鬼目），growing in mountains and valleys.

[Textual Research]

[In the book entitled] *Ming Yi Bie Lu*（《名医别录》，*Special Record of Great Doctors*），[it] says [that Shinan（石南，fruit of Chinese photinia，Fructus Photiniae Serrulatae）] grows in Huayin（华阴）. [Its] fruit [can be] collected in February and April，and dried in the shade.

Notes

1. Shinan（石南，fruit of Chinese photinia，Fructus Photiniae Serrulatae）is a herbal medicinal，pungent and bitter in taste，mild and slightly toxic in property，entering the liver meridian and the kidney meridian，effective in expelling wind and dampness，and strengthening sinews and bones. Clinically it is used to treat wind-dampness impediment and pain，headache due to wind attack，measles，ache and flaccidity of the waist and knees，impotence and seminal emission.

70．黄环

【原文】

味苦，平。

主蛊毒鬼注，鬼魅，邪气在脏中，除咳逆寒热。一名凌泉，一名大就。生山谷。

【考据】

1.《吴普》曰：蜀黄环，一名生刍，一名根韭，神农黄帝岐伯桐君扁鹊辛，一经，味苦有毒，二月生，初出，正赤，高二尺，叶黄，员端，大茎，叶有汗，黄白，五月实员，三月采根，根黄，从理如车辐，解，治蛊毒（《御览》）。

2.《名医》曰：生蜀郡，三月采根，阴干。

3. 案蜀都赋，有黄环，刘逵云：黄环出蜀郡。沈括补笔谈云：黄环即今朱藤也，天下皆有，叶如槐，其花穗悬紫色如葛，花，可作菜食，火不熟，亦有小毒，京师人家园圃中，作大架种之，谓之紫藤花者，是也。

70. Huanghuan（黄环，Chinese wisteria，Wisteria Sinensis）[1]

［Original Text］

［Huanghuan（黄环，Chinese wisteria，Wisteria Sinensis），］ bitter in taste and mild［in property］，［is mainly used］to treat ［disease caused by］worm toxin，［vicious pathogenic factors like］ ghost and evil-Qi in the Zang-organs，to eliminate cough with dyspnea and to treat cold-heat［disease］.［It is also］called Lingquan（凌泉）and Dajiu（大就），growing in mountains and valleys.

［Textual Research］

［In the book entitled］*Wu Pu Ben Cao*（《吴普本草》，*Wu Pu's Studies of Materia Medica*），［it］says［that］Huanghuan（黄环，Chinese wisteria，Wisteria Sinensis）［is also］called Shengchu（生刍）and Genjiu（根韭）.［According to］Agriculture God（神农），Yellow Emperor（黄帝），Qibo（岐伯），Tongjun（桐均）and Bianque （扁鹊），［it is］pungent［in taste］and may be bitter［in taste］and toxic［in property］.［It begins］to sprout in February and［is red］at the early period，about 2 *Chi*（尺）in height.［Its］leaves are yellow and round，［its］stalks are large.［It begins］to bear fruits in May. ［Its］root，yellow and like spokes，［can be］collected in March and ［used］to treat［disease caused by］worm toxin［according to the

【今译】

味苦,性平。

主治虫毒所致之病及鬼怪之邪所致之症,能祛除脏器中积聚的邪气,能消除咳嗽气逆,能治疗寒热病。又称为凌泉,又称为大就。该物生长在山谷之中。

book entitled] *Tai Ping Yu Lan* (《太平御览》, *Imperial Studies in Taiping Times*).

[In the book entitled] *Ming Yi Bie Lu* (《名医别录》, *Special Record of Great Doctors*), [it] says [that Huanghuan (黄环, Chinese wisteria, Wisteria Sinensis)] grows in Shujun (蜀郡). [Its] root [can be] collected in March and dried in the shade.

Liu Kui (刘逵) said, "Huanghuan (黄环, Chinese wisteria, Wisteria Sinensis) grows in Shujun (蜀郡)." [To supplement it], Shen Kuo (沈括) said, "Huanghuan (黄环) refers to Zhuteng (朱藤, Chinese wisteria, Wisteria Sinensis) [which can be] found everywhere. [Its] leaves are like [that of] the Chinese scholar tree; [its] spica is like [that of] kudzu vine; [its] flower can be used as vegetables. [If] not well cooked, [it is] also toxic. People living in the capital plant it in the garden with high frame and call it Zitenghua (紫藤花)."

Notes

1143

1. Huanghuan (黄环, Chinese wisteria, Wisteria Sinensis) is a herbal medicinal, sweet and bitter in taste, warm and mildly toxic in property, effective in removing toxin, ceasing vomiting, killing worms and relieving pain. Clinically it is used to treat wind impediment, oxyuriasis, vomiting, abdominal pain, diarrhea and pain of sinews and bones.

71. 溲疏

【原文】

味辛,寒。

主身皮肤中热,除邪气,止遗溺,可作浴汤。生山谷,及田野故邱虚地。

【考据】

1.《名医》曰:一名巨骨,生能耳山,四月采。

2. 案李当之云:溲疏,一名杨栌,一名牡荆,一名空疏,皮白中空,时时有节,子似枸杞,子冬日熟,色赤,味甘苦。

71. Soushu（溲疏，leaf and root of deutzia，Folium et Radix Deutziae）[1]

[Original Text]

[Soushu（溲疏，leaf and root of deutzia，Folium et Radix Deutziae），] pungent in taste and cold [in property]，[is mainly used] to expel heat in the body and skin，to eliminate evil-Qi and to treat enuresis. [It] grows in mountains，valleys and fields.

[Textual Research]

[In the book entitled] *Ming Yi Bie Lu*（《名医别录》，*Special Record of Great Doctors*），[it] says [that Soushu（溲疏，leaf and root of deutzia，Folium et Radix Deutziae）is also] called Jugu（巨骨），growing in Neng'er（能耳）mountain. [It can be] collected in April.

Li Dangzhi（李当之）said，"Soushu（溲疏，leaf and root of deutzia，Folium et Radix Deutziae）[is also] called Yanlu（杨栌），Mujing（牡荆）and Kongshu（空疏）. The bark is white，[the stalks are] hollow and the joints are various. [Its] seed is similar to Gouqi（枸杞，fruit of barbary wolfberry，Fructus Lycii），ripe in winter，red in color，sweet and bitter in taste."

【今译】

味辛,性寒。

主治身体和皮肤内发热,能清除邪气,能停止遗尿。可煎煮成洗浴用的汤剂。该物生长在山谷之中及田野故邱虚地里。

Notes

1. Soushu (溲疏, leaf and root of deutzia, Folium et Radix Deutziae) is a herbal medicinal, pungent and bitter in taste, slightly cold in property, effective in clearing heat, promoting urination, tonifying the kidney, removing toxin and invigorating bones. Clinically it is used to treat heat in the stomach, dysuria, nocturnal enuresis, malaria and fracture.

72. 鼠李

【原文】

主寒热瘰疬疮。生田野。

【考据】

1.《吴普》曰：鼠李，一名牛李(《御览》)。

2.《名医》曰：一名牛李，一名鼠梓，一名啤，采无时。

3. 案《说文》云：梗，鼠梓木。《尔雅》云梗，鼠梓。郭璞云：楸属也，今江东有虎梓。《毛诗》云：北山有梗.《传》云梗，鼠梓，据《名医》名鼠梓，未知是此否。《唐本》注云：一名赵李，一名皂李，一名乌槎。

【今译】

主治寒热病和瘰疬疮。该物生长在田野里。

72. Shuli（鼠李，davurian buckthorn fruit，Fructus Rhamni Davuricae）[1]

[Original Text]

[Shuli （鼠李，davurian buckthorn fruit，Fructus Rhamni Davuricae) is used] to treat cold-heat [disease]，scrofula and sore. [It] grows in fields.

[Textual Research]

[In the book entitled] *Wu Pu Ben Cao*（《吴普本草》，*Wu Pu's Studies of Materia Medica*），[it] says [that] Shuli （鼠李，davurian buckthorn fruit，Fructus Rhamni Davuricae) [is also] called Niuli （牛李）[according to the book entitled] *Tai Ping Yu Lan*（《太平御览》，*Imperial Studies in Taiping Times*）.

[In the book entitled] *Ming Yi Bie Lu*（《名医别录》，*Special Record of Great Doctors*），[it] says [that Shuli（鼠李，davurian buckthorn fruit，Fructus Rhamni Davuricae) is also] called Niuli （牛李），Shuzi（鼠梓） and Pi（啤）. [It can be] collected at any time.

Notes

1. Shuli （鼠 李，davurian buckthorn fruit，Fructus Rhamni Davuricae) is a herbal medicinal，bitter in taste，slightly cold and mildly toxic in property，effective in clearing heat，promoting defecation，enriching Yin，killing worms，removing toxin，nourishing the kidney and activating the blood. Clinically it is used to treat wind impediment，heat toxin in the skin，constipation，distension，edema，scrofula，hernia，conglomeration，scabies and ulcer.

73. 药实根

【原文】

味辛,温。

主邪气,诸痹疼酸,续绝伤,补骨髓。一名连木。生山谷。

【考据】

1.《名医》曰:生蜀郡,采无时。

2. 案《广雅》云:贝父,药实也。

73. Yaoshigen (药实根，herbal fruit and root，Radix et Fructus Herba)^[1]

［Original Text］

［Yaoshigen（药实根，herbal fruit and root，Radix et Fructus Herba），］pungent in taste and warm［in property］，［is mainly used］to treat various impediment and ache［caused by］evil-Qi，to heal traumatic injury and to tonify bone marrow.［It is also］called Lianmu（连木），growing in mountains and valleys.

［Textual Research］

［In the book entitled］*Ming Yi Bie Lu*（《名医别录》，*Special Record of Great Doctors*），［it］says［that Yaoshigen（药实根，herbal fruit and root，Radix et Fructus Herba）］grows in Shujun（蜀郡）and［can be］collected at any time.

［In the book entitled］*Guang Ya*（《广雅》，*The First Chinese Encyclopedic Dictionary*），［it］says［that Yaoshigen（药实根，herbal fruit and root，Radix et Fructus Herba）is also called］Beifu（贝父），referring to the fruit of herbs.

Notes

1. Yaoshigen（药实根，herbal fruit and root，Radix et Fructus Herba）is a herbal medicinal. This herbal medicinal was mentioned in many classics of traditional Chinese medicine and materia

【今译】

味辛,性温。

主治邪气所致之症,各种痹证和疼酸,能通过补益主治外伤所致之筋伤骨折,能补益骨髓。又称为连木。该物生长在山谷之中。

medica. But now it is difficult to understand what medicinal it actually is. When translating *Agriculture God's Canon of Materia Medica* (《神农本草经》), I have consulted a number of ancient and modern books about materia medica, but still unclear about what it is. According to ancient books about materia medica, it may refer to a number of herbal medicinals, such as Baiyaozi（白药子,root of oriental stephania，Radix Stephaniae Cepharanthae）, Hongyaozi（红药子,root of ciliatenerve knotweed，Radix Polygoni Ciliinervis）and Wuyaozi（乌药子,fruit of combined spicebush，Fructus Linderae）, etc.

74. 栾华

【原文】

味苦,寒。

主目痛泪出,伤眦,消目肿,生川谷。

【考据】

1.《名医》曰:生汉中,五月采。

2. 案《说文》云:栾木似栏。《山海经》云:云雨之山,有木名栾,黄木赤枝青叶,群帝焉取药。曰虎通云:诸侯墓树柏,大夫栾,士槐。《沈括补笔谈》云:栾有一种,树生,其实可作数珠者,谓之木栾,即本草栾花是也。

74. Luanhua (栾华, flower of paniculate goldraintree, Flos Koelreuteriae Paniculatae) [1]

[Original Text]

[Luanhua (栾华, flower of paniculate goldraintree, Flos Koelreuteriae Paniculatae),] bitter in taste and cold [in property], [is mainly used] to treat ocular pain with tearing and [disease that] damages the canthus, and to resolve oculars welling. [It] grows in mountain valleys and river valleys.

[Textual Research]

[In the book entitled] *Ming Yi Bie Lu* (《名医别录》, *Special Record of Great Doctors*), [it] says [that Luanhua (栾华, flower of paniculate goldraintree, Flos Koelreuteriae Paniculatae)] grows in Hanzhong (汉中) and [can be] collected in May.

[In] case [analysis in the book entitled] *Shuo Wen* (《说文》, *On Culture*), [it] says [that] Lianmu (栾木, paniculate goldraintree, Koelreuteriae Paniculatae) is like a baluster. [In the book entitled] *Shan Hai Jing* (《山海经》, *Canon of Mountains and Seas*), [it] says [that] in the mountains full of clouds and rain, there is a kind of yellow tree called Luan (栾, paniculate goldraintree, Koelreuteriae Paniculatae) with red branches and green leaves. All the emperors collected medicinals from it. [In] supplementing [it], Shen Kuo (沈括) said, "[The so-called] Luan

【今译】

味苦,性寒。

主治眼睛肿痛,泪流不止和眼角受伤,能消除眼睛肿胀,该物生长在山川河谷之中。

（栾）is a tree with various beads，known as Muluan（木栾）. [It] actually is Luanhua（栾华，flower of paniculate goldraintree，Flos Koelreuteriae Paniculatae）. "

Notes

1. Luanhua （栾 华，flower of paniculate goldraintree，Flos Koelreuteriae Paniculatae） is a herbal medicinal，bitter in taste，cold and non-toxic in property，entering the liver meridian，effective in clearing the liver，improving vision and resolving swelling. Clinically it is used to treat ocular pain，tearing and acute conjunctivitis.

75. 蔓椒

【原文】

味苦,温。

主风寒湿痹,疬节疼,除四肢厥气,膝痛。一名家椒。生川谷及邱家间。

【考据】

1.《名医》曰:一名猪椒,一名彪椒,一名狗椒,生云中,采茎根煮,酿酒。

2. 案陶宏景云:俗呼为樛,以椒竞小不香尔,一名稀椒,可以蒸病出汗也。

上木,下品一十七种,旧十八种,今移芜华入草。

75. Manjiao（蔓椒，root of shiny bramble，Radix Shinyleaf Pricklyash）[1]

[Original Text]

[Manjiao（蔓椒，root of shiny bramble，Radix Shinyleaf Pricklyash），] bitter in taste and warm [in property], [is mainly used] to treat wind-cold dampness impediment and acute arthritis, and to eliminate coldness of the four limbs and pain of the knees. [It is also] called Jiajiao（家椒），growing in mountain valleys，river valleys and courtyard.

[Textual Research]

[In the book entitled] *Ming Yi Bie Lu*（《名医别录》，*Special Record of Great Doctors*），[it] says [that Manjiao（蔓椒，root of shiny bramble，Radix Shinyleaf Pricklyash）is also] called Zhujiao（猪椒），Zhijiao（彘椒）and Goujiao（狗椒），growing in Yunzhong（云中）. [Its] stalks and roots [can be] collected to make wine.

Tao Hongjing（陶宏景）said，"[It is] popularly called Jiu（樛）because it is small and not fragrant. [It is also] called Xijiao（稀椒）and [can be used] to induce sweating to treat [bone] steaming disease."

Notes

1. Manjiao（蔓椒，root of shiny bramble，Radix Shinyleaf

【今译】

味苦,性温。

主治风寒湿邪所致痹证和关节疼痛,能祛除四肢厥气,能治疗膝部疼痛。又称为家椒。该物生长在山川河谷之中及百姓家中。

Pricklyash) is a herbal medicinal, pungent and bitter in taste, mild and slightly toxic in property, effective in expelling wind, activating the blood, ceasing pain and removing toxin. Clinically it is used to treat wind-dampness impediment, overstrained injury of the lumbar muscles, colic in the stomach and intestines, traumatic injury, pain caused by roundworms in the biliary tract, toothache and injury caused by snake bite.

76. 豚卵

【原文】

味苦,温。

主惊痫,瘨疾,鬼注,蛊毒,除寒热,贲豚,五癃,邪气,挛缩。一名豚颠。

悬蹄,主五痔,伏热,在肠,肠痈,内蚀。

【考据】

1. 案《说文》云:豚,小豕也,从彑省,象形,从又,持肉以给祭祀,篆文作豚。方言云:猪,其子或谓之豚,或谓之豯.吴扬之间,谓之猪子。

【今译】

味苦,性温。

主治惊风,癫痫,癫疾,鬼怪之邪所致之症及虫毒所致之病,能

76. Tunluan（豚卵，pig's testis，Sus Scrofa Domestica）[1]

[Original Text]

[Tunluan（豚卵，pig's testis，Sus Scrofa Domestica），] bitter in taste and warm [in property], [is mainly used] to treat convulsion, epilepsy, psychosis, severe disease [caused by vicious pathogenic factors like] ghost, [disease caused by] worm toxin, cold-heat [disease], running piglet, five [kinds of] dysuria and convulsion [due to] evil-Qi. [It is also] called Tundian（豚颠）.

Xuanti（悬蹄）[2] [can be used] to treat five [kinds of] hemorrhoids, retention of heat in the intestines, acute appendicitis and genital ulcer.

[Textual Research]

[In] case [analysis in the book entitled] *Shuo Wen*（《说文》，*On Culture*）, [it] says [that] the character refers to piglet. [According to] a popular explanation, piglet is called Tun（豚）or Xi（豨）. [In] the Wu（吴）[State] and Yang（扬）[State], [it is] called Zhuzi（猪子，pig's porkling）.

Notes

1. Tunluan（豚卵，pig's testis，Sus Scrofa Domestica）is an animal medicinal, sweet in taste and warm in property, entering the

治疗寒热病，贲豚，五种癃闭证以及邪气所引起的抽搐。又称为

豚颠。

　　悬蹄，能治疗五种痔疮，热邪隐藏在肠中，肠痈和阴部溃疡。

kidney meridian, effective in warming the kidney and dispersing cold, calming convulsion and arresting epilepsy. Clinically it is used to treat swelling and pain of testicle, pain caused by hernia, dysuria, pain of penis, convulsion and epilepsy.

77. 麋脂

【原文】

味辛,温。

主痈肿,恶疮,死肌,寒风,湿痹,四肢拘缓不收,风头,肿气,通凑理。一名官脂。生山谷。

【考据】

1.《名医》曰:生南山及淮海边,十月取。

2. 案《说文》云:麋,鹿属,冬至解其角。汉书云:刘向以为麋之为言迷也。盖牝兽之淫者也。

【今译】

味辛,性温。

主治痈肿,恶性疮,肌肉坏死,寒风湿邪所致痹证,四肢拘急不收,风邪袭头肿胀,能疏通腠理。又称为官脂。该物生长在山谷之中。

77. Mizhi（麋脂，fat of david's deer，Adeps Elaphuri Davidiani）[1]

[Original Text]

[Mizhi（麋脂，fat of david's deer，Adeps Elaphuri Davidiani），] pungent in taste and warm [in property]，[is mainly used] to treat abscess，severe sore，necrotic muscles，wind-cold and dampness impediment，spasm of the four limbs，[pain and] swelling of the head [due to invasion of] wind，and to regulate the interstices. [It is also] called Guanzhi（官脂），growing in mountains and valleys.

[Textual Research]

[In the book entitled] *Ming Yi Bie Lu*（《名医别录》，*Special Record of Great Doctors*），[it] says [that Mizhi（麋脂，fat of david's deer，Adeps Elaphuri Davidiani) can be] found in Nanshan（南山） and the sides of Huaihai（淮海）. [It can be] collected in October.

[In] case [analysis in the book entitled] *Shuo Wen*（《说文》，*On Culture*），[it] says [that] Mi（麋，elk) belongs to Lu（鹿，deer）. [Its] antlers [can be] collected on the Winter Solstice.

Notes

1. Mizhi（麋脂，fat of david's deer，Adeps Elaphuri Davidiani) is an animal medicinal. Its action and clinical application are the same as Lujiao（鹿角，antler，Cornu Cervi），Lujiaojiao（鹿角胶，antler glue Colla Cornus Cervi) and Lujiaoshuang（鹿角霜，powder of deglued antler，Cornu Cervi Degelatinatum）.

78. 鼺鼠

【原文】

主堕胎，令人产易。生平谷。

【考据】

1.《名医》曰：生山都。

2. 案《说文》云：鼺鼠形，飞走且乳之鸟也，籀文作鸓.《广雅》云。鸋鴂飞鸓也。

3. 陶宏景云是鼯鼠，一名飞生见,《尔雅》云鼺鼠夷由也。旧作鸓，非。

【今译】

主治堕胎，能使人分娩容易。该物生长在平谷中。

78. Leishu (鼺鼠, trogopterus, Petaurista Petaurista) [1]

[Original Text]

[Leishu (鼺鼠, trogopterus, Petaurista Petaurista) can be used] to induce abortion and to make it easy to deliver baby. [It] exists in plains and valleys.

[Textual Research]

[In the book entitled] *Ming Yi Bie Lu* (《名医别录》, *Special Record of Great Doctors*), [it] says [that Leishu (鼺鼠, trogopterus, Petaurista Petaurista)] exists in Shandu (山都).

Tao Hongjing (陶宏景) said, "Leishu (鼺鼠, trogopterus, Petaurista Petaurista) [is also] called Feishengxian (飞生见). [According to the book entitled] *Er Ya* (《尔雅》, *On Elegence*), Leishu (鼺鼠, trogopterus, Petaurista Petaurista) was originally brought from other tribes.

Notes

1. Leishu (鼺鼠, trogopterus, Petaurista Petaurista) is an animal medicinal, salty in taste, warm and toxic in property, entering the liver meridian and the kidney meridian, effective in delivering baby, ceasing pain and inducing abortion. Clinically it is mainly used to treat lumbago after delivery of baby, arthralgia and headache due to wind attack.

79. 六畜毛蹄甲（马、牛、羊、猪、狗、鸡）

【原文】

味咸，平。

主鬼注，蛊毒，寒热，惊痫，瘨痓，狂走，骆驼毛，尤良。

【考据】

1. 案陶宏景云：六畜，谓马、牛、羊、猪、狗、鸡也，蹄，即蹢省文。

上兽，下品四种，旧同。

【今译】

味咸，性平。

主治鬼怪之邪所致之症及虫毒所致之病，能治疗寒热病，惊风，癫痫，抽搐，狂奔乱跑。骆驼毛蹄的治疗效果更好。

79. Liuchu Maotijia（六畜毛蹄甲，hairy hoofs of six animals）[1]

［Original Text］

［Liuchu Maotijia（六畜毛蹄甲，hairy hoofs of six animals），］salty in taste and mild［in property］，［is mainly used］to treat［disease caused by vicious pathogenic factors like］ghost，［disease caused by］worm toxin，cold-heat［disease］，convulsion，epilepsy，psychosis and manic behavior. The hairy hoof of camel is more effective［in treating diseases］.

［Textual Research］

Tao Hongjing（陶宏景）said，"The six animals refer to horse，cow，sheep，pig，dog and chicken."

Notes

1. Liuchu Maotijia（六畜毛蹄甲，hairy hoofs of six animals）is an animal medicinal，salty in taste and mild in property. Clinically it is used to treat epilepsy，psychosis and other mental disorders. In ancient books，the explanation about Liuchu Maotijia（六畜毛蹄甲，hairy hoofs of six animals）is not the same. For example，camel was not mentioned in some ancient books.

80. 虾蟆

【原文】

味辛,寒。

主邪气,破症坚,血痈肿,阴疮。服之不患热病。生池泽。

【考据】

1.《名医》曰:一名蟾蜍,一名鼃,一名去甫,一名苦蚤,生江湖,五月五日,取,阴干,东行者良。

2. 案《说文》云:虾,虾蟆也,蟆,虾蟆也,黾,虾蟆也,蟾、詹诸也,其鸣詹诸,其皮蠢蠢,其行黾黾,或作鼃鼀,鼀詹诸也。夏水正《传》云:域也者,长股也,或曰屈造之属也。诗曰:鼃鼀得比,言其行鼀鼀,蜮鼀,詹诸,以鸣者,《广雅》云:蚁苦蚤胡鼀,虾蟆也。《尔雅》云:鼁鼀蟾诸,郭璞云:似虾蟆,居陆地,淮南谓之去蚊,又蝗。郭璞云:蛙类。

3.《周礼》云:蝈氏。郑司农云:蝈,读为蛙,蛙,虾蟆也,元谓蝈,今御所食蛙也。月今云:仲夏之月,反舌无声。蔡邕云:今谓之虾蟆。薛君韩诗注云:戚施蟾蜍。

4. 高诱注南子云:蟾蜍也,又蝈,虾蟆也,又蟾蜍,虾蟆,又鼓造,一

80. Xiamo（虾蟆，rice-paddy frog，Rana Limnocharis）[1]

[Original Text]

[Xiamo（虾蟆，rice-paddy frog, Rana Limnocharis），] pungent in taste and cold [in property], [is mainly used] to expel evil-Qi, to break hard lump and to treat abscess with bleeding and genital sore. Taking of it will not contract heat disease. [It] exists in lakes and swamps.

[Textual Research]

[In the book entitled] *Ming Yi Bie Lu*（《名医别录》，*Special Record of Great Doctors*），[it] says [that Xiamo（虾蟆，rice-paddy frog，Rana Limnocharis）is also] called Chanchu（蟾蜍），Qupu（去甫）and Ku（苦），existing in rivers and lakes. [It can be] collected on May 5 and dried in the shade. Those in the east region are better.

[In the book entitled] *Guang Ya*（《广雅》，*The First Chinese Encyclopedic Dictionary*），[it] says [that the so-called] Kuhu（苦胡）refers to Xiamo（虾蟆，rice-paddy frog，Rana Limnocharis）. Guo Pu（郭璞）said，"[It is] similar to Xiamo（虾蟆，rice-paddy frog，Rana Limnocharis），existing in land. [It is] called Wuwen（去蚊）and Youhuang（又蝗）in Huainan（淮南）."

曰虾蟆,《抱朴子·内篇》云:或问魏武帝曾收左元放而桎梏之,而得自然解脱。以何法乎。

5.《抱朴子》曰:以自解去父血。

【今译】

味辛,性寒。

主治邪气所致之症,能破除坚硬癥瘕,能消除血痛肿胀,能治疗阴部溃疡。服用了就不会患热病。该物生长在池泽中。

Notes

1. Xiamo (虾蟆, rice-paddy frog, Rana Limnocharis) is a ranidae medicinal, entering the heart meridian and the spleen meridian, effective in clearing heat and removing toxin, fortifying the spleen and resolving accumulation. Clinically it is used to treat abscess, febrile furuncle, oral ulcer, scrofula, diarrhea, dysentery and infantile malnutrition.

81. 马刀

【原文】

味辛,微寒(《御览》有补中二字,《大观本》,黑字)。

主漏下赤白,寒热,破石淋,杀禽兽贼鼠。生池泽。

【考据】

1.《吴普》曰:马刀,一名齐蛤,神农岐伯桐君咸有毒,扁鹊小寒大毒,生池泽江海,采无时也(《御览》)。

2.《名医》曰:一名马蛤,生江湖及东海,采无时。

3. 案《范子计然》云:马刀出河东,艺文类聚引本经云:文蛤表有文,又曰马刀,一曰名蛤,则,岂古本与文蛤为一邪。

81. Madao（马刀，gaper clam，Bivalvia et Mactridae） [1]

［Original Text］

［Madao（马刀，gaper clam，Bivalvia et Mactridae），］pungent in taste and slightly cold ［in property］, ［is mainly used］ to treat red and white vaginal bleeding and cold-heat ［disease］, to break stony stranguria, and to kill birds, beasts and thief-like mice. ［It］ exists in lakes and swamps.

［Textual Research］

［In the book entitled］ *Wu Pu Ben Cao*（《吴普本草》，*Wu Pu's Studies of Materia Medica*）, ［it］ says ［that］ Madao（马刀，gaper clam, Bivalvia et Mactridae）［is also］ called Qihe（齐蛤）. ［According to］ Agriculture God（神农），Qibo（岐伯）and Tongjun（桐均），［it is］ salty ［in taste］ and toxic ［in property］; ［according to］ Bianque（扁鹊），［it is］ mildly cold and severely toxic ［in property］. ［It］ exists in lakes, pools, rivers and seas, and ［can be］ collected at any time ［as mentioned in the book entitled］ *Tai Ping Yu Lan*（《太平御览》，*Imperial Studies in Taiping Times*）.

［In the book entitled］ *Ming Yi Bie Lu*（《名医别录》，*Special Record of Great Doctors*），［it］ says ［that Madao（马刀，gaper clam, Bivalvia et Mactridae）is also］ called Mage（马蛤），existing in rivers, lakes and Donghai（东海，East Sea）. ［It can be］ collected at

【今译】

味辛,性微寒。

主治阴道出血淋漓不断,赤白带下和寒热病,能破除石淋病症,能杀死禽兽和贼鼠。该物生长在池泽中。

神农本草经

any time.

〔In the book entitled〕 *Fan Zi Ji Ran* (《范子计然》, *Studies About Fan Li's Teacher*), 〔it〕 says 〔that〕 Madao (马刀, gaper clam, Bivalvia et Mactridae) exists in Hedong (河东). 〔According to〕 a book about arts, Wenge (文蛤, meretrix clam shell, Concha Meretricis) with texture in the superficies is also called Madao (马刀) and Mingge (名蛤). That is why in ancient books 〔Madao (马刀, gaper clam, Bivalvia et Mactridae)〕 and Wenge (文蛤, meretrix clam shell, Concha Meretricis) were the same one."

Agriculture
God's Canon of
Materia Medica

Notes

1. Madao (马刀, gaper clam, Bivalvia et Mactridae) is pungent in taste, slightly cold and mildly toxic in property, effective in relieving heat in the five Zang-organs, tonifying the middle (internal organs), resolving phlegm and dispersing stagnation. Clinically it is used to treat water goiter, Qi goiter, retention of fluid and phlegm, stranguria, red and white leucorrhea.

82. 蛇蜕

【原文】

味咸,平。

主小儿百二十种惊痫,瘛疭、瘨疾,寒热,肠痔,虫毒,蛇痫。火熬之良。一名龙子衣,一名蛇符,一名龙子单衣,一名弓皮。生川谷及田野。

【考据】

1.《吴普》曰:蛇蜕,一名龙子单衣,一名弓皮,一名蛇附,一名蛇筋,一名龙皮,一名龙单衣(《御览》)。

2.《名医》曰:一名龙子皮,生荆州,五月五日,十五日、取之良。

3. 案《说文》云:它,虫也,从虫而长,象冤,曲垂尾形,或作蛇蜕,蛇蝉所解皮也。《广雅》云:蝮蜻蜕也。《中山经》云:来山多空夺。郭璞云:即蛇皮脱也。

【今译】

味咸,性平。

主治小儿一百二十种惊风,癫痫,抽搐,癫证,寒热病,肠痔,虫

82. Shetuo（蛇蜕，snake slough，Periostracum Serpentis）[1]

[Original Text]

[Shetuo（蛇蜕，snake slough，Periostracum Serpentis），] salty in taste and mild [in property], [is mainly used] to treat one hundred and twenty infantile [diseases，such as] convulsion，epilepsy，convulsive limbs，epileptic disease，cold-heat [disease]，bloody stool，hemorrhoids，worm toxin and snake [-like] epilepsy. To be broiled in fire is better. [It is also] called Longziyi（龙子衣），Shefu（蛇符），Longzi Danyi（龙子单衣）and Gongpi（弓皮）. [It] exists in mountain valleys，river valleys and lands.

[Textual Research]

[In the book entitled] *Wu Pu Ben Cao*（《吴普本草》，*Wu Pu's Studies of Materia Medica*），[it] says [that] Shetuo（蛇蜕，snake slough，Periostracum Serpentis）[is also] called Longzi Danyi（龙子单衣），Gongpi（弓皮），Shefu（蛇附），Shejin（蛇筋），Shepi（龙皮）and Longdanyi（龙单衣）[according to the book entitled] *Tai Ping Yu Lan*（《太平御览》，*Imperial Studies in Taiping Times*）.

[In the book entitled] *Ming Yi Bie Lu*（《名医别录》，*Special Record of Great Doctors*），[it] says [that Shetuo（蛇蜕，snake slough，Periostracum Serpentis）is also] called Longzipi（龙子皮），existing in Jingzhou（荆州）. [It can be] collected on May 5 and 15.

毒,蛇痫等疾病。火熬后性存,疗效更好。又称为龙子衣,又称为蛇符,又称为龙子单衣,又称为弓皮。该物生长在山川河谷之中及田野里。

［It is］ better to collect ［at these two dates］.

Notes

1. Shetuo （蛇蜕, snake slough, Periostracum Serpentis） is sweet and salty in taste, mild and toxic in property, entering the liver meridian, effective in expelling wind, calming convulsion, removing toxin and resolving swelling. Clinically it is used to treat convulsion, infantile convulsive disease, epilepsy, impediment, swelling and pain of the throat, dysuria, scabies, ulcer, measles, chyluria and nebula.

Agriculture
God's Canon of
Materia Medica

83. 蚯蚓

【原文】

味咸,寒。

主蛇瘕,去三虫,伏尸,鬼注,蛊毒,杀长虫,仍自化作水。生平土。

【考据】

1.《吴普》曰:蚯蚓,一名白颈螳螾,一名附引(《御览》)。

2.《名医》曰:一名土龙,二月取,阴干。

3. 案《说文》云:螾,侧行者,或作蚓,螼螾也,《广雅》云:蚯蚓蜿蟺,引无也。

4.《尔雅》云:螼蚓紧蚕。郭璞云:即蟺也,江东呼寒蚓,旧作蚯,非,《吕氏春秋·淮南子》邱蚓出不从虫。又说山训云:蟮,无筋骨之强,高诱注:螾,一名蜷也,旧又有白颈二字,据《吴普》古本当无也。

【今译】

味咸,性寒。

83. Qiuyin（蚯蚓，earthworm，Pheretima）[1]

[Original Text]

［Qiuyin（蚯蚓，earthworm，Pheretima），］salty in taste and cold ［in property］，［is mainly used］to resolve abdominal mass and conglomeration，to eliminate three worms，unconsciousness ［like corpse］，［to treat］disease ［caused by vicious pathogenic factors like］ghost and ［disease caused by］worm toxin，and to kill roundworms.［It can］spontaneously transform into water.［It］exists in plains.

[Textual Research]

［In the book entitled］*Wu Pu Ben Cao*（《吴普本草》，*Wu Pu's Studies of Materia Medica*），［it］says ［that］Qiuyin（蚯蚓，earthworm，Pheretima）［is also］called Baijng Tangyin（白颈螳蟥）and Fuzi（附引）［according to the book entitled］*Tai Ping Yu Lan*（《太平御览》，*Imperial Studies in Taiping Times*）.

［In the book entitled］*Ming Yi Bie Lu*（《名医别录》，*Special Record of Great Doctors*），［it］says ［that Qiuyin（蚯蚓，earthworm，Pheretima）is also］called Tulong（土龙）.［It can be］collected in February and dried in the shade.

Notes

1. Qiuyin（蚯蚓，earthworm，Pheretima）is salty in taste and

主治蛇瘕，能祛除三种虫子，能治疗形若死尸之病，鬼怪之邪所致之症以及虫毒所致之病，能杀除长虫，又能自行化作为水。该物生长在平坦的土地上。

cold in property, entering the liver meridian, the spleen meridian and the lung meridian, effective in clearing heat, resolving convulsion, relieving panting, unobstructing collaterals, promoting urination and reducing blood pressure. Clinically it is used to treat high fever with vexation, convulsion, throat impediment, chronic bronchitis, asthma, eczema, paralysis, edema, jaundice, dysuria, hypertension, mumps, ulceration of the lower limbs, erysipelas, scald and fracture.

84. 蠮螉

【原文】

味辛,平。

主久聋,咳逆,毒气,出刺出汗。生川谷。

【考据】

1.《名医》曰:一名土蜂,生熊耳及牂柯,或人屋间。案《说文》云:蠮蠮蠃,蒲卢,细要土蜂也,或作螺蠃,螺蠃也。《广雅》云:土蜂,蠮螉也,《尔雅》土蜂。

2.《毛诗》云:螟蛉有子,螺蠃负之,《传》云螺蠃,蒲卢也。礼记云:夫政也者,蒲卢也。郑云:蒲卢,果蠃,谓土蜂也。方言云:蠮其小者谓之蠮螉,或谓之蚴蜕,《说文》无蠮字或当为医。

【今译】

味辛,性平。

主治长期耳聋,咳嗽气逆和毒气所伤,能拔出刺入人体之刺,能出汗。该物生长在山川河谷之中。

84. Yiweng（蠮螉，mud wasp，Delta seu Eumenes）[1]

［Original Text］

［Yiweng（蠮螉，mud wasp，Delta seu Eumenes），］pungent in taste and mild ［in property］，［is mainly used］ to treat deafness and cough with dyspnea，［to expel］ toxic Qi，to pull out thorns and to induce sweating．［It］exists in mountain valleys and river valleys.

［Textual Research］

［In the book entitled］ *Ming Yi Bie Lu*（《名医别录》，*Special Record of Great Doctors*），［it］says［that Yiweng（蠮螉，mud wasp，Delta seu Eumenes）is also］called Tufeng（土蜂），existing in the ears of bear and timber piles or houses．［In the book entitled］ *Guang Ya*（《广雅》，*The First Chinese Encyclopedic Dictionary*），［it］says［that the so-called］ Tufeng（土蜂）refers to Yiweng（蠮螉，mud wasp，Delta seu Eumenes）.

Notes

1. Yiweng（蠮螉，mud wasp，Delta seu Eumenes）is pungent in taste and mild in property，entering the heart meridian and the lung meridian，effective in ceasing cough and descending adverse flow of Qi．Clinically it is used to treat chronic deafness，cough with dyspnea，vomiting，stuffy nose and sore.

85．蜈蚣

【原文】

味辛，温。

主鬼注蛊毒，啖诸蛇虫鱼毒，杀鬼物老精，温虐，去三虫（《御览》引云：一名至掌，《大观本》在水蛭下）。生川谷。

【考据】

1.《名医》曰：生大吴江南，赤头足者良。

2. 案《广雅》云：蝍蛆，吴公也。

【今译】

味辛，性温。

主治鬼怪之邪所致之症及虫毒所致之病，能消除各种蛇毒、虫毒和鱼毒，能祛除鬼怪邪气所致之病，能治疗先热后冷的温虐，能杀除三种虫子。该物生长在山川河谷之中。

85. Wugong（蜈蚣，centipede，Scolopendra）[1]

[Original Text]

[Wugong（蜈蚣，centipede，Scolopendra），] pungent in taste and warm [in property], [is mainly used] to treat disease [caused by vicious pathogenic factors like] ghost and worm toxin, to eliminate various toxin of snakes, worms and fish, and to perish ghost-like vicious factors, to treat warm malaria and to expel three worms. [It] exists in mountain valleys and river valleys.

[Textual Research]

[In the book entitled] *Ming Yi Bie L u*（《名医别录》，*Special Record of Great Doctors*），[it] says [that Wugong（蜈蚣，centipede，Scolopendra）] exists in Dawu（大吴）and Jiangnan（江南）. [The one with] red head and claws is better.

[In the book entitled] *Guang Ya*（《广雅》，*The First Chinese Encyclopedic Dictionary*），[it] says [that the so-called] Jiqu（蛷蝫）refers to Wugong（蜈蚣，centipede，Scolopendra）.

Notes

1. Wugong（蜈蚣，centipede，Scolopendra）is pungent in taste, warm and toxic in property, effective in expelling wind, resolving convulsion and reducing toxin. Clinically it is used to treat wind stroke, convulsion, epilepsy, spasm, tetanus, facial paralysis, wind-dampness pain, whooping cough and scrofula.

86. 水蛭

【原文】

味咸,平。

主逐恶血瘀血,月闭(《御览》作水闭)。破血瘕积聚,无子,利水道。生池泽。

【考据】

1.《名医》曰:一名蚑.一名至掌,生雷泽,五月六月采,暴干。

2. 案《说文》云:蛭,蚑也,蟣,蛭蟣,至掌也。《尔雅》云:蛭蚑。郭璞云:今江东呼水中蛭虫入人肉者为蚑,又蛭蟣至掌。郭璞云未详,据《名医》,即蛭也。

【今译】

味咸,性平。

能祛除脓液,瘀血和经闭,能破除血瘕和积聚,能治疗不孕之症,能通利水道。该物生长在池泽中。

86. Shuizhi（水蛭，leech，Hirudo）[1]

[Original Text]

[Shuizhi（水蛭，leech，Hirudo），] salty in taste and mild [in property], [is mainly used] to eliminate blood stasis，[to resolve] amenorrhea，to break bloody conglomeration，accumulation and aggregation，[to treat] infertility，and to promote urination. [It] exists in lakes and swamps.

[Textual Research]

[In the book entitled] *Ming Yi Bie Lu* (《名医别录》，*Special Record of Great Doctors*)，[it] says [that Shuizhi（水蛭，leech，Hirudo) is also] called Ji（蚑）and Zhizhang（至掌），existing in Leize（雷泽）. [It can be] collected in May and June，and dried in the shade.

Notes

1. Shuizhi（水蛭，leech，Hirudo）is salty and bitter in taste，mild and toxic in property，entering the liver meridian and the bladder meridian，effective in expelling blood stasis，unobstructing meridians，resolving stagnation. Clinically it is used to treat amenorrhea due to blood stasis，abdominal conglomeration，accumulation and aggregation，traumatic injury，acute conjunctivitis and nebula.

87．班苗

【原文】

味辛，寒。

主寒热，鬼注，蛊毒，鼠瘘，恶疮，疽蚀，死肌，破石癃。一名龙尾。生川谷。

【考据】

1.《吴普》曰：斑猫。一名斑蚝，一名龙蚝，一名斑苗，一名胜发，一名盘蛩，一名晏青，神农辛，岐伯咸，桐君有毒，扁鹊甘有大毒，生河内川谷。或生水石。

2.《名医》曰：生河东，八月取，阴干。

3. 案《说文》云：螌，螌蝥，毒虫也。《广雅》云：螌蝥，晏青也，《名医》别出芫青条，非，芫晏音相近也，旧作猫，俗字。据吴氏云：一名斑苗，是也。

【今译】

味辛，性寒。

87. Banmiao（班苗，beetle of large blister，Mylabris）[1]

[Original Text]

[Banmiao（班苗，beetle of large blister，Mylabris），] pungent in taste and cold [in property]，[is mainly used] to treat cold-heat [disease]，disease [caused by vicious pathogenic factors like] ghost and worm toxin，tuberculosis，severe sore，ulceration and corrosion，necrotic muscles and stony dysuria. [It is also] called Longwei（龙尾），existing in mountain valleys and river valleys.

[Textual Research]

[In the book entitled] *Wu Pu Ben Cao*（《吴普本草》，*Wu Pu's Studies of Materia Medica*），[it] says [that] Banmao（斑猫，beetle of large blister，Mylabris）[is also] called Banhao（斑蚝），Longhao（龙蚝），Banmiao（斑苗），Shengfa（胜发），Panqiong（盘蛩）and Yanqing（晏青）. [According to] Agriculture God（神农），[it is] pungent [in taste]；[according to] Qibo（岐伯），[it is] salty [in taste]；[according to] Tongjun（桐均），[it is] toxic [in property]；[according to] Bianque（扁鹊），[it is] sweet [in taste] and severely toxic [in property]，existing in the mountains and valleys in Henei（河内）or in water and stones.

[In the book entitled] *Ming Yi Bie Lu*（《名医别录》，*Special Record of Great Doctors*），[it] says [that Banmiao（班苗，beetle of

主治寒热病,能治疗鬼怪病邪所致之病,虫毒所致之症,鼠瘘,恶性痈疮,疮肿溃烂和肌肉坏死,能破除石癃闭证。又称为龙尾。该物生长在山川河谷之中。

large blister, Mylabris)] exists in Hedong (河东). [It can be] collected in August and dried in the shade.

Notes

1. Banmiao (班苗, beetle of large blister, Mylabris) is pungent in taste, cold and severely toxic in property, entering the large intestine meridian, the small intestine meridian, the liver meridian and the kidney meridian, effective in removing toxin, dispersing stasis and foaming. Clinically it is used to treat psoriasis, neutral inflammation, distorted mouth and eyes, rheumatism, scrofula, bite by rabid dog and liver cancer.

88. 贝子

【原文】

味咸,平。

主目翳,鬼注,虫毒,腹痛,下血,五癃,利水道,烧用之良。生池泽。

【考据】

1.《名医》曰:一名贝齿,生东海。

2. 案《说文》云:贝,海介虫也,居陆名飙。在水名蜬,象形,《尔雅》云:贝小者。郭璞云:今细贝,亦有紫色,出日南,又鲼,小而椭。郭璞云:即上小贝。

【今译】

味咸,性平。

主治目中生翳,能治疗鬼怪病邪所致之症,虫毒所致之症,腹部疼痛,大便下血和五种癃闭证,能通利水道。火烧后使用,疗效更好。该物生长在池泽中。

88. Beizi（贝子，cowry shell，Concha Monetariae）[1]

[Original Text]

[Beizi（贝子，cowry shell，Concha Monetariae），] salty in taste and mild [in property], [is mainly used] to treat nebula, disease [caused by vicious pathogenic factors like] ghost, [disease caused by] worm toxin, abdominal pain, hematochezia and five [kinds of] dysuria, and to disinhibit waterway. [It is] better [when] broiled. [It] exists in lakes and swamps.

[Textual Research]

[In the book entitled] *Ming Yi Bie Lu*（《名医别录》，*Special Record of Great Doctors*），[it] says [that Beizi（贝子，cowry shell，Concha Monetariae）is also] called Beichi（贝齿）and exists in Donghai（东海，East Sea）.

Notes

1. Beizi（贝子，cowry shell，Concha Monetariae）is salty in taste and mild in property, effective in clearing heat, promoting urination and dispersing stagnation. Clinically it is used to treat dropsy due to retention of water, gonorrhea with pain and bleeding, dysuria, nasal discharge of pus and blood, nebula, dysentery, cold-heat disease and five kinds of stranguria.

89. 石蚕

【原文】

味咸,寒。

主五癃,破石淋,堕胎,内解结气,利水道,除热。一名沙虱。生池泽。

【考据】

1.《吴普》曰:石蚕亦名沙虱,神农雷公酸无毒,生汉中,治五淋,破随内结气,利水道,除热(《御览》)。

2.《名医》曰:生江汉。

3. 案《广雅》云:沙虱,蜻蛦也。淮南万毕术云:沙虱,一名蓬活,一名地脾。

4.《御览》虫豸部引李当之云:类虫,形如老蚕,生附石。广志云:皆虱,虱色赤,大过虮,在水中,入人皮中,杀人,与李似不同。

【今译】

味咸,性寒。

89. Shican（石蚕，phryganea larva，Larva Phryganeae）[1]

[Original Text]

[Shican（石蚕，phryganea larva，Larva Phryganeae），] salty in taste and cold [in property]，[is mainly used] to treat five [kinds of] gonorrhea，to break stony stranguria，to induce abortion，to relieve internal stagnation of Qi，to disinhibit waterway and to eliminate heat．[It is also] called Shashi（沙虱），existing in lakes and swamps.

[Textual Research]

[In the book entitled] *Wu Pu Ben Cao*（《吴普本草》，*Wu Pu's Studies of Materia Medica*），[it] says [that] Shican（石蚕，phryganea larva，Larva Phryganeae）[is also] called Shashi（沙虱）．[According to] Agriculture God（神农）and Leigong（雷公），[it is] sour [in taste] and non-toxic [in property]，existing in Hanzhong（汉中），treating five [kinds of] stranguria，breaking internal stagnation of Qi，disinhibiting waterway and eliminating heat [as mentioned in the book entitled] *Tai Ping Yu Lan*（《太平御览》，*Imperial Studies in Taiping Times*）.

[In the book entitled] *Ming Yi Bie Lu*（《名医别录》，*Special Record of Great Doctors*），[it] says [that Shican（石蚕，phryganea larva，Larva Phryganeae）] exists in Jianghan（江汉）.

主治五种癃闭证,能破解石淋病症,能堕胎,能消除体内积聚气结,能通利水道,能消除热邪所致之病。又称为沙虱。该物生长在池泽中。

Notes

1. Shican (石蚕, phryganea larva, Larva Phryganeae) is sweet and bland in taste, cool in property, effective in expelling wind and dampness, dispersing blood stasis, cooling the blood, removing toxin and ceasing pain. Clinically it is used to treat rheumatoid arthritis, lumbago, hepatitis, hematemesis, hematuria, sprain, breast abscess and erysipelas.

90. 雀瓮

【原文】

味甘，平。

主小儿惊痫，寒热，结气，蛊毒。鬼注。一名躁舍。

【考据】

1.《名医》曰：生汉中，采蒸之，生树枝间，蛅蟖房也。八月取。

2. 案《说文》云：蛅，蛅斯黑也。《尔雅》云蟔，蛅蟖。郭璞云：载属也，今青州人呼载为蛅蟖。按本经名为雀瓮者。瓮与蛹音相近，以其如雀子，又如茧虫之蛹，因呼之。

【今译】

味甘，性平。

主治小儿惊风，癫痫，寒热病，气机拘结，虫毒所致之病以及鬼怪病邪所致之症。又称为躁舍。

90. Queweng（雀瓮，cocoon of oriental moth，Incunabulum Cnidocampae Flavescentis）[1]

［Original Text］

［Queweng（雀瓮，cocoon of oriental moth，Incunabulum Cnidocampae Flavescentis），］sweet in taste ［and］ mild ［in property］，［is mainly used］ to treat infantile convulsion and epilepsy，cold-heat ［disease］，［disease caused by］ stagnation of Qi and worm toxin and disease ［caused by vicious pathogenic factors like］ ghost. ［It is also］ called Zaoshe（躁舍）.

［Textual Research］

［In the book entitled］ *Ming Yi Bie Lu*（《名医别录》，*Special Record of Great Doctors*），［it］ says ［that Queweng（雀瓮，cocoon of oriental moth，Incunabulum Cnidocampae Flavescentis）］ exists in Hanzhong（汉中）. ［It can be］ collected in August from among the twigs and branches of the tree and steamed ［for medical purpose］.

Notes

1. Queweng（雀瓮，cocoon of oriental moth，Incunabulum Cnidocampae Flavescentis）is sweet in taste，mild and non-toxic in property，entering the liver meridian，effective in extinguishing wind，stopping convulsion，removing toxin and resolving swelling. Clinically it is used to treat infantile convulsion，umbilical tetanus，epilepsy，cold-heat disease，stagnation of Qi and tonsillitis.

91. 蜣螂

【原文】

味咸,寒。

主小儿惊痫,瘈疭,腹张,寒热,大人瘨疾狂易。一名蛣蜣。火熬之良。生池泽。

【考据】

1.《名医》曰:生长沙,五月五日取,蒸藏之。

2. 案《说文》云:蜣,渠蜣,一曰天杜。《广雅》云:天杜,蜣螂也。《尔雅》云:蛣蜣,蜣螂,郭璞云:黑甲虫,啖粪土,玉篇,蜣螂同,《说文》无蜣字,渠蝪,即蛣蜣,音之缓急。

91. Qianglang（蜣蜋，dung beetle，Catharsius）[1]

[Original Text]

[Qianglang（蜣蜋，dung beetle，Catharsius），] salty in taste and cold [in property]，[is mainly used] to treat infantile，convulsion，epilepsy，clonic convulsion，abdominal distension，cold-heat [disease]，psychosis and mania in adults. [It is also] called Jieqiang（蛣蜣）. [It is] better [when] broiled in fire. [It] exists in lakes and swamps.

[Textual Research]

[In the book entitled] *Ming Yi Bie Lu* (《名医别录》，*Special Record of Great Doctors*)，[it] says [that Qianglang（蜣蜋，dung beetle，Catharsius）] exists in Changsha（长沙）. [It can be] collected on May 5，steamed and stored.

[In the book entitled] *Guang Ya* (《广雅》，*The First Chinese Encyclopedic Dictionary*)，[it] says [that the so-called] Tiandu（天杜）refers to Qianglang（蜣蜋，dung beetle，Catharsius）. [In the book entitled] *Er Ya* (《尔雅》，*On Elegance*)，[it] says [that the so-called] Jieqiang（蛣蜣）refers to Qianglang（蜣蜋，dung beetle，Catharsius）.

【今译】

味咸，性寒。

主治小儿惊风，癫痫，抽搐，腹部胀满，寒热病，成人癫痫及狂症。又称为蛄蟖。火熬后服之，疗效更好。该物生长在池泽中。

Notes

1. Qianglang (蜣螂, dung beetle, Catharsius) is salty in taste, cold and toxic in property, entering the liver meridian, the stomach meridian and the large intestine meridian, effective in resolving convulsion, breaking blood stasis, promoting defecation and removing toxin. Clinically it is used to treat infantile convulsion and epilepsy, clonic convulsion, abdominal distension, infantile malnutrition, abscess, scabies and hemorrhoids as well as to induce abortion.

92. 蝼蛄

【原文】

味咸,寒。

主产难,出肉中刺(《御览》作刺在肉中),溃痈肿,下哽噎(《御览》作咽),解毒,除恶疮。一名蟪蛄(《御览》作蟪蛄),一名天蝼,一名螜。夜出者良,生平泽。

【考据】

1.《名医》曰:生东城,夏至取,暴干。

2. 案《说文》云:蝼,蝼蛄也,蝼,蝼蛄也,姑,蝼蛄也。《广雅》云:炙鼠,津姑,蝼蛴,蟓蛉,蛞蝼,蝼蛄也,《夏小正》云:三月毂则鸣,毂,天蝼也,《尔雅》云:毂,天蝼,郭璞云:蝼蛄也。《淮南子·时则训》云:孟夏之月,蝼蝈鸣,高诱云:蝼,蝼姑也,方言云:蛞诣,谓之杜格,蝼蛄,谓之蝼蜂,或谓之蟓蛉,南楚谓之杜狗,或谓之蟓蝼。陆玑诗疏云:本草又谓蝼蛄为石鼠,今无文。

92. Lougu（蝼蛄，mole cricket，Gryllotalpa Africana）[1]

[Original Text]

[Lougu（蝼蛄，mole cricket，Gryllotalpa Africana），] salty in taste and cold [in property]，[is mainly used] to treat dystocia，to pull thorn out of the muscles，to resolve abscess，to remove obstruction of the throat，to expel toxin and to eliminate severe sore. [It is also] called Huigu（蟪蛄），Tianlou（天蝼）and Hu（螜）. [It] exists in lakes and pools. [Those] produced at night are better.

[Textual Research]

[In the book entitled] *Ming Yi Bie Lu*（《名医别录》，*Special Record of Great Doctors*），[it] says [that Lougu（蝼蛄，mole cricket，Gryllotalpa Africana）] exists in Dongcheng（东城）. [It can be] collected in summer and dried in the sun.

[In] case [analysis in the book entitled] *Shuo Wen*（《说文》，*On Culture*），[it] says [that the so-called] Du（蠹），Lou（蝼）and Gu（姑）refer to Lougu（蝼蛄，mole cricket，Gryllotalpa Africana）. [In the book entitled] *Guang Ya*（《广雅》，*The First Chinese Encyclopedic Dictionary*），[it] says [that the so-called] Zhishu（炙鼠），Jingu（津姑），Louhuo（蝼蝈），Xiangling（蟓蛉）and Kuolou（蛞蝼）all refer to Loulou（蝼蛄，mole cricket，Gryllotalpa Africana）.

【今译】

味咸,性寒。

主治产难,能拔出扎入肉中的刺,能消除痈肿溃破,能解除饮食不下对咽喉的阻塞,能排出毒气,能祛除恶性痈疮。又称为螻蛄。夜间出来的,疗效更好,该物生长在平川水泽之中。

Notes

1. Lougu (蝼蛄, mole cricket, Gryllotalpa Africana) is salty in taste and cold in property, entering the stomach meridian and the bladder meridian, effective in promoting urination and resolving swelling. Clinically it is used to treat edema, dysuria and tympanites.

93. 马陆

【原文】

味辛,温。

主腹中大坚症,破积聚,息肉,恶疮,白秃。一名百足。生川谷。

【考据】

1.《吴普》曰:一名马轴,(《御览》)。

2.《名医》曰:一名马轴,生元菟。

3. 案《说文》云:蠲,马蠲也,从虫皿,益声,勹象形。明堂月令曰:腐草为蠲。《广雅》云,蛆蝶,马蠖,马蚿也,又马践,蛆也。《尔雅》云:蛝,马践。郭璞云:马蠲匆,俗呼马蠸,《淮南子·时则训》云:季夏之月,腐草化为蚈。高诱云:蚈,马蚈也,幽冀谓之秦渠,又蚈论训云:蚈足众,而走不若蛇,又兵略训云:若蚈之足。高诱云:蠸,马蚿也,方言云,马蚿,北燕谓之蛆渠,其大者谓之马蚰。《博物志》云:马蚿,一名百足,中断成两段,名行而去。

93. Malu（马陆，diplopod，Millepeda）[1]

[**Original Text**]

[Malu（马陆，diplopod，Millepeda），] pungent in taste and warm [in property]，[is mainly used] to treat large and hard lump in the abdomen，to break accumulation and aggregation，and [to treat] polypus，severe sore and tinea tonsure．[It is also] called Baizu（百足）and exists in mountain valleys and river valleys．

[**Textual Research**]

[In the book entitled] *Wu Pu Ben Cao*（《吴普本草》，*Wu Pu's Studies of Materia Medica*），[it] says [that Malu（马陆，diplopod，Millepeda）is also] called Mazhou（马轴）[according to the book entitled] *Tai Ping Yu Lan*（《太平御览》，*Imperial Studies in Taiping Times*）．

[In the book entitled] *Ming Yi Bie Lu*（《名医别录》，*Special Record of Great Doctors*），[it] says [that Malu（马陆，diplopod，Millepeda）is also] called Mazhou（马轴），existing in Yuantu（元菟）．

Notes

1. Malu（马陆，diplopod，Millepeda）is pungent in taste，warm and toxic in property，entering the heart meridian and the lung meridian，effective in breaking accumulation，removing toxin and

【今译】

味辛,性温。

主治腹中坚硬巨大的癥瘕,能破解积聚,息肉,恶性痈疮和白秃。又称为百足。该物生长在山川河谷之中。

harmonizing the stomach. Clinically it is used to treat conglomeration, abdominal mass, stomachache, poor appetite, abscess, severe sore and scabies.

神农本草经

94. 地胆

【原文】

味辛,寒。

主鬼注,寒热,鼠蝼,恶疮,死肌,破症瘕,堕胎。一名蚖青,生川谷。

【考据】

1.《吴普》曰:地胆,一名元青,一名杜龙,一名青虹(《御览》)。

2.《名医》曰:一名青𧈭,生汶山,八月取。

3. 案《广雅》云:地胆蛇要,青蘁,青蠵也,陶宏景云:状如大马蚁,有翼,伪者即班猫所化,状如大豆。

94. Didan（地胆，all-grass of canton sonerila，Meloe coarctatus）[1]

[Original Text]

[Didan（地胆，beetle bile，Meloe coarctatus），] pungent in taste and cold [in property], [is mainly used] to treat disease [caused by vicious pathogenic factors like] ghost, cold-heat [disease], tuberculosis, severe sore and necrotic muscles, to break abdominal mass and conglomeration, and to induce abortion. [It is also] called Yuanqing（蚖青），existing in mountain valleys and river valleys.

[Textual Research]

[In the book entitled] *Wu Pu Ben Cao*（《吴普本草》，*Wu Pu's Studies of Materia Medica*），[it] says [that] Didan（地胆，beetle bile，Meloe coarctatus）[is also] called Yuanqing（元青），Dulong（杜龙）and Qinghong（青虹）[as mentioned in the book entitled] *Tai Ping Yu Lan*（《太平御览》，*Imperial Studies in Taiping Times*）.

1219

[In the book entitled] *Ming Yi Bie Lu*（《名医别录》，*Special Record of Great Doctors*），[it] says [that Didan（地胆，beetle bile，Meloe coarctatus）is also] called Qing（青）. [It] exists in Wenshan（汶山）and [can be] collected at August.

Tao Hongjing（陶宏景）said，"[Didan（地胆，beetle bile，Meloe coarctatus）is as] large as a big ant with wings. The pseudo-one is transformed from Banmao（斑猫，beetle of large blister，Mylabris），

【今译】

味辛,性寒。

主治鬼怪病邪所致之症,寒热病,鼠瘘,恶性痈疮以及肌肉坏死,能破除症瘕,能堕胎。又称为蚖青,该物生长在山川河谷之中。

like a big soybean. "

Notes

1. Didan (地胆, beetle bile, Meloe coarctatus) is pungent in taste, cold and toxic in property, effective in removing toxin, eliminating blood stasis, dispersing stagnation and resolving stagnation of Qi. Clinically it is used to treat severe sore, polypus, scrofula, abdominal mass and conglomeration, dysuria, hernia, stony stranguria, and scabies.

95. 鼠妇

【原文】

味酸,温。

主气癃,不得小便,女人月闭,血瘕,痫痉,寒热,利水道。一名负蟠,一名蚜蝛。生平谷。

【考据】

1.《名医》曰:一蟏蛸生魏郡及人家地上,五月五日取。

2. 案《说文》云:蛜蛜威,委黍,委黍,鼠妇也,蟠鼠负也。《尔雅》云:蟠,鼠负。郭璞云:瓮器底虫。又蛜威委黍。郭璞云:旧说,鼠妇别名。《毛诗》云:伊威在室。《传》云:伊威,委黍也。陆玑云:在壁根下,瓮底中生,似白鱼。

【今译】

味酸,性温。

主治气淋症,不得小便,经闭,血瘕,癫痫,抽搐以及寒热病,能通利水道。又称为负蟠,又称为蛜威。该物生长在平谷中。

95. Shufu (鼠妇, pillbug, Armadillidium) [1]

[Original Text]

[Shufu (鼠妇, pillbug, Armadillidium),] sour in taste and warm [in property], [is mainly used] to treat Qi stranguria, dysuria, amenorrhea with blood conglomeration, epilepsy with suffocation and cold-heat [disease], and to promote waterway. [It is also] called Fupan (负蟠) and Yiwei (蚜蝛), existing in plains and valleys.

[Textual Research]

[In the book entitled] *Ming Yi Bie Lu* (《名医别录》, *Special Record of Great Doctors*), [it] says [that Shufu (鼠妇, pillbug, Armadillidium)] exists in Weijun (魏郡) and in the homes of some people. [It can be] collected on May 5.

[In] case [analysis in the book entitled] *Shuo Wen* (《说文》, *On Culture*), [it] says [that the so-called] Weishu (委黍) refers to Shufu (鼠妇, pillbug, Armadillidium) and Panshu (蟠鼠). Lu Ji (陆玑) said, "[Shufu (鼠妇, pillbug, Armadillidium)] stays below the wall and behind the earthen jar, like whitefish."

Notes

1. Shufu (鼠妇, pillbug, Armadillidium), named differently in different places, is sour in taste and warm in property, effective in promoting urination, resolving stranguria, activating the blood, expelling blood stasis and ceasing suffocation. Clinically it is used to treat dysuria after delivery of baby, stranguria, infantile lockjaw, amenorrhea, abdominal mass and conglomeration, convulsion, toothache and various mycotic stomatitis.

96. 荧火

【原文】

味辛,微温。

主明目,小儿火疮,伤热气,蛊毒,鬼注,通神。一名夜光(《御览》引云,一名熠耀,一名即照,《大观本》,作黑字)。生池泽。

【考据】

1.《吴普》曰:荧火一名夜照,一名熠耀,一名救火,一名景天,一名据火,一名挟火(艺文类聚)。

2.《名医》曰:一名放光,一名熠耀,一名即照,生阶地,七月七日收,阴干。

3. 案《说文》云:粦,兵死及牛马之血为磷,鬼火也,从炎舛。《尔雅》云:荧水即照。郭璞云:夜飞,腹下有火。《毛诗》云:熠耀宵行,《传》云熠耀,磷也,磷,荧火也,月令云:季夏之月,腐草化为荧。郑元云:萤飞虫,萤火也,据毛苌以萤为磷,是也,《说文》无萤字,当以磷为之,《尔雅》作荧,亦是,旧作萤,非。又按月令,腐草为萤,当是蠲字假音。

96. Yinghuo（荧火，firefly，Lampyridae）[1]

[Original Text]

[Yinghuo（荧火，firefly，Lampyridae），] pungent in taste and slightly warm [in property], [is mainly used] to improve vision，[to treat] infantile scald，[to dispel] heat-Qi [in the viscera]，[to cure] disease [caused by vicious pathogenic factors like] ghost，and to invigorate the spirit. [It is also] called Yeguang（夜光），existing in lakes and swamps.

[Textual Research]

[In the book entitled] *Wu Pu Ben Cao*（《吴普本草》，*Wu Pu's Studies of Materia Medica*），[it] says [that] Yinghuo（荧火，firefly，Lampyridae）[is also] called Yezhao（夜照），Yiyao（熠耀），Jiuhuo（救火），Jingtian（景天），Juhuo（据火）and Jiahuo（挟火）.

[In the book entitled] *Ming Yi Bie Lu*（《名医别录》，*Special Record of Great Doctors*），[it] says [that Yinghuo（荧火，firefly，Lampyridae）is also] called Fangguang（放光），Yiyao（熠耀）and Zhao（照），existing in berms. [It can be] collected on July 7 and dried in the shade.

Notes

1. Yinghuo（荧火，firefly，Lampyridae）is pungent in taste，slightly warm and non-toxic in property，effective in improving

【今译】

味辛,性微温。

能使眼睛明亮,能治疗小儿因火烧所致的疮疡,热邪所伤而引发的疾病,虫毒伤害所致的病以及鬼怪病邪所致之症,能使神气通畅。又称为夜光。该物生长在池泽中。

vision and removing toxin. Clinically it is used to treat optic atrophy, infantile scald, disease caused by retention of heat in the body, convulsion and spasm due to worm toxin.

97. 衣鱼

【原文】

味咸,温,无毒。

主妇人疝瘕,小便不利(《御览》作泄利),小儿中风(览作头风),项强(《御览》作强),背起摩之。一名白鱼,生平洋。

【考据】

1.《吴普》曰:衣中白鱼,一名蟫(《御览》)。

2.《名医》曰:一名蟫,生咸阳。

3. 案《说文》云:蟫,白鱼也。《广雅》云:白鱼,蛃鱼也。《尔雅》云:蟫,白鱼。

4. 郭璞云:衣书中虫,一名蛃鱼。

上虫,鱼,下品一十八种,旧同。

97. Yiyu（衣鱼，silverfish，Lepisma Saccharina）[1]

[Original Text]

[Yiyu（衣鱼，silverfish，Lepisma Saccharina），] salty in taste，warm and non-toxic [in property]，[is mainly used] to treat hernia and conglomeration in women，dysuria，infantile wind stroke and stiffness of the neck involving the back [that can be regulated by] massage. [It is also] called Baiyu（白鱼），existing in rivers and seas.

[Textual Research]

[In the book entitled] *Wu Pu Ben Cao*（《吴普本草》，*Wu Pu's Studies of Materia Medica*），[it] says [that Yiyu（衣鱼，silverfish，Lepisma Saccharina) is also] called Yizhong Baiyu（衣中白鱼）and Yin（蟫）[according to the book entitled] *Tai Ping Yu Lan*（《太平御览》，*Imperial Studies in Taiping Times*）.

[In the book entitled] *Ming Yi Bie Lu*（《名医别录》，*Special Record of Great Doctors*），[it] says [that Yiyu（衣鱼，silverfish，Lepisma Saccharina) is also] called Yin（蟫），existing in Xianyang（咸阳）.

Notes

1. Yiyu（衣鱼，silverfish，Lepisma Saccharina）is salty in taste，warm and non-toxic in property，entering the bladder meridian，the

【今译】

味咸,性温,无毒。

主治妇人疝瘕,小便不利,小儿因感受风邪而导致的疾病,项强而牵引背部。又称为白鱼,该物生长于河流海洋之中。

small intestine meridian and the liver meridian, effective in promoting urination, resolving stranguria, expelling wind and removing toxin. Clinically it is used to treat stranguria, dysuria, sore, nebula, convulsion, epilepsy, heaviness of the tongue and cataract.

98. 桃核仁

【原文】

味苦,平。

主瘀血,血闭,癥瘕,杀小虫。桃花杀注恶鬼,令人好颜色。

桃凫,微温,主杀百鬼精物(初学记引云,枭桃在树不落,杀百鬼)。

桃毛,主下血瘕寒热,积寒无子,桃蠹,杀鬼邪恶不祥。生川谷。

【考据】

1.《名医》曰:桃核,七月采,取仁,阴干,花三月三日采,阴干,桃凫一名桃奴,一名枭景,是实着树不落,实中者,正月采之,桃蠹,食桃树虫也。生太山。

2. 案《说文》云:桃,果也。玉篇云:桃,毛果也。《尔雅》云:桃李丑核。郭璞云:子中有核仁。孙炎云:桃李之实,类皆有核。

【今译】

味苦,性平。

主治瘀血,经闭和癥瘕,能杀死小虫。

98. Taoheren（桃核仁，david peach seed，Semen Persicae）[1]

[Original Text]

[Taoheren（桃核仁，david peach seed，Semen Persicae），] bitter in taste and mild [in property], [is mainly used] to treat blood stasis，amenorrhea，abdominal mass and conglomeration，and to kill small worms.

Taohua（桃花，peach flower，david peach flower，Flos Persicae）[can] eliminate vicious [pathogenic factors like] ghost and luster facial expression.

Taofu（桃凫，immature fruit of peach，Fructus Persicae Immaturus）is slightly warm and [can] kill hundreds of [vicious pathogenic factors like] ghost and monster.

Taomao（桃毛 peach fluff，Fellis Persicae）[can] treat blood stasis，cold-heat [disease]，accumulation of cold and infertility.

Taodu（桃蠹，peach insect，Larva Persicae）[can] eliminate non-auspicious [pathogenic factors like] ghost.

[It] grows in mountain valleys and river valleys.

[Textual Research]

[In the book entitled] *Ming Yi Bie Lu*（《名医别录》，*Special Record of Great Doctors*），[it] says [that] Taohe（桃核，peach fruit，david peach fruit，Fructus Persicae）[should be] collected in July to

桃花,能杀除传染疾病的恶鬼恶邪,能使人面部色彩美丽。

桃凫,性微温,能杀除多种鬼怪病邪。

桃毛,能消除瘀血,能治疗瘕瘕,寒热病和不孕之症。

桃蠹,能杀除鬼怪病邪等不祥之物。

该物生长在山川河谷之中。

take the kernel. Taohua（桃花，peach flower，david peach flower，Flos Persicae）［should be］collected on March 3 and dried in the shade. Taofu （桃凫，immature fruit of peach，Fructus Persicae Immaturus）［is also］called Taonu（桃奴）and Xiaojing（枭景）.

Guo Pu（郭璞）said，"There is kernel in the fruit［of peach］." Sun Yan（孙炎）said，"There is kernel in all the fruits of peach."

Notes

1. Taoheren（桃核仁，david peach seed，Semen Persicae）is bitter and sweet in taste，mild in property，entering the heart meridian，the liver meridian and the large intestine meridian，effective in activating the blood，removing blood stasis，moistening dryness and the intestines. Clinically it is used to treat dysmenorrhea，amenorrhea，constipation due to intestinal dryness，blood-heat in the skin with itching，traumatic injury，pneumonia，enteritis，blood stagnation and wind impediment.

99. 杏核仁

【原文】

味甘,温。

主咳逆上气,雷鸣,喉痹下气,产乳,金属创伤,寒心,贲豚,生川谷。

【考据】

1.《名医》曰:生晋山。

2. 案《说文》云:杏,果也。《管子·地员篇》云:五沃之土,其木宜杏,高诱注《淮南子》云:杏有窍在中。

上果,下品二种旧同。

99. Xingheren（杏核仁，apricot seed；ansu apricot seed，Semen Armeniacae Amarum）[1]

[Original Text]

[Xingheren（杏核仁，apricot seed；ansu apricot seed，Semen Armeniacae Amarum），] sweet in taste [and] warm [in property], [is mainly used] to treat cough with dyspnea and upward counterflow of Qi, borborygum, thunderous sound [in the throat] and throat impediment，[disease after] delivery of baby, injury [caused by] metal，[pathogenic] cold [that damages] the heart[2] and running piglet, and to descend Qi.［It］grows in mountain valleys and river valleys.

[Textual Research]

[In the book entitled] *Ming Yi Bie Lu*（《名医别录》，*Special Record of Great Doctors*），[it] says [that Xingheren（杏核仁，apricot seed；ansu apricot seed，Semen Armeniacae Amarum）] grows in Jinshan（晋山）

[In] case [analysis in the book entitled] *Shuo Wen*（《说文》，*On Culture*），[it] says [that] peach means fruit. [In the book entitled] Guan Zi（《管子·地员篇》）about land，[it] says, "Fertile land in any place is appropriate for growing peach."．［In］explaining [the book entitled] *Huai Nan Zi*（《淮南子》，*A Philosophy Book Compiled by Liu An，King in Huainan*），Gao You

【今译】

味甘,性温。

主治咳嗽,呼吸困难和嗓内雷鸣之声,能治疗喉痹,能使气下行降逆,能治疗产妇病症,金属创伤,寒邪伤心及贲豚。该物生长在山川河谷之中。

（高诱）said，"There is orifice inside the peach."

Notes

1. Xingheren（杏核仁，apricot seed；ansu apricot seed，Semen Armeniacae Amarum）is bitter in taste，warm and mildly toxic in property，entering the lung meridian and the large intestine meridian，effective in expelling phlegm，ceasing cough，descending Qi，relieving panting and moistening the intestines. Clinically it is used to treat common cold with cough，rapid panting，fullness，vexation and oppression in the chest，constipation，dropsy，unsmooth urination，running piglet，hypertension and tetanus.

2. Heart here refers to the chest.

100. 腐婢

【原文】

味辛,平。

主痎疟,寒热,邪气,泄利,阴不起,病酒,头痛。生汉中。

【考据】

1.《吴普》曰:小豆花,一名腐婢(旧作付月,误),神农甘毒,七月采,阴干,四十日,治头痛止渴(《御览》)。

2.《名医》曰:生汉中,即小豆花也,七月采,阴干。

上米,谷下品一种,旧同。

100. Fubi（腐婢, stem or leaf of Japanese premna, Caulis seu Folium Premnae Microphyllae）[1]

[Original Text]

[Fubi（腐婢, stem or leaf of premna, Caulis seu Folium Premnae Microphyllae）,] pungent in taste and mild [in property], [is mainly used] to treat tension [at both sides of the abdomen], cold-heat [disease], [disease caused by] evil-Qi, diarrhea, impotence, disease [caused by] wine and headache. [It] grows in Hanzhong（汉中）.

[Textual Research]

[In the book entitled] *Wu Pu Ben Cao*（《吴普本草》, *Wu Pu's Studies of Materia Medica*）, [it] says [that the stem or leaf of premna is also] called Xiaodouhua（小豆花）and Fubi（腐婢）. [According to] Agriculture God（神农）, [it is] sweet [in taste] and toxic [in property], [can be] collected in July and dried in the shade for forty days for treating headache and ceasing thirst [as mentioned in the book entitled] *Tai Ping Yu Lan*（《太平御览》, *Imperial Studies in Taiping Times*）.

[In the book entitled] *Ming Yi Bie Lu*（《名医别录》, *Special Record of Great Doctors*）, [it] says [that Fubi（腐婢, stem or leaf of premna, Caulis seu Folium Premnae Microphyllae）], referring to the flower of red bean, grows in Hanzhong（汉中）, and [can be]

【今译】

味辛,性平。

主治瘕证和疟证,能治疗邪气所致的寒热病,泄泻,痢疾,阳痿不举以及醉酒所致头痛。该物生长在汉中。

collected in July and dried in the shade.

Notes

1. Fubi （腐婢, stem or leaf of premna, Caulis seu Folium Premnae Microphyllae) is bitter and slightly pungent in taste, cool in property, effective in clearing heat, removing toxin, resolving swelling and relieving pain. Clinically it is used to treat malaria, diarrhea, abscess, traumatic injury, abdominal pain, wasting-thirst, dysentery, appendicitis, headache, fire in the liver, bleeding due to external injury, snake bite and scald.

101. 苦瓠

【原文】

味苦,寒。

主大水,面目四肢浮肿,下水,令人吐。生川泽。

【考据】

1.《名医》曰:生晋地。

2. 案《说文》云:瓠匏,匏瓠也。《广雅》云:匏瓠也。《尔雅》云:瓠栖瓣。《毛诗》云:瓠有苦叶。《传》云:匏谓之瓠,又九月断壶。《传》云:壶瓠也。古今注云:瓠,壶芦也,壶芦,瓠之无柄者,瓠,有柄者。又云:瓢瓠也,其曰匏,瓠则别名。

【今译】

味苦,性寒。

主治水湿极度聚集,面部、眼睛和四肢浮肿,能使水液下行,能令人呕吐。该物生长在山川和平泽之中。

101. Kuhu（苦瓠，leaf of bottle gourd，Folium Lagenariae Sicerariae）[1]

[Original Text]

[Kuhu（苦瓠，leaf of bottle gourd，Folium Lagenariae Sicerariae），] bitter in taste and cold [in property]，[is mainly used] to treat severe edema and dropsy of the face，eyes and four limbs，[to induce] water to flow downwards and to induce vomiting. [It] grows in lakes and swamps.

[Textual Research]

[In the book entitled] *Ming Yi Bie Lu*（《名医别录》，*Special Record of Great Doctors*），[it] says [that Kuhu（苦瓠，leaf of bottle gourd，Folium Lagenariae Sicerariae）] grows in Jindi（晋地）.

Notes

1. Kuhu（苦瓠，leaf of bottle gourd，Folium Lagenariae Sicerariae）is bitter in taste，cold and toxic in property，effective in promoting urination，expelling dampness and killing worms. Clinically it is used to treat edema，stony stranguria，retention of phlegm，dysuria，jaundice，disease caused by worm toxin and scabies.

102. 水靳

【原文】

味甘,平。

主女子赤沃,止血养精,保血脉,益气,令人肥健,嗜食。一名水英,生池泽。

【考据】

1.《名医》曰:生南海。

2. 案《说文》云:芹,楚葵也,近菜类也。《周礼》有近菹。《尔雅》云:芹,楚葵。

3. 郭璞云:今水中芹菜。字林云:芹草生水中。根可缘器,又云芛菜,似蒜,生水中。

上菜,下品二种,旧同。

【今译】

味甘,性平。

102. Shuijin（水靳，javan waterdropwort herb，Herba Oenanthes Javanicae）[1]

[**Original Text**]

[Shuijin（水靳，javan waterdropwort herb，Herba Oenanthes Javanicae），] sweet in taste [and] mild [in property]，[is mainly used] to treat red and white leucorrhea，to cease bleeding，to nourish essence，to protect vessels，to replenish Qi and to enable people to be healthy with good appetite. [It is also] called Shuiying（水英），growing in lakes and swamps.

[**Textual Research**]

[In the book entitled] *Ming Yi Bie Lu*（《名医别录》，*Special Record of Great Doctors*），[it] says [that Shuijin（水靳，javan waterdropwort herb，Herba Oenanthes Javanicae）] grows in Nanhai（南海，South Sea）.

[In] case [analysis in the book entitled] *Shuo Wen*（《说文》，*On Culture*），[it] says [that the so-called] Qin（芹 celery）refers to Chukui（楚葵）[which is a kind of] vegetable. Guo Pu（郭璞）said，"[Shuijin（水靳，javan waterdropwort herb，Herba Oenanthes Javanicae）refers to] celery in waters now."

Notes

1. Shuijin（水靳，javan waterdropwort herb，Herba Oenanthes

主治女子赤白带下，能阻止出血，能滋养阴精，能保护血脉，能补益精气，能使人身体康健，食欲增加。又称为水英，该物生长在池泽中。

Javanicae) is sweet in taste and cool in property, effective in clearing heat, removing toxin, promoting urination, ceasing bleeding and reducing blood pressure. Clinically it is used to treat common cold with fever, lung heat with cough, whooping cough, jaundice, edema, stranguria, leucorrhea, hematuria, nosebleed, hematochezia, flooding and spotting (metrostaxis and metrorrhagia), and hypertension.

103. 彼子

【原文】

味甘,温。

主腹中邪气,去三虫,蛇螫,蛊毒,鬼注,伏尸。生山谷(旧在《唐本》退中)。

【考据】

1.《名医》曰:生永昌。

2. 案陶宏景云:方家从来无用此者,古今诸医,及药家子不复识,又一名熊子,不知其形何类也,掌禹锡云:树似杉子如槟榔。本经虫部云:彼子。

3. 苏注云:彼字合从木。《尔雅》云:彼一名棑。

【今译】

味甘,性温。

103. Bizi（彼子，seed of grand torreya，Semen Torreyae）[1]

[Original Text]

[Bizi（彼子，seed of grand torreya，Semen Torreyae），] sweet in taste [and] warm [in property]，[is mainly used] to expel evil-Qi in the abdomen，to eliminate three worms，to treat [injury caused by] snake bite，disease [caused by vicious pathogenic factors like] ghost and [unconsciousness like] corpse．[It] grows in mountains and valleys．

[Textual Research]

[In the book entitled] *Ming Yi Bie Lu*（《名医别录》，*Special Record of Great Doctors*），[it] says [that Bizi（彼子，seed of grand torreya，Semen Torreyae）] grows in Yongchang（永昌）．

Tao Hongjing（陶宏景）said，"Doctors have never used such a medicinal. From ancient times to the present，doctors and pharmacists know nothing about it and call it Xiongzi（熊子），unclear about what type it [belongs to]．"

Zhang Yuxi（掌禹锡）said，"Such a tree looks like Binglang（槟榔，areca，Areca Catechu）．"

　　主治腹中邪气所致之症，祛除三种虫子，能治疗蛇咬伤，虫毒所致之病，鬼怪病邪所致之症以及形若死尸之病。该物生长在山谷之中。

Notes

1. Bizi (彼子, seed of grand torreya, Semen Torreyae) is still unclear now. In the field of medicine, it is thought to be a sort of insect, or a sort of fruit, or a sort of wood.

图书在版编目（CIP）数据

汉英对照神农本草经：汉英对照/孙星衍考据；刘希茹今译；
李照国英译.—上海：上海三联书店，2017.9
ISBN 978－7－5426－5949－1

Ⅰ.①汉… Ⅱ.①孙…②刘…③李… Ⅲ.①《神农本草经》—
汉、英 Ⅳ.①R281.2

中国版本图书馆 CIP 数据核字(2017)第 157261 号

汉英对照神农本草经

考　　据／孙星衍
今　　译／刘希茹
英　　译／李照国
责任编辑／杜　鹃
特约编辑／周治华
装帧设计／一本好书
监　　制／姚　军
责任校对／张大伟

出版发行／上海三联书店
　　　　　(201199)中国上海市都市路 4855 号 2 座 10 楼
邮购电话／021－22895557
印　　刷／常熟市人民印刷有限公司

版　　次／2017 年 9 月第 1 版
印　　次／2017 年 9 月第 1 次印刷
开　　本／640×960　1/16
字　　数／1200 千字
印　　张／81.75
书　　号／ISBN 978－7－5426－5949－1/R·105
定　　价／269.00 元

敬启读者，如发现本书有印装质量问题，请与印刷厂联系 0512－52601369